TRENDS IN HELICOBACTER PYLORI INFECTION

Edited by **Bruna Maria Roesler**

Trends in Helicobacter pylori Infection
http://dx.doi.org/10.5772/57053
Edited by Bruna Maria Roesler

Contributors

Batool Mahdi, Amidou Samie, Nicoline F. Tanih, Roland Ndip, Siddalingam Rajinikanth, Mohammed Benghezal, Aleksandra Debowski, Hans-Olof Nilsson, Alma Fulurija, Jonathan Gauntlett, Barry James Marshall, Tomasz Brzozowski, Malgorzata Plonka, Aneta Targosz, Elżbieta Karczewska, Karolina Klesiewicz, Pawel Nowak, Edward Sito, Iwona Skiba, Alicja Budak, Malgorzata Zwolinska–Wcislo, Tomasz Mach, Aleksandra Sokic-Milutinovic, Dragan Popovic, Tamara Alempijevic, Sanja Dragasevic, Aleksandra Pavlovic Markovic, Snezana Lukic, Bruna Maria Roesler, José Murilo Zeitune, Shafiqul Alam Sarker, Elizabeth Maria Afonso Rabelo-Gonçalves, Carolina Negrei, Daniel Boda, Yousef Javadzadeh, Sanaz Hamedeyazdan, Florica Nicolescu

Published by InTech

Janeza Trdine 9, 51000 Rijeka, Croatia

Publishing Process Manager Iva Lipovic

Technical Editor InTech DTP team

Cover InTech Design team

First published April, 2014

Printed in Croatia

Additional hard copies can be obtained from orders@intechopen.com

Trends in Helicobacter pylori Infection , Edited by Bruna Maria Roesler

p. cm.

ISBN 978-953-51-1239-6

Meet the editor

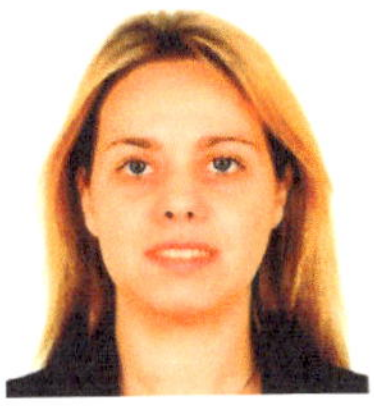

Dr. Bruna Maria Roesler is a pharmacist biochemist and holds a Master's Degree in Pharmacology and a Doctoral Degree in Basic Sciences – Internal Medicine from State University of Campinas (Campinas, SP, Brazil), where she has identified the principal genotypes of Helicobacter pylori in patients with chronic gastritis, peptic ulcer disease and early and advanced gastric adenocarcinoma through molecular biology techniques. She has published her work in several peer-reviewed journals and given oral and poster presentations at various congresses. She is a member of the Helicobacter pylori Research Group Study from State University of Campinas, including the study of etiology, epidemiology and physiopathology of gastrointestinal diseases. She has also participated in research that reports the possible relationship between H. pylori infection and idiopathic thrombocytopenic purpura, as well as between H. pylori infection and liver diseases. Her postdoctoral work includes the study of H. pylori in extradigestive manifestations, especially regarding pancreas and perigastric lymphonodes from patients with gastric adenocarcinoma.

Contents

Preface

The first successful isolation of *Helicobacter pylori* by Warren and Marshall has brought a new era in gastric microbiology. Although spiral microorganisms had been observed in the gastric mucus layer many years before, the isolation of *H. pylori* in conjunction with increased interest in the pathogenesis of gastrointestinal diseases, as well as the relatively frequent availability of clinical specimens via endoscopic biopsy, has led to important breakthroughs in medical care.

H. pylori remains one of the most common worldwide human infections and, although its colonization is not a disease in itself, it is a condition that affects the relative risk of developing various clinical disorders of the upper gastrointestinal tract, such as chronic gastritis, peptic ulcer disease, mucosa-associated lymphoid tissue (MALT lymphoma) and gastric adenocarcinoma. Besides, in the last two decades, *H. pylori* infection has been associated with the development of some extradigestive diseases, such as hepatobiliary, cardiovascular and pancreatic diseases, iron deficiency anemia and idiopathic thrombocytopenic purpura, among others.

Even though the routes of transmission of *H. pylori* are not completely clarified, infection is usually acquired during childhood and is characterized as being chronic, with greater prevalence in developing countries in all ages. Person-to-person transmission and intrafamilial spread seem to be the main route, based on the intrafamilial clustering. Children are often infected by a strain with a genetic fingerprint identical to that of their parents, and they maintain this genotype even after moving to a different environment. Besides, the waterborne infection remains possible.

All individuals with *H. pylori* infection have histological gastritis, which corresponds to classical chronic gastritis and is characterized by the infiltration of neutrophils and other inflammatory cells. However, most patients are asymptomatic for life, while only some will come to develop a digestive disease. Nevertheless, gastric cancer is a disease that continues to be a major global health problem and still remains the leading cause of cancer-related deaths in many parts of the world. Gastric cancer development involves the interaction of three major factors, the agent (in the most part of the cases, H. pylori) and its pathogenicity, the characteristics of the host, and the external environment. Specifically regarding *H. pylori* infection, there are some studies indicating that the eradication of the microorganism could reduce the incidence of gastric cancer in patients without precancerous lesions or, when lesions are present, the eradication may or may not reduce this incidence. Also, when the eradication is done after endoscopic mucosal resection in patients with early gastric adenocarcinoma, it could decrease the recurrence of metachronous gastric cancer in some patients.

Various guidelines for the management of *H. pylori* infection worldwide are available. Generally, the eradication of *H. pylori* in adults is recommended when the bacterium is present in the gastric mucosa. However, a discussion may arise about whether or not to recommend specific treatment in asymptomatic individuals that receive positive diagnoses for *H. pylori* in routine exams. In these cases, patients should be advised about the therapy, the adverse effects resulting from the use of the chosen medications, and the importance of *H. pylori* eradication in order to prevent some gastric diseases, such as peptic ulcer disease and gastric cancer. Nowadays, not only several drugs and regimens are in use, but also phytotherapy compounds have been associated with healing properties attributed, for instance, to the inhibition of cytokine-mediated inflammatory mechanism and to antioxidant activities. Besides, new systems of drug delivery systems have been developed and new regimens have been studied, considering the antimicrobial resistance.

All these aspects are considered in this book which is divided into following sections: Immunopathology and genetic diversity; Questions concerning possible routes of *H. pylori* transmission: water; *H. pylori* and gastric cancer: molecular epidemiology and possibilities of prevention; *H. pylori* infection in children and possible causes of iron deficiency anemia; Modern methods of bacterial DNA recovering; and Eradication therapy of *H. pylori* infection: new strategies.

Dr. Benghezal and colleagues present an interesting chapter regarding *H. pylori* genetic and epigenetic plasticity, discussing the hypothesis that this plasticity promotes *H. pylori* adaptation to individual human hosts by generating phenotypically diverse populations. A mathematical modeling of *H. pylori* chronic infection, its micro-evolution and related mechanisms for the generation of diversity including genetic and epigenetic diversity is also described. Finally, the chapter summarizes important alternatives to antibiotic treatment by targeting *H. pylori* persistence based on the urease enzymes.

Dr. Mahdi describes the important mechanisms of host immune response to *H. pylori* infection, which can be divided into innate and adaptive response, also describing the evasion of bacterium to the immune response. Besides, some aspects of vaccination against *H. pylori* infection are also considered.

Dr. Plonka and colleagues present a chapter that highlights the principal possible routes of *H. pylori* transmission, especially the evidence for water contamination. The principal sources and pathways of transmission are described as well as the methods used for the detection of bacterium in waterborne.

Dr. Roesler and Dr. Zeitune present a chapter that can be divided into two sections: the molecular characterization of *H. pylori* strains in Brazilian patients with early gastric adenocarcinoma through molecular techniques, specifically polymerase chain reaction, and the discussion of the principal aspects of *H. pylori* infection and the development of precancerous lesions and early gastric cancer properly, trying to highlight to what extent the microorganism eradication treatment could be important to preventing the disease progression.

Dr. Sokic-Milutinovic and colleagues describe the principal virulence factors of *H. pylori* that have been associated to gastric cancer development, considering that the outcome of the infection also depends on characteristics of the host and environmental factors. They also discussed these important aspects and considered them to suggest if *H. pylori* eradication is enough to prevent gastric cancer development.

Dr. Nicolescu describes the particulars of *H. pylori* infection in children, and summarizes important aspects of this infection, such as the rate of *H. pylori* infection, prevalence, possibility of transmission, principal diagnostic methods, incriminatory factors, pathophysiology and dissemination, among others, concluding the main text considering prospects studies.

Dr. Sarker presents a chapter concerning *H. pylori* infection, gastric physiology and iron deficiency anemia in children in developing countries. The main text brings aspects of hyperchlorhydria and hypochlorhydria and the role of *H. pylori* in gastric acid perturbation in children. After this, the chapter explains the possible relationship between *H. pylori* infection and iron deficiency anemia.

Dr. Rabelo-Gonçalves and colleagues present a research study describing the detection of *H. pylori* in liver tissue samples through laser capture microdissection technique (LCM), considering that this method can be extensively applied for bacterium identification in samples with small quantities of DNA.

Dr. Samie and colleagues describe the challenge of antimicrobial chemotherapy and the emergence of alternative treatments that have been used to eradicate *H. pylori* infection. Geographic differences in predominant *H. pylori* genotypes are delineated and the principal treatment regimens are discussed. Resistance mechanisms to metronidazole, clarithomycin, amoxicillin, tetracycline and fluoroquinolone are depicted. Potential treatments with medicinal plants are described, considering the principal plants used in Africa, Europe, South and North America, Asia and Australia. In addition, honey and probiotics are described as possible sources in the treatment and management of *H. pylori* infection.

Dr. Rajinikanth presents the current and future therapeutic strategies that can be used to eradicate *H. pylori* infection. First-line, second-line and third-line therapies are described as well as future therapeutic strategies, including novel drug delivery approaches, among them the floating drug delivery systems (FDDS) and the mucoadhesive drug delivery systems (MDDS). In addition, the development of vaccine against *H. pylori* and genome-based drug discovery are also depicted.

Dr. Javadzadeh and Dr. Hamedeyazdan present a chapter that discusses the importance of drug delivery systems in treatment of upper gastrointestinal diseases, especially peptic ulcer disease. The floating drug delivery systems are explained as well as the principal therapies that are currently used to *H. pylori* eradication.

Dr. Karczewska and colleagues describe a research concerning the empirical and the targeted treatment of *H. pylori* infection in Southern Poland according to the results of local antimicrobial resistance monitoring. The principal characteristics and virulence factors of *H. pylori* are explained as well as the treatment guidelines commonly used to eradicate its infection. Antimicrobial resistance in Poland is described and the results obtained suggest the need for constant monitoring of the resistance to a set of antimicrobial agents routinely used for empirical therapy.

Finally, Dr. Negrei and colleagues describe the mechanisms of action and resistance to fluoroquinolone in *H. pylori* infection, including the interaction with bacterial DNA gyrase and topoisomerase IV, the SOS gene network response and the plasmid mediated resistance, among other resistance mechanisms. In addition, the clinical and social implications of fluoroquinolone resistance are depicted.

"Trends in Helicobacter pylori Infection" will certainly provide an updated set of information in all the principal aspects of *H. pylori* infection, enriching the knowledge of the whole scientific community.

The editor expresses her thankfulness for the excellent work of the contributing authors. The editor thanks Ms. Danijela Duric, head of production at InTech, for her invitation to edit this book. In addition, the editor is especially thankful for the excellent support given by Ms. Iva Lipovic, as well as the entire InTech Open Access publishing team.

Dr. Bruna Maria Roesler
Pharmacist Biochemist
Department of Internal Medicine, Center of Diagnosis of Digestive Diseases,
Faculty of Medical Sciences, State University of Campinas,
Campinas, São Paulo, Brazil

Section 1

Immunopathology and Genetic Diversity

Chapter 1

Persistence of *Helicobacter pylori* Infection: Genetic and Epigenetic Diversity

Mohammed Benghezal, Jonathan C. Gauntlett,
Aleksandra W. Debowski, Alma Fulurija,
Hans-Olof Nilsson and Barry James Marshall

Additional information is available at the end of the chapter

http://dx.doi.org/10.5772/57428

1. Introduction

Helicobacter pylori is a Gram negative bacterium found on the luminal surface of the gastric epithelium. Infection is generally acquired during childhood and persists life-long in the absence of antibiotic treatment. *H. pylori* has a long period of co-evolution with humans, going back at least since human migration out of Africa about 60, 000 years ago [1, 2]. This co-evolution is reflected in DNA sequence signatures observed in *H. pylori* strains of different geographic origin and has enabled the mapping of human migration out of Africa. This prolonged and intimate relationship is likely to have shaped the large and diverse repertoire of strategies which *H. pylori* employs to establish robust colonization and persist in the gastric niche. Key challenges that *H. pylori* encounters are fluctuation of acidic pH of the gastric lumen, peristalsis of the mucus layer leading to washout in the lower intestine, nutrient scarcity, and the innate and adaptive immune responses promoting local inflammation or gastritis [3-8]. These challenges, particularly host immune responses, are likely to represent the selective pressure driving *H. pylori* micro-evolution during transmission leading to persistence in the human host.

Host defences against *H. pylori* have been extensively studied including mechanisms which *H. pylori* uses to avoid or inhibit an effective host immune response and review of these related studies is beyond the scope of this chapter (see reviews [9-24]). Instead, key strategies of *H. pylori* immune escape with emphasis on regulation of inflammation are succinctly presented in the context of *H. pylori* persistence. *H. pylori* has evolved to avoid detection by pattern recognition receptors of the innate immune system, such as toll-like receptors and C-type lectins. Indeed, the TLR4 determinant of *H. pylori* lipopolysaccharide is a very weak stimulus as a result of its altered and highly conserved lipid A structure [25, 26]. In addition, the lipopolysaccharide O-antigen mimics Lewis antigen expressed on host cells and has been shown to regulate dendritic cell function through its binding of DC-SIGN [27-32]. Mutation of the TLR5 recognition site in the flagellin and the sheath protecting the flagella prevent strong activation of the TLR5 signalling pathway [33-35]. *H. pylori* inhibits the adaptive immune response by blocking T-cell proliferation at different levels via at least three different factors, the gamma-glutamyltranspeptidase [36], the cytotoxin VacA [37] and its unique glucosyl cholesterol derivatives [38] (produced from the cholesterol *H. pylori* extracts from host cells). A recent study on the role of the inflammasome during *H. pylori* infection unveiled the pro-inflammatory and regulatory properties of caspase-1 mediated by its substrates IL-1β and IL-18, respectively [39]. In light of the acid-suppressive properties of IL-1β [40], the latter observation exemplifies how seamlessly adapted *H. pylori* is to its human host in its ability to balance gastric pH, inflammation and avoid overt gastric pathology to maintain the physiology of its niche and persist for decades. It would therefore be interesting to note the higher risk for atrophic gastritis in patients with IL-1β polymorphisms that leads to increased expression of IL-1β [41-43] as elevated IL-1β levels might interfere with the dual role of caspase-1 and promote overt inflammation during *H. pylori* chronic infection. Further studies on the activation/regulation of the inflammasome are warranted to gain new insights into gastric cancer caused by *H. pylori* infection.

The scope of this chapter is to review *H. pylori* genetic and epigenetic plasticity and discuss the hypothesis that this plasticity promotes *H. pylori* adaptation to individual human hosts by generating phenotypically diverse populations. Emphasis has been put on mathematical modelling of *H. pylori* chronic infection [44], its micro-evolution and related mechanisms for the generation of diversity including genetic [45-49] and epigenetic diversity [50, 51]. Mechanisms of horizontal gene transfer and the generation of intra-strain genetic diversity are reviewed and the implication of phasevarion-mediated epigenetic diversity is discussed in the context of bacterial population and adaption.

Examples of experimental strategies to study and decipher *H. pylori* persistence are presented and include bacterial genetics combined with the use of animal models as well as *H. pylori* comparative genomics during chronic and acute infection in humans. The chapter summarises the mechanism of *H. pylori* micro-evolution, in particular the tension between generation of genetic diversity to adapt and genome integrity. Finally, alternatives to antibiotic treatment by targeting *H. pylori* persistence are discussed based on the urease enzyme.

2. *H. pylori* persistence: Mathematical modelling

H. pylori survive in the gastric niche in a dynamic equilibrium of replication and death by manipulating the host immune system to keep a favourable balance that allows for persistence and transmission. Blaser and Kirschner developed an elegant mathematical model of *H. pylori* persistence based on the Nash equilibrium, specifically that *H. pylori* uses the evolutionary stable strategy based on cross-signalling and feedback loop regulations between the host and the bacteria [44]. In this model, a set of interactions between bacteria and the host is defined as well as their corresponding rate parameters. Two populations are considered, the non-replicating free swimming bacteria in the mucus and the adherent bacteria replicating in a nutrient-rich site. This model predicts clearance of the bacteria in the presence of a strong host immunological response and persistence if the host response is weaker. However, this model does not take into account random fluctuations for stochastic phenotype transitions. *H. pylori* is likely to exhibit phenotypic and genetic plasticity to adapt to changing gastric environments but it has relatively few sensors of gastric environment change (e.g. pH, immunological responses, receptor availability, and nutrients). *H. pylori*'s apparently limited gene regulation and its small genome suggest alternative adaptive mechanisms, different from exclusive maintenance of active sensory machinery that is costly. Possibilities include small RNA regulation [52], automatic random genetic switches for generating diverse adaptive phenotypes [53], exemplified by the frameshift-prone repetitive sequences at the beginning of certain phase variable genes [47, 50, 51], and the numerous duplicate and divergent outer membrane genes, which could be part of a more general gene regulation network, so far unidentified. Thus further refinement of this model is required to understand the mechanisms involved in establishing the optimal balance between sensing changes and random phenotype switching. Introducing random fluctuations for stochastic phenotype transitions in this model is highly relevant to phase variation and phasevarion, two mechanisms *H. pylori* uses to generate phenotypic changes and adapt.

3. Genetic diversity

The above mentioned mathematical model based on cross-signalling and feedback loop regulation between the host and the bacteria predicts a unique *H. pylori* population in every human host. In other words, *H. pylori* transmission results in adaptation to a specific host during the acute phase of transmission as well as in the chronic phase. The Nash equilibrium model for *H. pylori* colonization is in line with the genetic diversity of *H. pylori* populations as the result of human migration out of Africa and with vertical transmission. Indeed, *H. pylori* strains transmitted within families are genetically less diverse than strains from unrelated infected persons. This highlights the isolation of *H. pylori* strains within a host and genetic adaptation to human subpopulations. Multi-locus sequence typing analysis has identified 6 ancestral populations of *H. pylori* named ancestral European 1, ancestral European 2, ancestral East Asia, ancestral Africa1, ancestral Africa2 [2], and ancestral Sahul [1].

3.1. Intra-strain generation of genetic diversity

Adaptive evolution of species relies on a balance between genetic diversity and genome stability promoted by genome maintenance mechanisms and DNA repair preventing mutations and ensuring cell viability. Intra-strain or intracellular genetic changes have several origins including spontaneous chemical instability of DNA such as depurination and deamination, errors during DNA replication and the action of DNA damaging metabolites, either endogenous or exogenous. The DNA repair machinery is essential to all living organisms and has been best studied for the model organism *Escherichia coli*. The advances in DNA sequencing technologies and comparative genomics provided a unique opportunity to better understand genome maintenance beyond *E. coli* model organism by comparing the DNA repair gene content in different bacterial species. This is of particular interest for bacterial pathogens that have to overcome immune responses and associated DNA damaging oxidative stress [54]. Comparative genomics of nine human pathogens (*Helicobacter pylori, Campylobacter jejuni, Haemophilus influenza, Mycobacterium tuberculosis, Neisseria gonorrhoea, Neisseiria meningitidis, Staphylococcus aureus, Streptococcus pneumonia and Streptococcus pyogenes*) revealed a reduced number of genes in DNA repair, recombination and replication compared to *E. coli* [54].

During replication DNA polymerase encountering DNA damage could either be blocked or continue and introduce a mutation into the daughter strand. Maintenance of the template for DNA replication before the replication fork reaches the DNA lesion is therefore an effective DNA repair strategy employed by the cell to avoid mutation or replication arrest. A blocked replication fork requires the homologous recombination machinery to repair the damaged DNA and to resume replication. DNA template maintenance is achieved through several mechanisms pre- and post-replication:

- Direct repair that reverses base damage.
- Excision repair that removes the lesion from the DNA duplex. There are three types of excision repair:
    - Base excision repair (BER) – PolI dependent [54].
    - Nucleotide excision repair (NER) – PolI dependent [54].
    - Alternative excision repair (AER) has been described in a limited number of organisms such a *Schizosaccharomyces pombe* and *Deinococcus radiodurans* – Endonuclease and DNA ligase dependent [55].
- Mismatch repair (MMR) is a post-replication mechanism which contributes to the DNA polymerase fidelity by identifying mismatched bases and removing them from the daughter strand [54].
- Recombinational repair that exchanges the isologous strands between the sister DNA molecules.

Table 1 shows that nucleotide excision repair is the only fully conserved repair pathway amongst the nine pathogens mentioned above and that the SOS response related genes are completely missing from *H. pylori* [46, 54]. Direct repair and mismatch repair are often completely absent whereas base excision repair, recombinational repair and replication (*dnaA, dnaB, dnaG, gyrA, gyrB, parC, parE, priA, rep, topA* and *polA*) are often missing one or several genes. This absence of DNA repair and replication genes suggests either that functional homologs remain to be discovered or that specific genome dynamics and genome integrity maintenance strategies are at play in different microbial pathogens to adapt to their niche.

http://dx.doi.org/10.5772/57428

Pathway	Protein	*H. pylori* gene	Protein function	Bacterial species	
				Ec	Hp
Direct repair					
	Ada		Methyltransferase	+	-
	AlkB		Oxidative demethylase	+	-
	Ogt	HP0676	Methyltransferase	+	+
	Phr/Spl		Photolyase	+	-
Base excision repair					
	MutY	HP0142	Glycosylase (adenine)	+	+
	MutM		Glycosylase (8-oxoG)	+	-
	Nei		Endonuclease VIII	+	-
	Nth	HP0585	Endonuclease III	+	+
	Tag		Glycosylase I (adenine)	+	-
	AlkA		Glycosylase II (adenine)	+	-
	Ung	HP1347	Glycosylase (uracil)	+	+
	Xth	HP1526	Exonuclease III	+	+
	Mpg		Glycosylase (purine)	+	-
	YgjF		Glycosylase (thymine)	+	-
	Nfo		Endonuclease IV	+	-
	MagIII	HP0602	Glycosylase (adenine)	-	+
Nucleotide excision repair					
	UvrA	HP0705	DNA damage recognition	+	+
	UvrB	HP1114	Exinuclease	+	+
	UvrC	HP0821	Exinuclease	+	+
	UvrD	HP1478	Helicase II	+	+
	Mfd	HP1541	Transcription-repair coupling factor	+	+
Mismatch excision repair					
Mismatch recognition	MutS1		Mismatch recognition	+	-
	MutS2	HP0621	Repair of oxidative DNA damage	-	+
	MutL		Recruitment of MutS1	+	-
	MutH		Endonuclease	+	-

Pathway	**Protein**	***H. pylori* gene**	**Protein function**	**Bacterial species**	
				Ec	**Hp**
Recombinational repair					
	RecA	HP0153	DNA strand exchange and recombination	+	+
RecBCD pathway	RecB (AddA)	HP1553	Exonuclease V, β subunit	+	+
	RecC (AddB)	HP0275	Exonuclease V, γ subunit	+	+
	RecD		Exonuclease V, α subunit	+	-
RecFOR pathway	RecF		Gap repair protein	+	-
	RecJ	HP0348	5□3□ssDNA exonuclease	+	+
	RecO	HP0951	Gap repair protein	+	+
	RecR	HP0925	Gap repair protein	+	+
	RecN	HP1393	ATP binding	+	+
	RecQ		3'-5'DNA helicase	+	-
Branch migration	RuvA	HP0883	Binds junctions; helicase (with RuvB)	+	+
	RuvB	HP1059	5'-3'junction helicase (with RuvA)	+	+
	RecG	HP1523	Resolvase, 3'-5'junction helicase	+	+
Resolvase	RuvC	HP0877	Junction endonuclease	+	+
Chromosome dimer resolution					
	XerC		Recombinase	+	-
	XerD		Recombinase	+	-
	XerH	HP0675	Recombinase	-	+

Adapted from References Kang and Blaser, Nat Rev Microbiol. 2006; 4(11):826-36 and Ambur et al., FEMS Microbiol.Rev. 2009; 33:453-470. AP, apurinic/apyrimidinic; ds, double stranded; ss, single stranded.

Table 1. Comparative analysis of DNA repair and recombination pathways in *E. coli* and *H. pylori*

H. pylori specific DNA repair and replication pathways and their potential role in colonization, virulence and persistence are discussed below based on experimental evidence.

3.1.1. DNA repair and mutagenesis

The most striking feature of *H. pylori* DNA repair gene content is the absence of the mismatch repair. A distant homolog of *mutS* was identified [56, 57] and phylogenetic analysis revealed that MutS belongs to the MutS2 subfamily of proteins [58] that are not associated with MMR. Functional analysis of *H. pylori* MutS2 identified a role of this protein in repair of oxidative DNA damage and Muts2 is required for robust colonization in the mouse model of *H. pylori* infection [59]. Deficiency in MMR activity leads to an increase in mutation rate and is known as the mutator phenotype in Enterobacteriaceae and *Pseudomonas aeruginosa* [60, 61]. The apparent lack of MMR is in line with *H. pylori* mutation rate that is about 2 orders of magnitude higher than in *E. coli* [45]. *H. pylori* mutator phenotype could confer genetic diversity and a selective advantage to adapt and persist in the changing gastric niche. Alternatively, the mutator phenotype of *H. pylori* might promote transmission as postulated for *Neisseria meningitidis* based on the observation of high prevalence of mutations in MMR genes in a *N. meningitidis* epidemic [62].

Numerous reports have confirmed *H. pylori* dependence on DNA repair to establish robust colonization and to persist, suggesting that the human gastric niche induces bacterial DNA lesions [63].

Four of the base excision repair proteins only (MutY, Nth, Ung and Xth) are present in *H. pylori* [54, 64-67] in addition to a novel 3-methyladenine DNA glycosylase (MagIII) that defines a new class within the endonuclease III family of base excision repair glycosylases resembling the Tag protein [68, 69]. *magIII* and *xth* mutants were identified in a signature-tagged mutagenesis screen based on the mouse model of *H. pylori* infection suggesting a role during colonization [70]. Deletion mutants *mutY*, *ung* and *xth* exhibited higher spontaneous mutation frequencies compared to wild-type, with a *mutY* mutant displaying the highest frequency of spontaneous mutation. *mutY* mutants colonized the stomach of mice less robustly compared to wild-type, demonstrating a role for MutY in base excision repair *in vivo* to correct oxidative DNA damage [64]. The presence of an adenine homopolymeric tract in *mutY* suggests that MutY phase varies. This raises an interesting question whether *H. pylori* can vary its mutation rate to adapt to its gastric niche, and highlights the tension between mutation and repair. Deletion of the *nth* gene also led to hypersensitivity to oxidative stress, reduced survival in macrophages and an increased mutation rate compared to wild-type [71]. The *nth* mutant also colonized the mouse stomach poorly 15 days post challenge and was almost cleared after 60 days [71].

Mutants in nucleotide excision repair genes *uvrA*, *uvrB*, *uvrC* and *uvrD* have been constructed in *H. pylori* [49, 72, 73] and their UV sensitivity phenotype confirmed their role in DNA repair. Although surprisingly *uvrA* and *uvrB* mutants had lower mutation rate and recombination frequencies [49]. This phenomenon can be explained by nucleotide exchange of undamaged DNA and was hypothesized to be another mechanism *H. pylori* uses to generate genetic diversity [49]. Furthermore, *uvrC* mutation led to an increase in the length of DNA import, suggesting that NER influences homologous recombination. UvrD limited homologous recombination between strains [49, 73]. A mutant deficient in Mfd, the transcription repair coupling factor, was found to be more sensitive to DNA damaging agents [74], suggesting that *H. pylori* may also detect blocked RNA polymerase as a damage recognition signal in addition to the DNA distortion recognition properties of UvrA and UvrB. In summary, NER has opposite dual functions; maintenance of genome integrity by excision repair versus generation of genetic diversity by increasing the spontaneous mutation rate and controlling the rate of homologous recombination and corresponding import length of DNA. Full conservation of the NER pathway in *H. pylori* contrasts with other lacunar DNA repair pathways and highlights the importance of the dual role of NER for *H. pylori* during its replication cycle to balance genetic diversity and genome integrity. To date, the role of NER in genetic diversification has not been tested *in vivo*. Only the *mfd* mutant was identified in a signature-tagged mutagenesis screen based on the mouse model of *H. pylori* infection, suggesting a role of NER during colonization [70].

Finally, recombinant *H. pylori* overexpressing DNA polymerase I displays a mutator phenotype suggesting a role of replication in generating genetic diversity. Bacterial DNA polymerases I participates in both DNA replication and DNA repair. *H. pylori* DNA PolI lacks a proofreading activity, elongates mismatched primers and performs mutagenic translesion synthesis. Conversely, the DNA polymerase I deficient mutant exhibited lower mutation frequency compared to wild-type.

3.1.2. DNA recombination

3.1.2.1. Homologous recombination

Recombination between similar sequences is called homologous recombination (HR). HR participates in DNA repair of double strand breaks and stalled replication forks. It is dependent on RecA, a protein that binds and exchanges single stranded DNA. As depicted in Figure 1, HR is a three-step process involving presynapsis, synapsis and postsynapsis. The presynapsis pathway is dictated by the nature of the DNA substrate. Two categories of proteins prepare the single stranded DNA for binding by RecA. A linear DNA duplex with a double-strand end (that could arise during partial replication of incoming single stranded DNA during conjugation, transduction, or DNA damage) is processed by RecBCD. Gapped DNA (that may form during replication) is processed to single-stranded DNA by RecQ and RecJ, whereas RecFOR inhibits RecQ and RecJ activities to allow RecA binding. The result is a nucleoprotein filament that is ready for the search of homologous sequence in the DNA duplex and RecA-mediated strand exchange once that homologous sequence is found. This synapsis step leads to the formation of a structure termed the D-loop. Postsynapsis involves D-loop branch migration and Holliday junction formation catalysed by RuvAB prior to resolution by RuvC or RusA. RecG has also been shown to be involved in recombination and to catalyse branch migration, in addition to its role in replication fork reversal. Interestingly, RuvC-mediated Holliday junction resolution is biased towards non-crossover, avoiding the formation of a chromosome dimer that requires the Xer/*dif* machinery for resolution.

H. pylori expresses most of the HR proteins of *E. coli* including; RecA, AddAB instead of RecBCD, RecOR (lacking RecF and RecQ), RuvABC (lacking RusA), RecG, and XerH/dif_H for chromosome dimer resolution. The presence of most HR genes in *H. pylori* suggests that HR plays an important role in *H. pylori* gastric colonization. Intragenomic recombination in families of genes encoding outer membrane proteins leads to *H. pylori* cell surface remodelling to adapt to the human host by adjusting bacterial adhesive properties, antigen

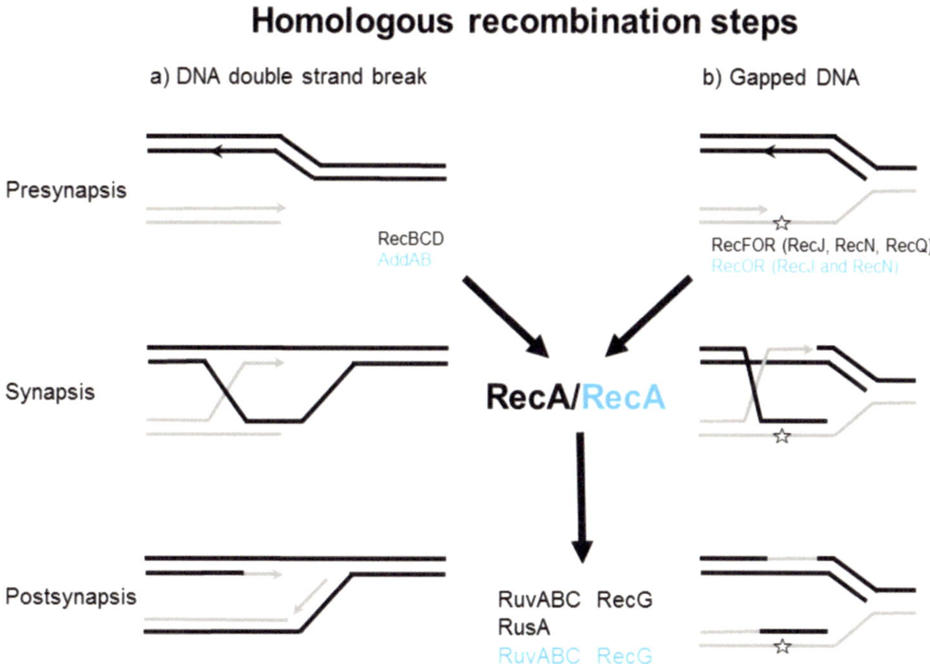

Figure 1. Homologous recombination. Two DNA substrates can be processed by the HR machinery **a)** double strand break DNA **b)** gapped DNA. Three stages of HR are presented starting with presynapsis (DNA processing to ssDNA for RecA loading), synapsis (search of the homologous sequence in the DNA duplex and RecA-mediated strand exchange leading to the formation of a structure termed D-loop) and postsynapsis (D-loop branch migration and Holliday junction formation catalysed by RuvAB before resolution by RuvC or RusA). Proteins involved at the different steps are indicated in black for the model organism *E. coli* and in blue for *H. pylori*.

mimicry [75, 76] and modulation of the immune system [76]. HR was suggested to be the underlying recombination mechanism for *homA/homB* and *galT/Jhp0562* allelic diversity [77, 78], whereas gene conversion (non-reciprocal recombination) is responsible for *sabA* diversity [79]. Mutants in *recA*, *addA* or *recG* had lower rates of *sabA* adhesin gene conversion suggesting that RecA-independent gene conversion exists and that this recombination may be initiated by a double-strand break [79].

The RecA deficient mutants are sensitive to DNA damaging agents such as UV light, methyl methanesulfonate, ciprofloxacin, and metronidazole [80, 81]. RecA was the first HR protein to be characterized in *H. pylori* and it was found not to complement an *E. coli* RecA deficient mutant [80]. Lack of cross-species complementation was first attributed to the putative post-translational modification of RecA [80], however, studies showed that the lack of complementation was due to species specific interaction of RecA with proteins involved in presynapsis such as RecA loading on the single stranded DNA by AddAB [82]. RecA's role *in vivo* is supported by poor colonization of a RecA deficient mutant [82]. Interestingly, RecA was shown to integrate the transcriptional up-regulation of DNA damage responsive genes (upon DNA uptake) and natural competence genes (upon DNA damage) in a positive feedback loop. The interconnection of natural competence and DNA damage through RecA highlights the role of HR in persistence and in generating genetic diversity. Alternatively, and not exclusive to a role in generation of genetic diversity, RecA-mediated genetic exchange might represent a mechanism for genome integrity maintenance in an extreme DNA-damaging environment.

Several gene deletion studies have shown that *H. pylori* has two separate and non-overlapping presynaptic pathways, AddAB and RecOR, contrasting with the redundancy of RecBCD and RecFOR in *E. coli* [83, 84]. The single *addA* mutant and double mutant *addA recO* exhibit similar sensitivity to double strand break inducing agents, suggesting that AddAB is involved in the double strand break repair pathway, and RecOR in gap repair. Finally, RecOR is involved in intragenomic recombination and AddAB in intergenomic recombination. Both pathways are required *in vivo* for robust colonization and persistence based on the lower colonization loads of single *addA*, *recO*, and *recR* mutants in the mouse model of *H. pylori* infection with the double *addA recO* mutant displaying the lowest bacterial load. As expected for recombinational repair proteins, RecN mediated DNA double strand break recognition and initiation of DNA recombination is also required *in vivo* for robust colonization [85].

Resolution of the Holliday junction formed by the action of RecA is performed by RuvABC in *H. pylori* and *recA*, *ruvB*, or *ruvC* mutants exhibited similar UV sensitivities [86, 87]. Colonization of the recombinational repair mutant, *ruvC*, was affected and 35 days post-infection the *ruvC* mutant was cleared by mice. Thus, although dispensable for the initial colonization step, recombinational DNA repair and HR are essential to *H. pylori* persistent infection. Furthermore, the *ruvC* deletion mutant elicited a Th1 biased immune response compared to a Th2 biased response observed for wild-type, highlighting the role of homologous recombination in *H. pylori* immune modulation and persistence [88].

Unexpectedly, the RecG homolog in *H. pylori* limits recombinational repair [86] by competing with the helicase RuvB. Mutation of RecG increased recombination frequencies in line with a role of RecG in generating genetic diversity. The term 'DNA antirepair' was coined to highlight the tension between the generation of diversity and genome integrity maintenance for *H. pylori* adaptation to its niche. Further regulation of homologous recombination is mediated by the MutS2 protein that displays high affinity for DNA structures such as recombination intermediates thus inhibiting DNA strand exchange and consequent recombination [89]. MutS2 deficient cells have a 5-fold increase in recombination rate [90].

3.1.2.2. Non-homologous recombination

XerH/dif_H machinery for chromosome dimer resolution was found to be essential for *H. pylori* colonization [87]. Deletion of *xerH* in *H. pylori* caused: (i) a slight growth defect in liquid culture, as is typical of *xer* mutants of *E. coli* [91], (ii) markedly increased sensitivity to DNA breakage inducing and homologous recombination stimulating UV irradiation and ciprofloxacin, (iii) increased UV sensitivity of a *recG* mutant [86], and (iv) a defect in chromosome segregation. The inability of the *xerH* mutant to survive in the gastric niche contrasts with *ruvC* mutant colonization and further supports the idea that XerH is not involved in DNA repair but in chromosome maintenance such as chromosome dimer resolution, regulation of replication and possibly in chromosome unlinking. This, in turn, suggests that slow growing *H. pylori* depends on unique chromosome replication and maintenance machinery to thrive in their special gastric niche.

Rearrangement of the middle region of the *cagY* gene, independent of RecA [92], leads to in frame insertion or deletion of CagY and gain or loss of function of the CagA type IV secretion system. Recombination of *cagY* was proposed to be a mechanism to regulate the inflammatory response to adapt and persist in the gastric niche [93]. To date the exact recombination mechanism involving direct repeats in the middle region of *cagY* remains unknown.

3.1.3. Phase variation

Host adapted human pathogens, such as *H. influenzae*, *Neisseria* species and *H. pylori*, have evolved genetic strategies to generate extensive phenotypic variation by regulating the expression of surface bound (or secreted) protein antigens that directly (or indirectly) interact with host cells. Phenotypic variation of the bacterial external composition will alter the appearance of the bacterium as sensed by the host immune system. One common regulatory mechanism to achieve antigen diversity within a bacterial population is known as phase variation [94, 95].

In pathogens, simple sequence repeats (SSRs) are tandem iterations of a single nucleotide or short oligonucleotides that, with respect to their length, are hypermutable (Figure 2). Reversible slipped strand mutation/mispairing of SSRs within protein coding regions cause frame shifts, resulting in the translation of proteins that vary between being in-frame (on), producing functional full-length proteins, and out-of-frame (off), where a truncated or non-sense polypeptide is produced [96]. Additionally, SSRs may occur in the promoter region of genes where variation in their length may affect promoter strength by mechanisms such as alteration of the distance between -10 and -35 elements.

In *H. pylori*, phase variation regulates the expression of genes that are likely to be important for adaptation in response to environmental changes and for immune evasion in order to establish persistent colonization of the host. Analysis of DNA sequence motifs based on annotated genomes of *H. pylori* strains 26695 [57] and J99 [97] revealed substantial occurrence, intra- and intergenic, of homopolymeric tracts and dinucleotide repeats. Certain categories of genes (or their promoter region) were particularly prone to contain SSRs, such as those coding for LPS biosynthesis enzymes, outer membrane proteins and DNA restriction/modification systems, and thus have been identified as possible candidates regulated by phase variation [98].

Further genome analysis of *H. pylori* strains 26695 and J99 demonstrated an expanded repertoire of candidate phase-variable genes. In addition to previous sequence motif analyses of the annotated genomes by Tomb and Alm, 13 novel putative phase-variable antigens were identified *in silico* [99]. Poly-A and poly-T repeats were almost exclusively found in intergenic regions whereas poly-C and poly-G repeats were mostly intragenic. Five classes of gene function were described; i) LPS biosynthesis (seven genes), ii) cell surface associated proteins (22 genes), iii) DNA restriction/modification systems (nine genes), iv) metabolic or other proteins (three genes), and v) hypothetical ORFs with unidentified homology (five genes). This

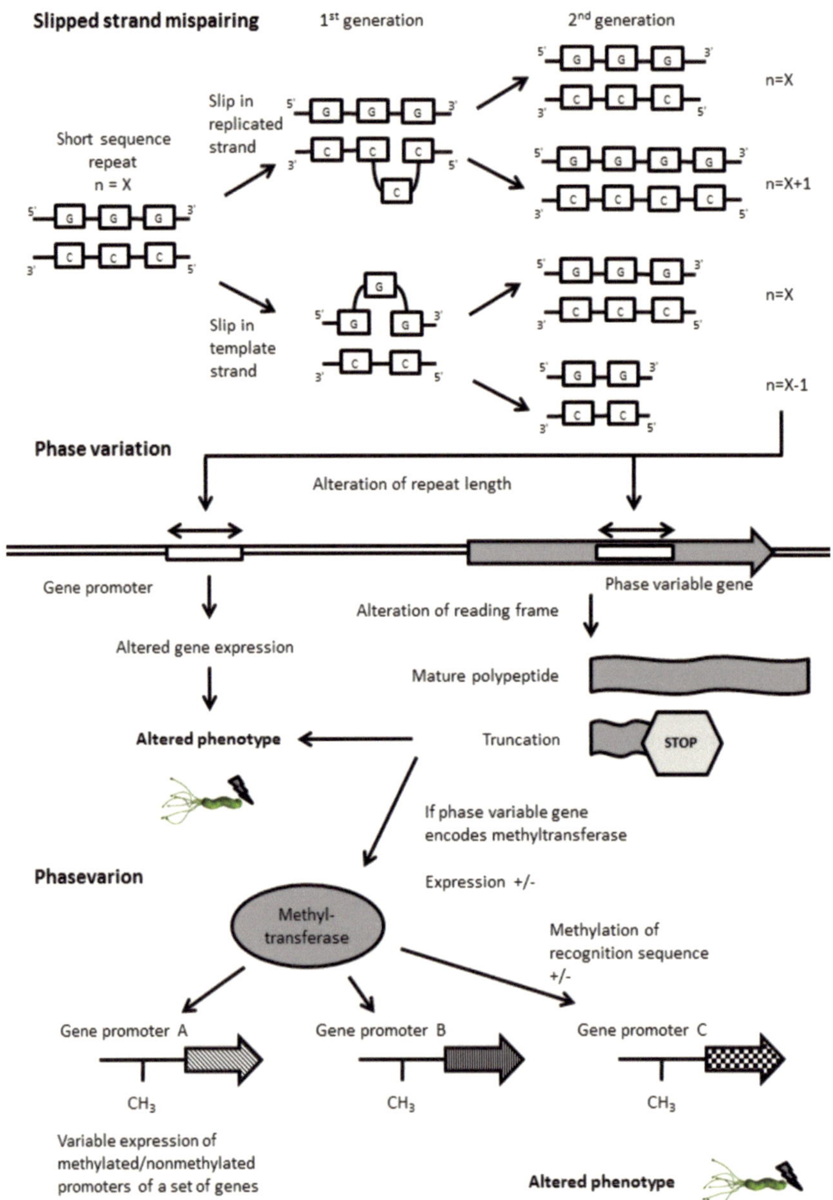

Figure 2. Phase variation and generation of epigenetic diversity by phasevarions. Slipped strand mispairing of short sequence repeats during DNA replication results in alteration of repeat length in descendants. Figure adapted from Thomson *et al*. [316]. Repeat sequences, represented by a white box, may be present in gene promoters or within the coding sequence of a gene where variation in repeat length alters gene expression, or changes the reading frame leading to the generation of a premature stop codon, respectively. This leads to phenotypic variation due to the presence or absence of the encoded protein. In instances where the phase varying gene encodes a methyltransferase, phase variable expression of the methylase results in either the methylation, or absence of methylation, of target DNA sequences of the enzyme. In instances where methylation affects gene promoter activity this results in varied gene expression. A set of genes, referred to as a phasevarion, may be regulated in this manner resulting in rapid, reversible epigenetic generation of phenotypic diversity.

analysis highlights the importance for a bacterial species such as *H. pylori* to be able to regulate cell surface antigen expression that is responsible for direct interaction with a changing environment.

Multi locus sequence typing (MLST) analysis was then applied for analysis of sequence motif variation in 23 *H. pylori* strains selected on the basis of ethnicity and country of origin (Table 2). Four strain types were investigated, i) hpEastAsia, ii) hpLadakh, iii) hpEurope, and iv) hpAfrica1 and hpAfrica2. In conclusion, approximately 30 genes have been identified as likely phase-variable and it has been postulated that a much higher degree of recombination occurs for genes under constant selective pressure as opposed to more neutral genes such as those encoding 'housekeeping' functions [99]. DNA sequence analysis of *H. pylori* strains indicated that recombination of LPS biosynthesis genes may reflect genetic exchange within the population lineage and that phase variable gene evolution occurs at a high rate [100].

Gene function	**CDS**		**Repeat**	**Strain variation**[1]		
	26695 (HP)	J99 (jhp)		+[2]	-[3]	Abs[4]
LPS biosynthesis						
α-1, 3-fucosyltransferase*	0651	0596	A	7	16	0
			C	10	13	0
α-1, 3-fucosyltransferase*	0379	1002	A	12	11	0
			C	14	9	0
FutC (α-1, 2-fucosyltransferase)*	0093-4	0086	C	23	0	0
			A	19	4	0
Lex2B	0619	0563	C	20	0	3
RfaJ (α-1, 2-glycosyltransferase)	0208	0194	GA	20	0	3
RfaJ (α-1, 2-glycosyltransferase)	NH[5]	0820	C	8	11	4
β-1, 4-*N*-acetylgalactoamyl transferase*	0217	0203	G	21	2	0
			G	3	20	0
RfaJ homologue	0159		-	Putative[6]		
RfaJ homologue	1416		-	Putative		
OMP[7]						
FliP (flagellar protein)	0684-5	0625	C	6	16	1
OM adherence protein	1417	1312	GA	14	0	9
Streptococcal M protein	0058	0050	C	12	2	9
HopH (OipA)	0638	0581	CT	16	7	0
TlpB (chemotaxis protein)	0103	0095	G	20	0	3
BabA (Leb binding protein)	1243	0833	CT	Putative		

Gene function	CDS		Repeat	Strain variation[1]		
	26695 (HP)	J99 (jhp)		+[2]	-[3]	Abs[4]
BabB (Leb binding protein homologue)	0896	1164	TC	22	0	1
SabA (sialic acid binding adhesion)	0725	0662	TC	17	2	4
SabB (sialic acid binding adhesion)	0722	0659	TC	7	16	0
HopZ (adhesion)	0009	0007	TC	22	0	1
Oxaluglutarate	0143	0131	A	23	0	0
PldA (phospholipase A)	0499	0451	G	20	3	0
HcpA (cysteine rich protein)	0211	0197	-	Putative		
HcpB (cysteine rich protein)	0335	0318	G	13	0	10
DNA Restriction/modification						
Methyltransferase*	1353-4	1272	G	15	0	8
			G	15	0	8
Type III restriction enzyme	1369-70	1284	G	18	3	2
Type II R/M enzyme	1471	1364	G	14	1	8
Type III R/M enzyme	1522	1411	G	6	0	17
HsdR (type I restriction enzyme)*	0464	0416	C	23	0	0
			A	2	21	0
MboIIR (type II restriction enzyme)	1366	1422	A	6	12	5
Metabolic proteins						
FrxA (NADPH flavin oxidoreductase)	0642	0586	G	6	15	2
Hypothetical ORFs						
Hypothetical protein	0744	0681	AG	18	0	5
Hypothetical protein	1433	1326	C	18	2	3
Hypothetical protein	0767	NA[8]	G	7	0	16
Hypothetical protein	NH	0540	A	20	0	3

[1]Phase variation investigated for 30 genes in 23 *H. pylori* strains. Adapted from Salaün et al [99, 122]

[2]Gene present with repeat

[3]Gene present with repeat absent or stabilized

[4]Gene absent

[5]No homolog in genome

[6]Putative phase variable gene

[7]Outer membrane protein

[8]Not annotated

*'on'-'off' gene status directed by more than one repeat

Table 2. Phase variation in *H. pylori* strains from different geographic regions

3.1.3.1. Lipopolysaccharide (LPS) biosynthesis

All Gram-negative bacterial outer membranes contain a structurally important component called LPS (or endotoxin). *H. pylori* LPS consists of three major moieties; a lipid A membrane anchor, a core- and an O-polysaccharide antigen. Although structurally similar to many other Gram-negative bacteria, *H. pylori* LPS has low immunological activity [101]. The O-polysaccharide chain of the LPS of most *H. pylori* strains contains carbohydrates that are structurally related to human blood group antigens, such as Lewis a, b, x and y. The structural oligosaccharide pattern of the LPS of some pathogenic bacteria, including *H. pylori*, is regulated by phase variable fucosyl- and glycosyltranferases; enzymes that transfer sugar residues to its acceptor.

H. pylori strain NCTC 11637 (ATCC 43504, CCUG 17874) expresses the human blood group antigen Lewis x (Le^x) in a polymeric form $(Le^x)_n$ on its core antigen. However, Le^x expression is not stable and can lead to different LPS variants in single cell populations. Loss of α1, 3-linked fucose resulted in a non-fucosylated $(\text{lactosamine})_n$ core antigen, known as the i antigen, that was reversible. Other LPS variants lost the $(Le^x)_n$ main chain resulting in the expression of monomeric (Le^y)-core-lipid A or had acquired α1, 2-linked fucose expressing polymeric Le^x and Le^y simultaneously. Most *H. pylori* isolates have been shown to be able to switch back to the parental phenotype but with varying frequency [102].

Moreover, poly-C tract length variation causes frame shifts in *H. pylori* α3-glycosyltransferases that can inactivate gene products in a reversible manner. Serological data suggested that LPS structural diversification arises from phase variable regulation of glycosyltransferase genes, provisionally named *futA* and *futB* [103]. Phase variation of *futA* and *futB* genes independently has been confirmed and genetic exchange between these loci was shown to occur in single colonies from the same patient and also during *in vitro* passage [104].

H. pylori strain NCTC 11637 also has been shown to express blood group antigen H type I. This epitope demonstrated high frequency phase variation that was reversible. Insertional mutagenesis of gene jhp563 (a poly-C tract sequence containing an ORF homologous to glycosyltransferases) in NCTC 11637 showed that LPS then lacked the H type I epitope. DNA sequence analysis confirmed gene-on and gene-off variation. In *H. pylori* strain G27 mutagenesis of jhp563 yielded a mutant expressing Le^x and Le^y as opposed to wild-type [H type 1, Le^a, Le^x and Le^y]. Jhp563 may encode a β3-galactosyltransferase involved in H type I synthesis that phase varies due to poly-C tract changes [105].

H. pylori ORF HP0208, and its homologues HP0159 and HP1416, show homology to the *waaJ* gene that encodes a α1, 2-glycosyltransferase required for core LPS biosynthesis in *Salmonella typhimurium*. HP0208 contains multiple repeats of the dinucleotide 5'GA at its 5' end and transcription of its gene product has been predicted to be controlled by phase variation. Most strains examined, including strains 26695, J99 and NCTC 11637, had repeat numbers inconsistent with expression of the gene; i.e. placing the translational initiation codon out-of-frame with the full length ORF. A 'phase-on' HP0208 was constructed in the genome of strain 26695. Tricine gel and Western blot analysis demonstrated a role for HP0208 as well as HP0159 and HP1416 in the biosynthesis of core LPS [106]. It is likely that the biosynthesis machinery of not only the *H. pylori* LPS O-antigen side chain but also the core oligosaccharide of *H. pylori* LPS is subject to phase variation. These complex processes possibly give rise to the diversification of LPS observed in clonal populations of *H. pylori*.

3.1.3.2. Lewis expression in vitro

The α1, 2-fucosyltransferase (*futC*) of *H. pylori* catalyses the conversion of Le^x to Le^y, the repeating units of the LPS O-antigen. *futC* is subjected to phase variation through slipped strand mispairing involving a poly-C tract. Single colonies (*n*=379) from *in vitro* cultures have been examined for Lewis expression and demonstrated equal distribution of Le^x and Le^y expression and the phenotypes correlated with *futC* frame status. The founding population remained, since phenotypes did not change significantly over additional hundreds of generations *in vitro* [107].

Two single colonies of the same isolate of *H. pylori* that expressed Le^y of different molecular weights demonstrated wild-type Lewis phenotype after 50 *in vitro* passages after expansion of a larger cell mass; however after 50 *in vitro* passages of single colonies, ~5% of the analysed strains also expressed considerable levels of Le^x in addition to low levels of Le^y, suggesting reduced expression of *futC*. Successive *in vitro* passaging of single colonies introduced a much more frequent phenotypic diversification in terms of O-antigen size and Le^x expression [104].

3.1.3.3. Lewis expression in vivo

With a limited number of passages of strains in the laboratory, analysis of the phenotypic diversity of Lewis antigen expression from 180 clonal *H. pylori* populations from primary cultures of 20 gastric biopsies indicated a substantial difference in Lewis expression in 75% of the patients. The variation of Lewis expression was unrelated to the overall genetic diversity. In experimentally infected rodents however, Lewis expression was highly uniform [108]. Intra population diversity of Lewis expression has since been confirmed. *H. pylori* isolates with identical DNA signatures (arbitrary primed PCR) from the same chronically infected patient demonstrated variations in the amount and size (length) of the O-antigen and immunoassays detected exclusively the presence of Le^y, suggesting simultaneous expression of both α1, 2- and α1, 3-fucosyltransferases. LPS diversification has also been investigated in transgenic mice expressing Le^b on gastric epithelial cells. The challenging strain expressed a high molecular weight O-antigen and showed a strong antibody response against Le^y. More than 90% of the mouse output isolates produced glycolipids of low molecular weight compared with the input strain. Subsequent immunoblot analysis demonstrated decreased or no Le^y expression [104].

3.1.3.4. Adhesins and cell surface proteins

Expression of bacterial outer membrane proteins can be regulated by environmental changes through signal transduction as well as the generation of genetic changes controlling protein function. Cell surface associated proteins are the most abundant group of *H. pylori* proteins that is subject to phase variation. Such proteins include so called adhesins, flagellar and flagellar hook proteins, pro-inflammatory proteins, cysteine-rich proteins as well as some other categories. With exception of adhesins, most proteins in this group remain uncharacterized.

The outer membrane of *H. pylori* partially comprises adhesins, which bind to host gastric epithelial cell surface receptors. Gene functions of *H. pylori* adhesins, many of which belong to the so called *hop* gene family, are regulated through phase variation.

The sialic acid binding adhesin (SabA) of *H. pylori* adhere to glycosphingolipids that display sialyl Lewis x antigens. Such antigens have been shown to be upregulated on human epithelial cell surfaces as a result of gastric inflammation [109]. DNA sequence analysis demonstrated that locus HP0725 (*sab*A) of *H. pylori* strain 26695 contained repetitive CT dinucleotides at the 5' end of the ORF [57]. Translational modification may encounter premature termination (non-functional protein) or a full length functional adhesion protein. *sab*A has promoter poly-T as well as ORF 5' end CT tract repeats. Multiple length alleles have been shown to occur in single colonies isolated from the same individual and genome sequence analyses of isolates of *H. pylori* strains demonstrated genetic and phenotypic variation of SabA [110].

The *H. pylori* protein HopZ is a candidate to be involved in the adherence to host gastric epithelial cells and *hopZ* is likely phase variable due to a CT dinucleotide repeat in the signal sequence of the gene [111]. Human volunteers have recently been challenged with a *H. pylori* strain with *hopZ* 'off' status. Out of 56 re-isolated strains (from 32 volunteers at 3 month post inoculation) 68% had switched to a *hopZ* 'on' status. After 4 years, paired isolates had 54% *hopZ* 'on' status. Sequence analysis of *hopZ* 'on' and 'off' status in 54 *H. pylori* strains representing seven different phylogeographic populations (hpAsia2, hpEurope, hpNEAfrica, hpAfrica1, hpAfrica2, hpEastAsia and hpSahul) and 11 subpopulations, demonstrated variability between and within most populations; only two subpopulations (hspAfrica2SA and hspAmerind) were exclusively *hopZ* 'off' [112].

Many *H. pylori* strains bind to the human blood group antigen Le^b. This adherence is mediated by the blood group antigen binding adhesin BabA. Some strains contain two alleles; *babA1* which is 'silent' and *babA2* that expresses the adhesin [113]. Although BabA expression has not been identified to be phase variable by DNA sequence analysis [99], experimental infection of rhesus macaques showed that, in some animals, compared with its parent challenge strain, output strains lost BabA expression due to an alteration in dinucleotide CT repeats in the 5' coding region. Output strains from other macaques that also had lost Le^b binding, had *babA* exchanged for *babB*. Duplication of *babB* has also been observed in human clinical *H. pylori* isolates [75]. *babB* and *babA* have very similar 5' and 3' end sequences but *babB* lacks the mid region that codes for the Le^b binding epitope. BabB is an uncharacterized outer membrane protein and *babB* contains repetitive sequence motifs and is likely subject to frameshift-based phase variation [57, 97].

Gene function of *hopH* (*oipA*) depends on slipped strand mispairing in a CT dinucleotide repeat in the signal sequence of the gene. HopH has been associated with increased interleukin-8 (IL-8) production in epithelial cells and gastric epithelial adherence *in vitro* [114, 115]. *H. pylori* isolates with a *hopH* 'in-frame' status were more common than 'out-of-frame' strains in patients with chronic gastritis, a feature that correlated with the virulence factor status of the strains, particularly *cagA* [114]. In a patient setting, *hopH* (*oipA*) 'in-frame' status was associated with a higher colonization density of *H. pylori* and clinical presentation regarding gastric inflammation and mucosal IL-8 production [116].

3.1.3.5. Acid adaptation

H. pylori can reversibly change its membrane phospholipid composition, producing variants with differing concentrations of lysophospholipids. Lysophospholipid-rich cells are more adherent, secrete more VacA and are more haemolytic. As opposed to neutral culture conditions, growth at low pH (3.5) renders an accumulation of membrane lysophospholipids. This variation in lipid composition is mediated by phase variation in the phospholipase A (*pldA*) gene. A change in the C-tract length of the ORF results either in a functional full-length or a truncated non-functional gene product [117].

The structure and composition of LPS adapts to an acid environment. Under acidic growth conditions (pH 5) *in vitro*, the LPS core and lipid A moieties seem not to be altered. However, the O-side chain backbone is partially fucosylated forming Le^x, whereas the terminal sugar residues on the O-side chain are modified differently and terminate with Le^y instead of Le^x [118].

3.1.3.6. Immune modulation

H. pylori genomes contain a family of genes coding for proteins designated Helicobacter cysteine rich proteins (Hcp). HcpA, a secreted protein, has partially been characterized. Recombinant HcpA, as opposed to HcpC, induced maturation of non-adherent human Thp1 monocytes into macrophages (star-like morphology with filopodia) with phagocytic ability and surface adherent properties [119].

Surfactant protein D (SP-D), a component of innate immunity, is expressed in human gastric mucosa. SP-D has an affinity for simple sugars and likely functions as a mucosal receptor that recognizes pathogen associated molecular patterns (PAMPs). SP-D induces aggregation of microorganisms facilitating pathogen clearance by neutrophil and macrophage phagocytosis. Some *H. pylori* strains lack a ligand for SP-D and this 'escape' mechanism is associated with phase variation of the LPS structure. Fucosylation of the O-side chain, determined by slipped strand mispairing in a fucosyltransferase gene leading to terminal Le^x (SP-D binding) or Le^y (escape), controls the *H. pylori* ligand recognized by SP-D [120].

DC-SIGN, a C-type lectin, is a surface receptor expressed on dendritic cells that captures and aids the internalization of microbial antigens. *H. pylori* strains that express Lewis antigens on their LPS bind DC-SIGN and thereby block T helper cell (Th) 1 development, whereas some strains that do not express Lewis antigens escape binding to dendritic cells and promote a Th 1 response. Phase variation of LPS in terms of Lewis expression may influence host immunity through the dendritic cell pathway. Clonal populations of *H. pylori*, with high frequency of subclone phase variation in LPS biosynthesis genes, are proposed to manipulate the Th response for optimal persistence that prevents severe atrophy and destruction of the ecological niche [29, 121].

3.1.3.7. Experimental infections

Phase variable OMP gene switch status of *H. pylori* have been investigated in an experimental mouse model of infection. The gene switch status of several OMPs (*hopH, hopZ, hopO* and *hopP*) influenced *H. pylori* density in gastric tissue and its ability to colonise mice. If two or more of the genes were in the switch 'off' mode, the colonization ability was markedly reduced. These results correlated well with observations in humans; i.e. patients with strains whose *hop* genes were in the 'off' mode had lower bacterial load [115].

In a murine model of infection, repeat length and function of 31 phase variable genes of several *H. pylori* strains were followed for up to one year. At endpoint, 15 genes had a change in repeat length. However, a third of these did not lead to an alteration in protein expression. Ten genes demonstrated a frame shift to an 'on' mode of the encoded protein. At early time points (3 and 21 days), mixed *pldA* phenotypes rapidly and exclusively changed to 'on' status, followed by LPS biosynthesis genes modifying terminal sugars. Glycosyltransferases modifying LPS core structures remained in 'off' configuration throughout the study. From 21 days onward some OMPs (*babB* and *hopZ*) switched from 'on' to 'off'. Restriction/modification systems did not show a particular pattern over time [122].

BabA expression has been shown to be lost during experimental infection in rhesus macaques, either by allele replacement with *babB*, or phase variation. A follow up study investigated this phenomenon in other animal hosts using additional *H. pylori* strains. Murine and gerbil experimental infection models further demonstrated loss of Le^b binding (as a result of *babA* recombination) of output strains by varying mechanisms. In the mouse, BabA expression was lost due to phase variation in a 5' CT repeat region of *H. pylori* strain J166 [123].

To conclude, *H. pylori* randomly exhibits phase variation in sets of genes that directly interact with the environment. These include LPS biosynthesis genes, adhesins and genes with an impact on the structural composition of the bacterial outer membrane. Phase variation also influences the expression of some genes affecting host immune responses. Taken together, these traits are likely to aid a continuous adaptation to the ecological niche and persistence of the bacterium.

Selection pressure in terms of host niche physiology and maturation of host immune response likely contributes to the genetic regulation and diversification of bacterial adherence properties as well as the composition of the outer membrane. For bacteria such as *H. pylori* that may cause life-long colonization, surface antigen diversity likely requires parallel evolution with host cell subsets over time for continuous adaptation to a dynamic host environment.

3.1.4. Epigenetic diversity: phasevarion

As previously described, phase variation via the high-frequency reversible ON/OFF switching of gene expression is beneficial to pathogenic bacteria, including *H. pylori,* as a means of rapidly generating the genotypic and phenotypic diversity required for adaptation to the host environment and evasion from the immune system [124]. However, certain evolutionary advantages arise when expression of a repertoire of genes is brought under the influence of a single phase-variable gene as is the case for a phase-variable regulon or "phasevarion" (Figure 2).

The phasevarion is an epigenetic regulatory system whereby the expression of a set of genes is randomly switched as coordinated by the activity of the modification (Mod) component of a restriction-modification (R-M) system [51]. R-M systems share two components; the restriction (Res) component that specifically cleaves unmethylated DNA at a recognition sequence, and the Mod component that methylates the same recognition sequence to prevent cleavage by the Res component [125]. Most R-M systems fall within one of three major families (Type I, II, III). Type II and type III Mod proteins recognise specific DNA sequences whereas type I Mod proteins require an additional specificity subunit [126]. A role for R-M systems in host-pathogen interaction was unexpected, as these systems generally function to protect the genome integrity of bacteria from invasion by foreign DNA by restriction of DNA that does not share the same modifications as that of the host. However, where the Res component is absent or not functional, phase variation of the Mod component results in the random switching of methylation of DNA sequences recognized by the *mod* encoded methyltransferase. For genes where DNA methylation by the phase-variable Mod affects promoter activity, either by altering the DNA binding affinity of regulatory proteins for promoters [127], or by other mechanisms, differential gene expression results.

Although phase-variable R-M systems had previously been identified in a number of bacteria [128], the first experimental evidence for the phasevarion was from *H. influenzae*, a pathogen of the upper respiratory tract [51]. The *mod* gene of the sole type-III R-M system of *H. influenza* contains tetranucleotide repeats consistent with an ability to phase vary. Microarray analysis of a mutant in this gene revealed differential expression of 16 genes, including genes implicated in pathogenicity, in the absence of *mod*. The differential expression of these genes was shown by reporter gene fusions to be dependent on the phase variation of *mod*. Hence the phase variation of a single gene, *mod*, was shown to influence the expression of multiple genes, suggesting the presence of a phase-variable regulon, or "phasevarion."

Phasevarion mediated gene switching has now been confirmed in *H. influenzae* [51], *N. gonorrhoeae* and *N. meningitidis* [129], and *H. pylori* [50]. This wide distribution, and the allelic diversity of phase-variable methyltransferases, indicates that there is strong selective pressure on phasevarions. It has been postulated that it may be simpler for a gene to evolve to join a phasevarion than become phase variable. The evolution of phase-variation requires the generation of repeat sequences without destroying either promoter or gene function, whereas joining a phasevarion requires only a few key point mutations to generate the methyltransferase recognition site in a region where methylation would affect gene expression [51]. A further evolutionary advantage of the phasevarion may be that it represents an extension of the regulation achieved by phase variation. Rather than randomly reversibly switching a single gene, the phasevarion switches a whole set of genes, thereby differentiating a bacterial population into two different cell types based on many phenotypic characteristics [50, 130]. This switching between different physiological states, rather than merely individual proteins, may assist the bacterium in taking advantage of microenvironments within the host.

Genome sequencing of *H. pylori* 26695 [57] and J99 [97] revealed a surprisingly large number of R-M systems (22 in 26695) when compared to other sequenced bacterial and archaeal genomes. Each strain of *H. pylori* contains its own complement of R-M systems, some of which may have the potential to phase vary due to the presence of repeat regions [47, 97, 131, 132]. Typically multiple *mod* genes may be present in any given strain and there may be multiple different *mod* alleles for each *mod* gene within a given species [128]. Diversity of *mod* genes can be driven by recombination of DNA recognition domains between non-orthologous genes and horizontal gene transfer [133, 134]. Phylogenetic analysis of clinical isolates of *H. pylori* revealed a diverse set of 17 alleles of the *modH* gene that differed in the DNA recognition domain and phase-varying repeat region. This diversity in *mod* genes indicates corresponding diversity in the set of genes regulated by Mod and also indicates that there may be many phasevarions present in *H. pylori* [50]. Any R-M system present within the genome with an inactive Res may represent a phasevarion. Phasevarions may therefore represent common epigenetic mechanisms for generating rapid reversible phenotypic diversity in bacterial host-adapted pathogens such as *H. pylori*.

Functional analysis of the Type-II R-M systems in J99 and 26695 revealed that less than 30% were fully functional (with both Res and Mod functional) and that there were many functional Mod enzymes with no apparent functional Res partner [132, 135], indicative of these *mod* genes regulating a phasevarion. Repeat sequences and homopolymeric tracts, indicative of phase variation, where identified in a number of R-M systems (both type-II and type-III) in *H. pylori* [47, 57, 97, 98, 130]. Direct experimental evidence of phase variation within an R-M system was first given by *lacZ* reporter fusions to a type-III R-M system [136]. An R-M system has also been shown to phase vary in the mouse model, suggesting a role for these systems in host-adaptation [122].

Given that *H. pylori* contains a diverse repertoire of R-M systems that phase vary and R-M systems with orphaned Mod proteins, it is likely that many of these systems regulate a phasevarion. The first evidence that the activity of a phase-variable Mod influenced the transcription of other genes in *H. pylori* came from the analysis of the type-II methyltransferase M.HpyAIV in 26695. M.HpyAIV was found to phase vary due to the presence of homopolymeric tract of adenine residues. Analysis of the genomes of 26695 and J99 revealed 60 genes common to both strains where the M.HpyAIV DNA-methylation sites occurred in the intergenic region upstream of ORFs, indicating a possible role for these sites in regulating gene expression. Differential expression of these genes was studied by qPCR and the expression of catalase encoding *katA* was shown to be significantly decreased in a 26695 mutant of M.HpyAIV [137].

Further evidence of the presence of phasevarions in *H. pylori* came from deletion of the *modH5* type-III methyltransferase from *H. pylori* P12. Microarray analysis of the mutant strain revealed six genes, including outer membrane protein HopG and flagellar associated proteins, that were differentially expressed compared to wild-type [50].

A phasevarion regulated by *hpyAVIBM* may also be present in *H. pylori*. The presence of AG repeats in this type-II methyltransferase indicates that this gene may have the potential to phase vary, although this has not been experimentally demonstrated. Deletion of *hpyAVIBM* from *H. pylori* SS1 and clinical isolate AM5 resulted in differential regulation in a diverse set of genes, including outer membrane proteins, genes involved in motility, pathogenicity, LPS biosynthesis, and R-M systems, when compared to WT by microarray analysis. Further analysis revealed corresponding alterations in phenotype of the *hpyAVIBM* mutant such as altered motility, increased expression of CagA as determined by Western blot, altered LPS profile, improved ability to induce IL-8 production in human AGS cells, and a decrease in transformation efficiency. Differences observed in gene expression and phenotype due to deletion of *hpyAVIBM* varied between the two strains investigated potentially due to different distribution of the methylation recognition site of HpyAVIBM across the genome of the two strains. The occurrence of the *hpyAVIBM* allele in *H. pylori* strains isolated from individuals with duodenal ulcer and healthy individuals revealed that the methyltransferase was present in most strains isolated from symptomatic patients but absent in most strains isolated from healthy individuals, indicating that *hpyAVIBM* expression may be clinically relevant [138]. Even if *hpyAVIBM* does not phase vary, this study demonstrates the wide ranging regulatory capabilities of DNA methyltransferases.

3.2. Inter-strain generation of diversity

3.2.1. Natural transformation

H. pylori is naturally competent, it is able to be transformed by the uptake and incorporation of foreign DNA into its genome [139]. Potential reasons for natural competence in bacteria are a matter of discussion. It is postulated that bacteria may utilize the uptake of foreign DNA for nutrition, for DNA repair, for evolution via horizontal gene transfer, or that DNA-uptake is an evolutionary spandrel of adhesion and twitching motility [140, 141]. As we will discuss, it is becoming increasingly clear that natural transformation plays an important role in *H. pylori* genome evolution and host adaptation.

3.2.1.1. Quick overview of players in uptake and recombination

A complete picture of the process of DNA uptake followed by integration into the genome in *H. pylori* is beginning to emerge, although many details remain to be clarified. Uptake of foreign DNA into the bacterial cell is achieved by a two-step mechanism as shown in Figure 3. Firstly, dsDNA is taken up through the outer membrane by the ComB type-IV secretion system [142]. The ComEC system is then responsible for DNA uptake through the inner membrane [143, 144]. Transport of DNA by ComEC likely results in the entry of single-stranded DNA into the cytoplasm based on the function of ComFA in *Bacillus subtilis*, although this has not been directly experimentally demonstrated in *H. pylori*. Incoming DNA is at some point subjected to the activity of restriction endonucleases [145]. Once in the cytoplasm DprA and RecA cooperatively bind the incoming ssDNA forming a heterodimer [146]. During recombination RecA mediates strand invasion of incoming DNA with chromosomal DNA and this process is subject to interference from UvrD and MutS2 [49, 73, 90, 147]. RecA mediated synapsis with chromosomal DNA results in the formation of four-way branched DNA intermediate structures referred to as Holliday junctions whose migration and resolution are mediated by DNA processing enzymes. Branch migration of Holliday junctions is mediated by either the competing RuvAB or RecG helicases [86]. Resolution of the Holliday junction is primarily by DprB in instances of natural transformation with homeologous DNA from other *H. pylori* strains, although RuvC, the DNA-repair resolvase, can partially compensate for a loss of DprB [148].

3.2.1.2. Structure of the uptake system

In contrast to other bacterial species where DNA-uptake occurs via systems related to type IV pili, the ComB system *of H. pylori* is related to type IV secretion systems and its components have been named for their homologues in the *Agrobacterium tumefaciens* VirB type IV secretion apparatus [142, 149]. The genes encoding ComB are organized in two separate loci with an operon consisting of *comB6 – 10* and a second operon consisting of *comB2 – 4* [142, 150-152]. All the *comB* and *comEC* genes are essential for competence with the exception of *comB7* which is postulated to play a stabilizing role for the comB complex [142, 143, 151]. Sequence homology with the VirB type IV secretion system and topological mapping of the ComB proteins has given some insight into the structure of the ComB apparatus [151, 153]. ComB2 is postulated to be located as a "stump structure" in the external membrane and have a role in initial DNA-uptake. It has also been associated with adhesion to human gastric tissue [152]. ComB7 is also associated with the outer membrane and may serve to stabilize ComB9, which is present in the periplasm with an anchor to the outer membrane via a disulphide bond. ComB8 contains a large periplasmic domain and spans the inner membrane and may interact with ComB9 and/or ComB10 which is postulated to be anchored in the inner membrane where it may be present as a homodimer. ComB4 is cytoplasmic and serves as the ATPase that energises the ComB machinery. A role for ComB3 is largely unknown although it is predicted to contain one transmembrane domain.

3.2.1.3. Process of DNA uptake

The process of DNA uptake by *H. pylori* has been studied using fluorescently labelled DNA and single molecule analysis with laser tweezers [143]. The initial step in transformation is the binding of extracellular DNA to the surface of the bacterium. The ComB machinery may play a role in DNA-binding to the cell as mutants lacking inner-membrane components of the ComB machinery showed impaired DNA-binding [151]. Once bound, DNA was found to be rapidly taken into the periplasm of the cell through ComB via an ATP-dependent mechanism likely driven by the ATPase ComB4. Multiple DNA-uptake complexes were found to be simultaneously active. Uptake of DNA through the outer membrane by ComB appears to be non-specific as uptake of DNA was not distinguished on the basis of DNA sequence. Following transport of DNA into the periplasm by ComB, ssDNA enters the cytoplasm via ComEC. Transport of DNA by ComB and ComEC appears to be spatially and temporally uncoupled. The identity of any motor driving uptake of DNA by comEC remains to be uncovered. Transport of DNA by ComEC appears to be more discriminating than ComB, as covalently labelled DNA transported by ComB could not enter the cytoplasm via ComEC. As DNA sequence does not seem to play a role in the initial uptake of DNA by *H. pylori*, discrimination of incoming DNA and protection from the potentially hazardous consequences of the incorporation of foreign DNA may come from the numerous restriction-modification systems of *H. pylori*.

3.2.1.4. The restriction barrier - frequency

The fate of incoming DNA is either one of restriction or recombination. Restriction of foreign DNA forms the most significant barrier to natural transformation in *H. pylori* [145]. Like other bacteria, *H. pylori* discriminates the DNA of self from non-self by the modification of bases by methylation. Restriction modification systems (R-M) consist of a methyltransferase that methylates specific DNA sequences and a restriction endonuclease that cleaves non-methylated DNA at the same sequence. Incoming foreign DNA that does not share the same methylation pattern as that of the host is thus digested. In this manner, many R-M systems function to prevent transformation and protect the host from foreign DNA [125]. The number and diversity of R-M systems in the *H. pylori* genome is notable, with many being strain specific [57]. The diversity of R-M systems can be driven by deletion and acquisition of such systems by horizontal gene transfer [154]. These strain specific R-M systems may be responsible for the observation that competence of different *H. pylori* strains varies [155]. The barrier posed by R-M systems to competency has been experimentally demonstrated by assessing transformation frequency in the presence and absence of R-M systems. The removal of four active type-II restriction endonucleases from *H. pylori* 26695 lead to higher transformation efficiency both of donor DNA from *E. coli* and other *H. pylori* strains [156]. The removal of two active type-II restriction endonucleases from NSH57 greatly reduced the barrier to transformation resulting in greater transformation frequency with DNA from a J99 donor [145].

3.2.1.5. The restriction barrier – integration length

In addition to transformation frequency, restriction of incoming DNA also influences the length of incoming DNA that is integrated into the host chromosome. It has been proposed that although *H. pylori* takes up long DNA fragments by natural transformation, only shorter fragments are integrated into the genome. Genomic sequencing of isolates revealed that sequences recombined with imported DNA varied in length from 261 to 629 bp and were clustered. This observation was suggested to be consistent with the uptake of long stretches of DNA, corresponding to the length of the region in which recombination sites were clustered, that has subsequently been broken up and partially integrated [157]. Mutants of *H. pylori* NSH57 lacking active type-II restriction endonucleases where found to integrate longer DNA fragments into their genome following natural transformation than the WT strain [145].

3.2.1.6. DrpA overcomes restriction

Although restriction presents a barrier to transformation, *H. pylori* achieves a balance between restriction and recombination. It has been proposed that the concentration of restriction enzymes in the cell may be limited to produce only partial cleavage of incoming DNA in order to allow a basal level of transformation [145]. In addition to this proposal, the DNA processing protein A (DrpA), has been shown to lower the barrier to recombination in a number of bacterial species and is widely conserved [146]. Deletion of *drpA* in *H. pylori* has been reported to result in either a significant decrease [158, 159], or abrogation of transformation frequency [145]. In *H. pylori* DprA has a polar localisation and interacts with incoming DNA, binding ssDNA and also dsDNA to a lesser extent. DprA protects incoming DNA from restriction by both preventing the access of type-II restriction endonucleases to DNA and enhancing methylation of incoming DNA by direct interaction with methyltransferases. It thus appears to play a key role in the balance between restriction and recombination [160]. However, the temporal and spatial aspects of restriction endonuclease cleavage and DprA activity are not yet clearly understood. Single-stranded DNA is thought to enter the cytoplasm following uptake by ComEC and DprA binds preferentially to ssDNA, yet restriction enzymes, which contribute the most significant barrier to transformation, find ssDNA a poor substrate in preference to dsDNA.

3.2.1.7. DNA processing enzymes and competence

As depicted in Figure 3, following entry into the cytoplasm, incoming DNA is co-operatively bound by DrpA and RecA. RecA acts to mediate strand invasion of foreign DNA with the host chromosome and promotes homologous recombination. The nucleotide excision repair helicase, UvrD, likely disrupts this process by removal of RecA from DNA, preventing potential recombination events. Mutants in RecA therefore are unable to undergo recombination whereas mutants in UvrD display a hyper-recombination phenotype [49, 73]. MutS2 is also proposed to interrupt RecA-mediated strand invasion. Deletion of MutS2 from *H. pylori* results in an increase in transformation efficiency suggesting a role of MutS2 in regulation of homologous recombination. Analysis of MutS2 indicates that it is not a member of the mismatch repair pathway but rather has a distinct function in strand displacement of incoming DNA from RecA-mediated D-loop formation during stand invasion of incoming DNA with the host chromosome. This function is independent of the degree of homology of the two strands [90, 147]. Thus in addition to the restriction barrier, enzymes involved in determining the outcome between formation or dissolution of the D-loop also appear to play a role in determining the fate of foreign DNA. The influence on transformation of other DNA processing enzymes acting during the recombination event is less clear. Reports regarding transformation efficiency of a *recG* mutant vary [145, 161] and integration length in a *recG* mutant was reported to be decreased [145]. In contrast to an initial report where deletion of *ruvC* resulted in a decrease in transformation frequency [162], two reports have found no decrease in transformation frequency [145, 148] but an increase in integration length in a *ruvC* mutant was noted [145]. Reports regarding the phenotype of a mutant in *dprB*, the recombination specific Holliday junction resolvase, are consistent that deletion of *dprB* results in a decrease in transformation frequency but does not influence integration length [145, 148].

3.2.1.8. Other factors

A further factor required for competence that appears to be unique to *H. pylori* is ComH. Mutants in *comH* could not be transformed with chromosomal or plasmid DNA [163, 164]. ComH is a surface-exposed outer membrane protein that binds ssDNA but whose function in competence remains to be further characterized [165].

The role of the nuclease NucT in *H. plyori* competence is also unclear. NucT is an outer membrane bound nuclease that preferentially cleaves ssDNA. The observation that transformation rates are reduced in a *nucT* mutant leads to the proposal that NucT functions either in

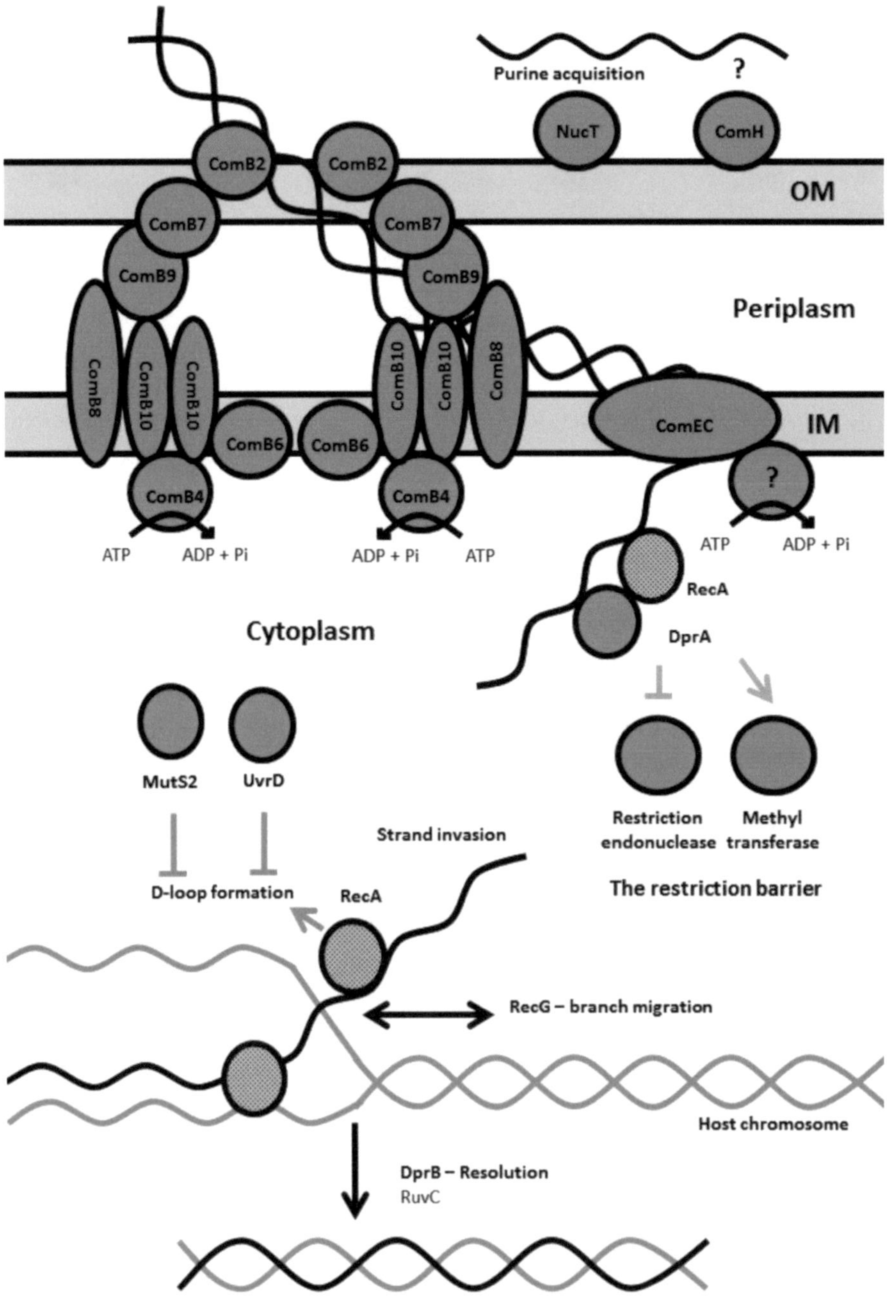

Figure 3. Natural transformation in *H. pylori*. Schematic representation of the uptake of foreign DNA and its integration into the host chromosome in *H. pylori*. Double stranded DNA is taken up through the outer membrane by the ComB machinery and through the inner membrane by ComEC. Following DNA uptake ssDNA is bound by RecA and DprA, which affects the activity of restriction endonucleases and methyltransferases. Strand invasion of the host chromosome by foreign DNA is mediated by RecA and this process is inhibited by MutS2 and UvrD. Branch migration and resolution are mediated by RecG and DprB, respectively. NucT may function as a nuclease for the acquisition of purines and the exact role of ComH in competence has yet to be determined.

initial DNA binding, or translocation into the cell [166]. In contrast, a later study found that deletion of *nucT* did not influence transformation efficiency, but did result in an increase in the length of DNA integrated into the chromosome [145]. The presence of NucT as a stable outer membrane nuclease and the requirement of *H. pylori* to scavenge purines for growth as a result of its inability to synthesise purines *de novo* led to an investigation of the role of NucT in purine acquisition [167]. NucT was found to be required for growth when exogenous DNA is the only purine source, indicating that the primary function of NucT is the digestion of human DNA in the gastric mucosa as a purine source. Digestion of dsDNA in the absence of its preferred ssDNA substrate *in vitro* could be responsible for the conflicting results obtained in assays of transformation efficiency.

3.2.1.9. Regulation of competence is by DNA damage

Competence is usually a tightly regulated and transient feature in bacteria. *H. pylori* is unusual in that it displays very high levels of competence. Competence was found to vary across stages of growth with each strain displaying a different pattern of peaks in transformation efficiency in different growth phases. The pattern observed was independent of the type of donor DNA [168]. Competence is upregulated in response to DNA damage by the induction of the transcription and translation of competence machinery. A marginal increase in transformation frequency was observed after UV induced DNA damage [73]. Transcription of several genes involved in competence were found to be upregulated in both cDNA microarrays of cells where acute double strand break DNA damage had been induced by ciprofloxacin treatment and in cells where chronic DNA damage had accumulated in *addA* mutants deficient in double-strand break repair. These genes include components of the ComB system and a lysozyme proposed to function by lysing neighbouring cells to provide DNA for uptake. This transcriptional response was dependent on both *recA* and the ability to uptake DNA. The authors proposed a RecA-dependent positive feedback loop in the induction of DNA damage responsive genes that is initiated by DNA damage and amplified by DNA uptake. This system was found not to be important in initial mouse colonization but may be of relevance to persistence. These results demonstrate that unlike other bacteria, *H. pylori* does not mount an SOS response to DNA damage but relies on homologous recombination for maintenance of genome integrity [169]. It seems plausible that *H. pylori* responds to stress induced by the immune system during persistence in the human host by increasing competence to not only repair DNA damage but also to increase genetic diversity in order to continually adapt to a changing host-mediated niche [63].

3.2.2. Competence in vitro

3.2.2.1. Substrate requirements for transformation

The characteristics of natural transformation in *H. pylori in vitro* have been studied in detail. Investigations into the influence of the properties of substrate DNA on natural transformation of *H. pylori* 26695 revealed a number of interesting features [155]:

- Transformation efficiency decreases with shorter DNA fragments although transformants could be obtained with fragments as short as 50 bp.
- Although uptake of DNA occurs within minutes of exposure, transformation efficiency increases with increasing time prior to transformant selection to allow time for uptake, recombination, and expression of a new phenotype.
- Transformation frequency of selectable alleles decreases with decreasing length of flanking sequences, although transformants were obtained with as little as 5 bp flanking sequence.
- Transformation frequencies are higher with chromosomal DNA than PCR products.
- Transformants could be obtained with both single stranded and double stranded DNA but with 1000-fold greater efficiency for double stranded DNA.
- Transformation efficiency is greater with homologous DNA than homeologous DNA.
- Different *H. pylori* strains vary in their competence.
- DNA uptake could be saturated at high DNA concentrations.

3.2.2.2. Length of insertions

Study of transformation *in vitro* has also revealed that *H. pylori* typically imports fragments of short length into the chromosome in comparison to other bacteria and that these imports are regularly interrupted by wild-type recipient sequences. Mean lengths of between 1294 and 3853 bp of integrated DNA were observed from transformations of rifampicin sensitive recipient strains with DNA from resistant donors with different import lengths observed with different donor/recipient combinations [170]. Transformation of streptomycin sensitive strains with DNA of streptomycin resistant strains obtained a mean length of integration of 1300 bp. Furthermore the effect of the restriction barrier may have been observed, as endpoints of integration were found to be clustered, consistent with restriction of incoming DNA at those sites [171]. Short length of imported fragments has also been recorded *in vivo* [157].

3.2.2.3. Why are insertions interspersed?

The region of integrated DNA is commonly reported to be interrupted by short interspersed sequences of the recipient (ISR) and multiple explanations for this observation are present in the literature. Lin *et al.* have suggested ISR could result from two separate but neighboring strand invasion events that would be consistent with the restriction of an invading strand prior to recombination [171]. Conversely, Kulick *et al.* reported that overexpression of the base excision repair glycosylase MutY increased the occurrence of ISR within imported regions, implicating it in their formation. MutY was also found to influence integration length. It was proposed that MutY-mediated DNA repair at impaired bases following recombination results in the insertion of host sequence within recombined regions [170]. The allelic variation generated by ISR is a further mechanism increasing genotypic variation.

3.2.2.4. Promiscuity of DNA uptake

H. pylori is very promiscuous as it does not require incoming DNA sequences for transformation to be as closely related as what other bacterium do. This may be due to the absence of a mismatch repair system, a lack of DNA sequence specificity in DNA uptake machinery, absence of DNA uptake sequences, and a relaxed restriction barrier. Recombination between unrelated strains in co-infected hosts has been observed. Analysis of synonymous distance between recombined alleles within the genomes of *H. pylori* isolates from two South African families revealed recombination with sequences from unrelated strains, in contrast to studies of *S. enterica, E. coli,* and *B.cereus* where recombination only occurred between members of the same lineage [172]. Recombination can also occur between different *Helicobacter* species. Transformation of *H. pylori* 26695 with both homologous and homeologous streptomycin resistance conferring *rpsL* DNA derived from 26695 and *H. cetorum* respectively, yielded transformants, although with 1.5 $\log_{10}$ greater efficiency with homologous DNA. No transformants could be obtained with DNA from *C. jejuni.* Competition between DNA from different sources for transformation revealed that *H. pylori* DNA could compete with *H. pylori* DNA but DNA from unrelated sources could not compete with *H. pylori* DNA, indicating that *H. pylori* can distinguish DNA from different sources on the basis of DNA sequence [155, 173]. This discrimination does not occur at the level of DNA uptake by ComB/ComEC, as cytoplasmic uptake of λ-phage DNA was comparable to *H. pylori* DNA [143], but is likely a consequence of the restriction barrier. Thus although transformation of *H. pylori* is efficient with DNA from unrelated strains, and even to a lesser degree with DNA of other *Helicobacter* species, it has not been observed with DNA from other bacterial genera.

H. pylori displays considerable allelic diversity and genetic variability. The high degree of competence facilitates frequent horizontal transfer of genetic material to the extent that the genome has been found to be in linkage equilibrium [174, 175]. Although genetic variability typifies *H. pylori,* with populations being regarded as panmictic, clonality is observed in the natural transmission of strains within closely related and co-habitating individuals [176]. Also, *H. pylori* populations can be grouped according to geographic location as strains located within a region are more closely related to each other than to strains outside the region [2]. The uptake of foreign DNA by natural transformation and resulting recombination generates a considerable portion of the genetic diversity observed in *H. pylori.*

3.2.3. Plasmids and mobilizable transposons conjugation

In many bacterial species plasmid transfer by conjugation is a significant contributor to the acquisition of genetic material by horizontal gene transfer and often mediates the dissemination of genes of particular phenotypic importance such as antibiotic resistance, virulence determinants, and the ability to utilize certain substrates. Bacterial conjugation can generate chromosomal rearrangements due to plasmid insertion and excision and can also transfer chromosomal genetic material when errors in excision occur. Although diversity exists in bacterial conjugative mechanisms, a generalized overview of the process can be formed. Initially a mating pair of cells must make contact and be brought into proximity. This is typically achieved by the expression of the sex pilus, an elongated tubular appendage, by the donor cell. Once in contact a conjugative pore or some other mechanism for the transfer of DNA to the recipient must be established. This is commonly achieved by a type-IV secretion system. In order to transfer plasmid DNA, a relaxase and accessory proteins, the relaxosome, bind to the plasmid origin of transfer (*oriT*) where they cleave a single strand. The single strand and bound relaxase is recognized by a coupling protein and transferred into the recipient cell in tandem with the rolling circle replication of the intact strand of the plasmid. The relaxase then circularizes the single strand which is replicated to form an intact plasmid within the recipient [177].

H. pylori commonly carry plasmids of varying sizes [178], often of low copy number, which can be divided into two groups [179, 180]. The first are homologous to Gram positive vectors that replicate via the rolling circle mechanism. The second, more common group, are proposed to replicate via the theta mechanism predominately utilising the replication protein, RepA, which binds to short tandem repeats in the plasmid origin of replication. There are several reports characterising the properties of various plasmids in *H. pylori* [180-185].

Plasmid transfer has been demonstrated to occur between different strains of *H. pylori* [186, 187]. Mating experiments with *H. pylori* P8 and P12 revealed that transfer of two conjugative *H. pylori* plasmids could occur through three distinct routes. Firstly, natural transformation, which was dependent on the ComB type-IV secretion system and was DNaseI sensitive, secondly, DNaseI insensitive mobilisation which was dependent on both ComB and the plasmid encoded relaxase (*mobA*), and finally, an alternative DNaseI resistant (ADR) pathway that is independent of ComB. No evidence was found for the involvement of chromosomal relaxases in any pathway [187]. Backert *et al.* also demonstrated conjugative plasmid transfer in *H. pylori* but used two mobilizable vectors containing a broad host range *oriT* [186]. In this instance transfer was insensitive to DNaseI and dependent on viable cell contact, indicative of a conjugative process. No role was found for ComB, indicating that natural transformation was not taking place, but both the chromosomally encoded TraG coupling protein homolog and relaxase *rlx1* were required. The mechanism of transfer thus appears similar to the ADR pathway observed by Rohrer *et al.* It may be that the ADR pathway is a minor pathway for conjugative plasmids with an endogenous relaxase as utilized by Rohrer *et al.*, but may be the only pathway for transfer of mobilizable plasmids via the utilization of chromosomal mobilisation genes. Transfer of *H. pylori* conjugative plasmids was found to occur at a rate orders of magnitude higher than that for the introduced mobilizable plasmids (10^{-4} vs 10^{-7}). The observation that *H. pylori* is capable of transferring plasmids with a broad-host range *oriT* utilising a chromosomal mobilisation system indicates that *H. plyori* may be promiscuous in its ability to uptake foreign plasmids. In both studies the *cagPAI* and *tfs3* type-IV secretion systems were found to play no role in plasmid transfer. Given that no type-IV secretion apparatus has been implicated in the ADR pathway, the mode of DNA transfer by this route has yet to be determined.

The high rate of plasmid occurrence and the presence of three pathways for plasmid acquisition indicate that genes carried by plasmids may assist in host adaptation and be an important source of genetic diversity amongst *H. pylori* strains. The observation of chromosomal sequences in *H. pylori* plasmids indicates that they are capable of acquiring genetic material from the chromosome [181, 188]. Additionally, the presence of genes, displaying homology to chromosomal genes of unknown function, flanked by repeat and IS sequences on pHel4 and pHel5 gave rise to the proposal that *H. pylori* plasmids have a modular structure where genes can be integrated from the chromosome or other plasmids at repeat sequences by recombination or IS sequences by transposition events. Such shuffling of genes could represent a mechanism generating inter-strain diversity in *H. pylori* [180].

A role for plasmid encoded genes in virulence or host adaptation has yet to be clearly demonstrated as most plasmids characterized to date carry predominately only elements required for replication and hypothetical genes of unknown function [179]. Genes with homology to the *E. coli* microcin toxin operon have been identified in plasmids pHel4 and pHPM8. These genes function in *E. coli* to block protein biosynthesis in closely related bacteria, but their function has yet to be demonstrated in *H. pylori*. Similarly, both plasmids also contain a gene with homology to the tetracycline resistance determinant, *tetA*, but which has been demonstrated not to confer tetracycline resistance to host cells and thus remains of unknown function [179, 180, 188].

Plasmids are not the only entities transferred by conjugation in *H. pylori*. Initial evidence that *H. pylori* may be capable of transferring chromosomal elements by conjugation came from mating experiments in the presence and absence of DNaseI [189]. Subsequently, the transfer of chromosomally encoded streptomycin resistance by conjugation was demonstrated from *H. pylori* into *C. jejuni*. The transfer required cell to cell contact and was independent of any known type-IV secretion system [190].

More recently, the horizontal transfer of *H. pylori* plasticity zones has been investigated. Comparison of the first two genome sequences of *H. pylori* revealed the presence of chromosomal regions, termed plasticity zones, which contained strain specific genes. These regions vary from the rest of the genome in their G+C content, indicating possible acquisition from a foreign source [56]. Plasticity zones have been found to contain genes of interest, including DNA processing enzymes, type IV secretion systems [191, 192], and genes implicated in disease outcome. Plasticity regions have been found to be diverse in their gene content and presence in *H. pylori* strains [191, 193-195]. A large number of studies have implicated plasticity region localized genes, particularly JHP947 and surrounding genes, as virulence determinants in *H. pylori*. The presence or absence of these genes in clinical isolates have variously been correlated with gastric carcinoma and duodenal ulcer disease status and have been associated with variations in inflammatory cytokines [194-202]. The plasticity zones of *H. pylori* have been found to be able to horizontally transfer as conjugative transposons [191, 193].

Conjugative transposons are a form of integrative and conjugative elements (ICEs). These elements reside within, and are replicated by, the host chromosome and contain the elements required for their excision and integration. Following excision they circularize, are replicated and transferred to a recipient cell by conjugation. Following transfer, the ICE integrates into the recipient chromosome and the copy remaining in the donor also reintegrates. Many plasticity zones and genomic islands present in many bacterial species may be functional ICEs or remnants of mobile elements [203]. Given the importance of genomic and pathogenicity islands in the physiology of many bacteria, in particular the *cag* pathogenicity island and genes implicated in disease within the plasticity zones of *H. pylori*, ICEs may represent a rapid means of generating genetic diversity of clinical relevance between different *H. pylori* strains. Deletion of plasticity zones has been found to decrease the fitness of some strains *in vivo* and mediate the induction of inflammatory cytokines in human AGS cells [193].

An investigation into the nature of plasticity zones by sequencing *H. pylori* strains to identify their gene content and genomic location lead to the proposal that they were conjugative transposons termed 'transposon plasticity zone' (TnPZ) [193]. The plasticity zones in the sequenced strains could be classified according to their gene content and arrangement. Plasticity zones of a particular class could be identified at different genomic contexts in different strains, indicating their ability to move as a discrete unit. The plasticity zones were often found to be flanked by direct repeats and contained terminal inverted sequences, characteristic of transposable elements. There was also evidence of recombination occurring between different classes of TnPZs and many strains appeared to contain vestigial remnants TnPZs including J99 and 26695 whose plasticity regions were described as 'complex mosaics of TnPZ remnants'. Full length TnPZs were found to contain DNA processing enzymes, including a candidate transposase, *xerT,* which displays homology with the recombinases XerC and XerD of *E. coli* and the *H. pylori dif*-specific XerH recombinase. Transfer of TnPZ1 of *H. pylori* strain P12 was demonstrated by co-cultivation experiments performed with both WT and mutant donor and recipient strains [191]. Transfer of the plasticity zone was observed by a conjugative mechanism that could occur, although at reduced frequency, in the absence of the TnPZ-encoded type-IV secretion system and was dependent on the TNPZ-encoded *xerT*. Circular DNA intermediates from donor strains could be visualised by PCR. Excision of the TnPZ was found to leave one copy of the direct repeat in the donor chromosome while the circular intermediate contained the second.

The genes present on TnPZ may represent a pool of genes that can be quickly acquired as a set, as the conjugative method of transfer is not subjected to the same restriction barrier as transformation. It seems that plasticity zones have been present in *H. pylori* for a long time as similar zones are also found in other *Helicobacter* species including *H. acinonychis* and *H. cetorum* and many have been subject to gene deletion and recombination over that time. Plasticity zones are widely present in *H. pylori* strains with each strain having a unique combination of such zones and the strain specific genes found within, they thus contribute significantly to the *Helicobacter* pan-genome [191]. The transfer of TnPZs may represent a further method utilized by *H. pylori* to generate a diverse population that displays fitness in a diverse set of niches. The physiological function of genes in plasticity zones requires further investigation to clarify their potential roles in host adaptation and disease outcome. Although conjugative transfer of TnPZs, other chromosomal elements, and plasmids does occur in *H. pylori,* the precise mechanisms of such transfer and their regulation are not completely understood. The contribution of conjugative processes to genetic diversity in *H. pylori* may not be as significant as that contributed by natural transformation but is still of evolutionary significance.

3.2.4. Transduction of bacteriophage

Phages are often important drivers of genetic diversity and host adaptation. Phages represent a significant mode of horizontal gene transfer responsible for a large portion of strain-specific genetic diversity in many bacterial species. The action of temperate phages may play a significant role in the evolution of bacterial genomes by the disruption of host genes during insertion events, delivery of bacterial DNA for recombination by transduction, or the introduction of new genes (morons) that are carried, but not required, by an integrating phage. This has phenotypic consequences and the presence of prophages in the bacterial genome may alter bacterial fitness and influence host-bacterial interactions. This is particularly significant in many instances where morons encode virulence factors such as bacterial toxins [204]. Despite the significance of phages in the evolution of other bacterial species, the presence of phages in *Helicobacter* has drawn little attention until recently.

Bacteriophages are relevant to the physiology of *H. pylori in vivo*. Early observations of *H. pylori* noted the presence of bacteriophage-like particles within cells in electron microscope images of gastric biopsies [205]. Similarly, electron microscopy of clinical isolate SchReck 290 [206] revealed the presence of the bacteriophage HP1 that could be propagated in a lytic cycle *in vitro* [207]. Active *H. pylori* bacteriophages can be isolated from human faeces [208].

More recently, several bacteriophages have been characterised in *H. pylori*. Genome sequencing of clinical isolate, B45, revealed the presence of a 24.6 kb prophage within the genome [209]. The phage was found to be similar to a previously identified phage in *H. acinonychis* [210] and could be induced by UV irradiation, producing phage particles. Screening of a further 341 clinical strains from different geographical regions by PCR revealed that the phage was widespread, being detected in 21.4% of isolates. This high prevalence could indicate that bacteriophages play a role in *Helicobacter* evolution [209].

The bacteriophage 1961P was isolated from a clinical isolate of *H. pylori*. It has a genome of 27 kb containing 33 genes. Sequence comparison revealed that prophages or prophage remnants similar to 1961P are likely present in six other sequenced *H. pylori* strains. Interestingly, 1961P was demonstrated to be a transducing phage demonstrating that transduction of *H. pylori* by bacteriophages does occur [211].

The sequence of two phages isolated from East-Asian-type isolates from Japanese patients has been reported [212] and one, KHP30, has been characterized further [213]. The phage did not appear to be integrative and may represent a novel category of bacteriophage.

Although it is becoming clear that bacteriophages may be widely present in *H. pylori*, with some recently well characterized, a potential role for bacteriophages in genomic evolution and host-adaptation in *H. pylori* remains largely unexplored. Genomic sequencing revealed the presence of two prophages within the feline-associated *H. acinonychis* genome which account for 26% of genes present in the sequenced *H. acinonychis* but absent in *H. pylori* J99 and 26695. Although most of these genes appear to have been acquired after the divergence of the two species and largely encode hypothetical proteins, three genes from one of the two prophages were implicated by the authors as potentially having played a role in enabling the host jump of the *H. acinonychis* ancestor into felines [210].

Lehours *et al*. have raised the hypothesis that plasticity zones in *H. pylori* could have a phage origin much as phages mediate the transfer of pathogenicity islands in *Staphylococcus* [214]. Kersulyte *et al*. have proposed that plasticity zones transfer as conjugative transposons [193]. Further research will be required to determine if the bacteriophages in *Helicobacter* have played any significant role in the evolution of its genome.

4. Small RNAs and regulation

To date only a limited number of transcriptional regulators have been discovered in the small 1.67 Mbp genome of *H. pylori*, including a mere three sigma factors, namely RpoD, FliA and RpoN [57]. Consequently *H. pylori* was thought not to have any extensive regulatory networks. However, a recent comprehensive analysis of the *H. pylori* primary transcriptome has revealed that the compact genome produces an abundant number of antisense and small RNA (sRNA) transcripts portending a great potential for the use of riboregulation by *H. pylori* in gene expression [215].

Small RNAs have emerged as essential regulators that allow organisms to cope with environmental changes and stresses [216, 217]. Like transcription factors, sRNA can modulate the expression of multiple target genes and thereby function as key regulators of metabolic pathways and stress responses. In bacteria, sRNAs have been discovered to regulate processes as varied as carbon metabolism, iron homeostasis, RNA polymerase function, virulence, quorum sensing, biofilm formation, as well as response to stresses such as oxidation and outer membrane perturbation [216, 218-220].

Bacterial sRNAs exhibit a diverse range of molecular mechanisms of action. One class of bacterial sRNA acts by binding directly to protein targets and modulating their activity [221, 222]. Another group of sRNAs known as riboswitches consist of RNA sequences located in the 5' untranslated regions (UTRs) of mRNAs. Riboswitches regulate gene expression through their capacity to adopt different conformations that are mediated by factors such as temperature or small molecule metabolites that specifically bind to the riboswitch [223, 224].

The most extensively studied class of sRNAs are those that act through antisense base pairing with target mRNAs. These sRNAs are classified as either *cis*-encoded, because they are transcribed from the strand of DNA opposite their mRNA targets and so have extensive complementarity to their target, or as *trans*-encoded sRNAs, which are transcribed from a genomic location different from those of their targets. The base pairing interactions of *trans*-encoded sRNAs tend to involve less complementarity with their targets, permitting the regulation of multiple genes [217]. Furthermore many *trans*-encoded sRNAs in enteric bacteria require binding to Hfq, a chaperone protein that aids in sRNA stability and base pairing with target mRNAs [225]. Antisense base pairing of sRNAs can exert either negative or positive regulatory effects on their mRNA targets including RNA degradation, termination of transcription, inhibition of translation and the relief of intrinsic translation-inhibitory structure formation in the mRNA's 5' UTR (For detailed reviews of basepairing sRNAs and their regulatory mechanisms, refer to [220, 226-228]).

The discovery of substantial antisense transcription as well as a high number (>60) of sRNAs which included potential regulators of *cis*- and *trans*-encoded mRNA targets has revealed a new class of molecules that should to be considered for their role in mediating *H. pylori* persistence. Since sRNAs in *H. pylori* were discovered only recently, knowledge regarding their target genes and the mechanism by which they regulate them is still very limited. The current literature on riboregulation for *H. pylori* has been recently reviewed [229]. When corrected by genome size, the sRNA repertoire of *H. pylori* rivals that of *E. coli*, the model organism of bacterial RNA research [220], and thus the mechanisms of sRNA action in *H. pylori* are likely to be much more diverse than what is currently known.

With the exception of a handful of housekeeping RNAs, none of the enterobacterial sRNAs are conserved in *H. pylori* [215]. *H. pylori* has no Hfq homolog, an RNA chaperone shown to be important for mediating sRNA function in enteric bacteria, and *H. pylori* lacks homologs of endonucleolytic RNases E/G and other common processing factors of stable RNAs [57, 230]. It has been hypothesized that antisense-mediated processing by double-strand specific ribonuclease RNase III may compensate for this paucity and act as the major regulator as has been recently suggested for *S. aureus* [229, 231]. To date the only sRNA shown to be essential in *H. pylori* and required for stress response is tmRNA, which is involved in the rescue of stalled ribosomes [232].

One of the most abundant transcripts identified in *H. pylori* is a homolog of 6S RNA [215], a ubiquitous riboregulator which mimics an open promoter complex and thereby sequesters RNA polymerase [233, 234]. In *E coli*, deletion of 6S RNA has no obvious phenotype during exponential growth, however altered growth phenotypes are observed during stationary phase and under extreme stress conditions [222]. Whether 6S RNA has a similar role during stress response, stationary growth, or if it impacts on virulence as seen for *Legionella* [235] and therefore has implications in *H. pylori* persistence in the host still needs to be investigated.

Antisense transcripts have been identified for one third of the putative phase-variable genes with functions in lipopolysaccharide biosynthesis, surface structure and DNA restriction/modification [215], raising the possibility of antisense regulation of surface structure and host interactions. Furthermore, acid-stress-induced antisense RNAs opposite to known acid-stress-repressed genes have also been detected, suggesting that antisense regulation would also play an important role in adapting to changing environmental pH. To date only a few physiological effects of sRNA regulation have been demonstrated in *H. pylori*. The *ureAB* operon has been shown to be negatively regulated by a *cis*-encoded antisence 5′ *ureB*-sRNA which is induced by unphosphorylated ArsR under neutral conditions [236]. The chemotaxis receptor TlpB, which is involved in pH-taxis, quorum sensing, colonization and gastric mucosa inflammation, has been shown to be negatively regulated by the *trans*-encoded HPnc5490 sRNA [237-239].

It has become increasingly clear that sRNAs serve as diverse regulators that impact almost every aspect of bacterial physiology in response to changes in the environment. It is therefore highly likely that riboregulation may have a very important role in *H. pylori* persistence. The stomach is a highly dynamic environment undergoing constant changes in pH, due to long periods of fasting interspaced with the intake of various food material, while continual shedding of gastric mucus, where a majority of the bacteria reside [240], leads to washout into the lower intestine where the bacteria are exposed to an anaerobic environment and greater exposure to the host immune system through Peyer's patches. Here riboregulation may be very important for the quick changes and modulation, such as initiation of peptidoglycan remodelling and alterations in the lipid content [241, 242], necessary to transition from the spiral to coccoid form that is phagocytosed by dendritic cells in Peyer's patches [243].

5. Experimental strategies to study *Helicobacter pylori* persistence

A multidisciplinary approach is required to study persistence *in vivo*, through the combination of microbiology, immunology, genetics and clinics. Although powerful techniques in cellular microbiology as well as the flurry of transgenic mouse strains have been instrumental in investigating *H. pylori* pathogenesis, *in vivo* studies are limited to loss of function mutants based on gene deletion. This prevents the distinction between colonization and/or persistence functions of the gene of interest. Furthermore, deletion mutants also suffer the drawback of potential rapid genetic adaption in case of a strong selective pressure (which might often be the case already *in vitro*) *in vivo*, and this is particularly relevant in view of *H. pylori*'s genome plasticity.

5.1. Gene deletion

Both bacterial and host genetics have led to a tremendous progress in our understanding of *H. pylori* pathogenesis. However, the mechanisms of persistence of *H. pylori* have not yet been rigorously tested in animal models due to the difficulty in assessing the temporal requirement of virulence factor expression for colonization and/or persistence. Only a few genes have been strictly shown to be required for persistence based on the inability of mutant strains to colonize in the long-term despite identical short-term colonization loads compared to wild-type. For example, the peptidoglycan deacetylase (*pgdA*) mutant displayed significant attenuation in its ability to colonize mouse stomachs at 9 weeks infection although it is dispensable for up to 3 weeks during the initial colonization [244]. Furthermore, compared to wild-type *H. pylori*-infected mice, elevated levels of MIP-2, IL-10 and TNFα were observed in mice infected with the *pgdA* mutant, indicating that peptidoglycan deacetylation modulates the host immune system [244]. Another study reported the DNA repair *ruvC* mutant to be spontaneously cleared from the gastric mucosa of mice between 36 to 67 days of the initial challenge of mice [88]. Interestingly, the *ruvC* mutant was less efficient in modulating the murine immune system, suggesting that DNA recombination is critical for immune modulation and persistence of *H. pylori* [88]. Catalase (KatA) and the catalase associated proteins (KapA) have also been implicated in persistence of *H. pylori* infection [245]. KapA and KatA were proposed to promote survival of *H. pylori* in the inflamed gastric mucosa where the concentration of reactive oxygen species, particularly hydrogen peroxide, is high [245]. Very recently, a comparative analysis of the colonization loads between wild-type *H. pylori* and the *lpxE* isogenic mutant, harbouring a partial TLR4 determinant restoration, was conducted in C57/BL6J and the corresponding TLR4 knockout transgenic mice [26]. This two-sided genetic approach demonstrated that although LpxE-mediated avoidance of TLR4 recognition had little effect on the early colonization phase 15 days) *lpxE* mutant was prevented from persisting for more than 45 days due to TLR4 activation [26] that likely led to sterilizing adaptive immunity.

The natural competence of *H. pylori* has also recently been demonstrated to promote chronic colonization. A competition experiment between wild-type and *comB10* or *drpA* mutant strains showed that mutation of either the Com apparatus or a cytosolic competence factor resulted in reduced persistence despite normal initial colonization [246]. This recent data strongly suggests that the exchange of DNA between a heterogeneous population and genome plasticity and integrity are important for *H. pylori* to maintain chronic infection.

5.2. Gene mutagenesis: The urease example

As an alternative to gene deletion, protein engineering was applied to the urease complex to investigate its role in the host-pathogen interaction without affecting the enzymes ureolytic activity which is essential for colonization [247]. Surface exposed loops that display high thermal mobility were targeted for in-frame insertion mutagenesis (Figure 4). *H. pylori* expressing urease with insertions at four different sites retained urease activity and were able to establish robust infections. Bacteria expressing one of these four mutant ureases, however, had reduced bacterial loads after longer term (3 to 6 months) colonization. These results indicate that a discrete surface region of the urease complex, distinct from the ureolytic activity *per se*, is important for *H. pylori* persistence during gastric colonization [247].

H. pylori urease consists of a ball-like supramolecular structure of about 1000 kDa. It is composed of twelve UreA-UreB subunits (26.5 and 61.7 kDa, respectively), assembled in a high molecular weight complex of four alpha/beta trimers [248, 249]. Urease is an abundantly expressed enzyme (10% of the cell weight) that decreases the acidity of *H. pylori*'s immediate environment by generating ammonia and carbonate from the urea we secrete as metabolic waste and is one of the first characterized factors identified as essential for colonization by *H. pylori* [250-252]. The majority of the urease is localized in the bacterial cytoplasm, however, urease is also present on the cell surface and in the extracellular medium. The secretion of urease is still a matter of debate as both autolysis and specific secretion [250, 253, 254] have been postulated to be responsible for the release of urease.

Uptake of urea into the cytoplasm is controlled by an acid gated urea channel, UreI, that does not open until the periplasmic pH decreases below pH 6.5 to avoid alkalization of the cytoplasm [255-257]. The recruitment and interaction of the urease complex with UreI at the inner membrane is hypothesized to enable coupling of urea transport and urease activity for efficient pH homeostasis of the periplasm [258]. It is tempting to postulate that the surface properties of urease plays a key role in the intrabacterial regulation of its enzymatic activity by docking of the urease complex to the urea channel (UreI) to maintain periplasmic pH.

Although such local control of gastric acidity is considered essential, urease-negative *H. pylori* strains were unable to colonize piglets whose acid secretion had been suppressed, suggesting an additional role for urease [259]. Possible explanations include the utilization of urease generated ammonia by *H. pylori* to synthesize essential metabolites, especially amino acids [260]; protection from peroxynitrite [261], enhanced survival in macrophages [262],

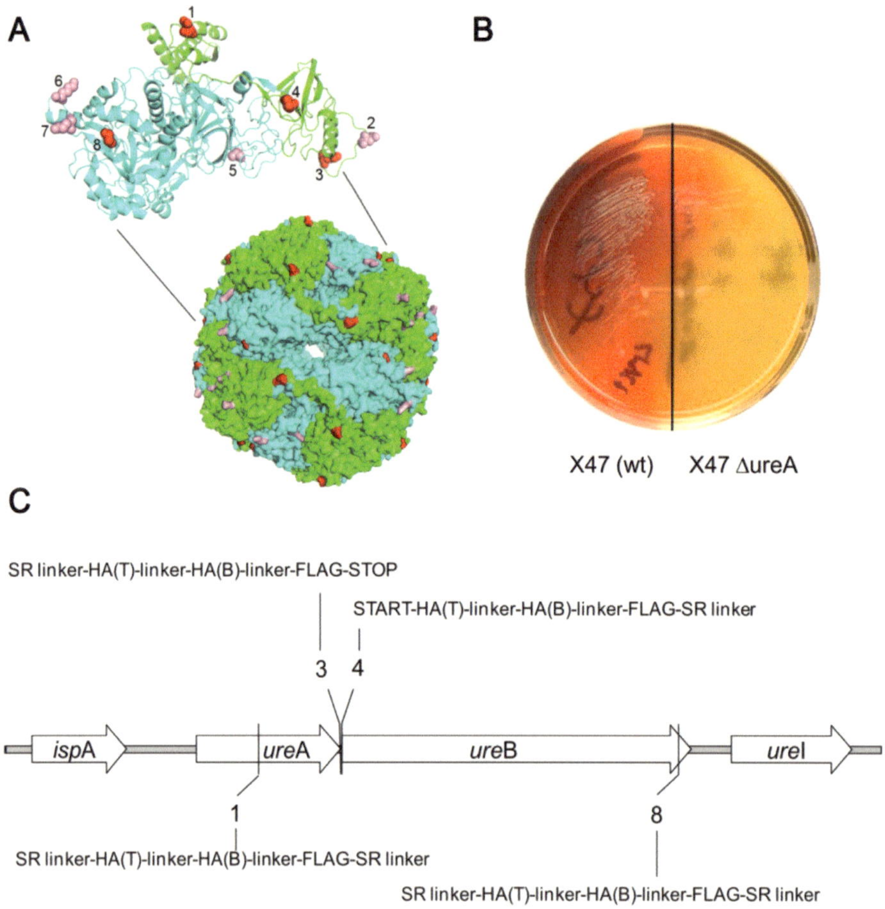

Figure 4. Recombinant regions of urease and selection for enzyme function (Figure adapted from [247]). **a)** Molecular structure of urease showing insertion sites on the surface of urease. Urease subunit A (green) and subunit B (blue) associate to form a dodecameric supramolecular molecule [248, 249]. Sites 1 to 8 correspond to residues 102, 231 and 238 from UreA and residues 1, 66, 326, 541 and 549 from UreB, respectively. Insertion sites 1, 3, 4, and 8 are indicated in red. Urease activity could not be retained when altered at sites 2, 5, 6, and 7 (pink). **b)** Selection of bacteria producing functional urease on acidified media supplemented with the urease substrate, urea. Left side: X47 wild type; the colour change observed on the left side indicated that bacterial colonies were producing functional urease and growing. Right side: X47 Δ*ureA*: there was no colour (X47 wild-type). Colour change did not occur on the right side, indicating that inoculated colonies were unable to grow or functional urease was not being produced (X47 Δ*ureA*). **c)** A schematic showing insertion sites at the urease locus of DNA coding epitopes and linkers. Insertions were made in DNA corresponding to insertion after amino positions 102 (site 1) and 238 (site 3) of UreA (GenBank AAD07144.1), and amino acid positions 1 (site 4) and 549 (site 8) of UreB (GenBank AAD07143.1). Insertions at sites 3 and 4 correspond to the C- and N-termini of UreA and UreB, respectively. DNA coded HA(T): hemagglutinin T cell eptitope; HA(B) hemagglutinin B cell epitope; SR linker: semi-random linker; linker: GPSL linker; FLAG: FLAG epitope; STOP: STOP codon.

evasion of phagocytosis [263], complement mediated opsonisation [264], and decreased viscosity in gastric mucin at high pH facilitating *H. pylori* motility [265]. An alternative explanation invokes the existence of urease-host tissue interactions, that are independent of urease enzymatic activity, and is based on *in vitro* studies that detected urease mediated activation of macrophages [266], monocytes [267] and blood platelets [266, 267], dysregulation of gastric epithelial tight junctions [268] and induction of cytokine production from gastric epithelial cells [269] through binding to CD74 (MHC class II invariant chain) [270].

The above examples highlight the importance of studying the kinetics of colonization so as to gain deeper insights into the *H. pylori* persistence mechanisms and revisit the role of well-known and studied virulence factors such as urease.

5.3. Conditional mutants

The use of conditional *H. pylori* mutants makes it possible to investigate genes for their role in persistence by turning off target gene expression *in vivo* once colonization has been established. Several *H. pylori* conditional knockouts based on the *lac* operon have been constructed to study essential genes *in vitro* [271, 272]. So far however, this system has not been tested in the mouse model of *H. pylori* infection. Due to certain limitations, including leakiness of transgene expression and limited bioavailibility of the IPTG transgene-inducers, this *lac* operon-based system is not very well suited for *in vivo* studies. On the contrary, the tetracycline-mediated gene expression regulation has been extensively used to construct mouse conditional knock-outs as well as to study host-pathogen interactions using tetracyline-regulated bacterial conditional knockouts [273, 274]. Tetracycline gene regulation has recently been developed in *H. pylori* [275-277] (Figure 5) and successfully applied *in vivo* to monitor changes in colonization load upon the down regulation of *ureB* gene expression [277].

This system will enable study of the temporal requirements of specific genes during *H. pylori* colonization as well as during persistence. More importantly, tetracycline-mediated *H. pylori* gene regulation will allow for subtle characterization, *in vivo* and ex *vivo,* of changes in the innate and adaptive immune responses by monitoring the activation of antigen presenting cells and T cell proliferation, respectively.

The tetracycline gene regulation combined with host genetics will facilitate the investigation of *H. pylori* persistence mechanisms and may allow for the discovery of new markers for cancer risk and for novel therapeutic interventions specifically targeting persistence.

6. Comparative genomics

The genome era created the possibility to study gene contents of individual *H. pylori* strains, allelic diversity and related genetic plasticity. The first *H. pylori* strain, 26695, was sequenced in 1997 and was isolated from an English patient with chronic gastritis. The chromosome of strain 26695 is circular and composed of 1 667 867 base pairs [57]. J99, isolated from an American patient with a duodenal ulcer, was sequenced in 1999 and for the first time, a comparison of two unrelated genomes was made [97]. Compared to 26695, J99 has a slightly smaller circular chromosome (1 643 831 base pairs). *H. pylori* is believed to possess a large degree of genomic diversity but the overall genomic organization, gene order and predicted proteomes of the two sequenced strains was found to be similar. The two genomes displayed

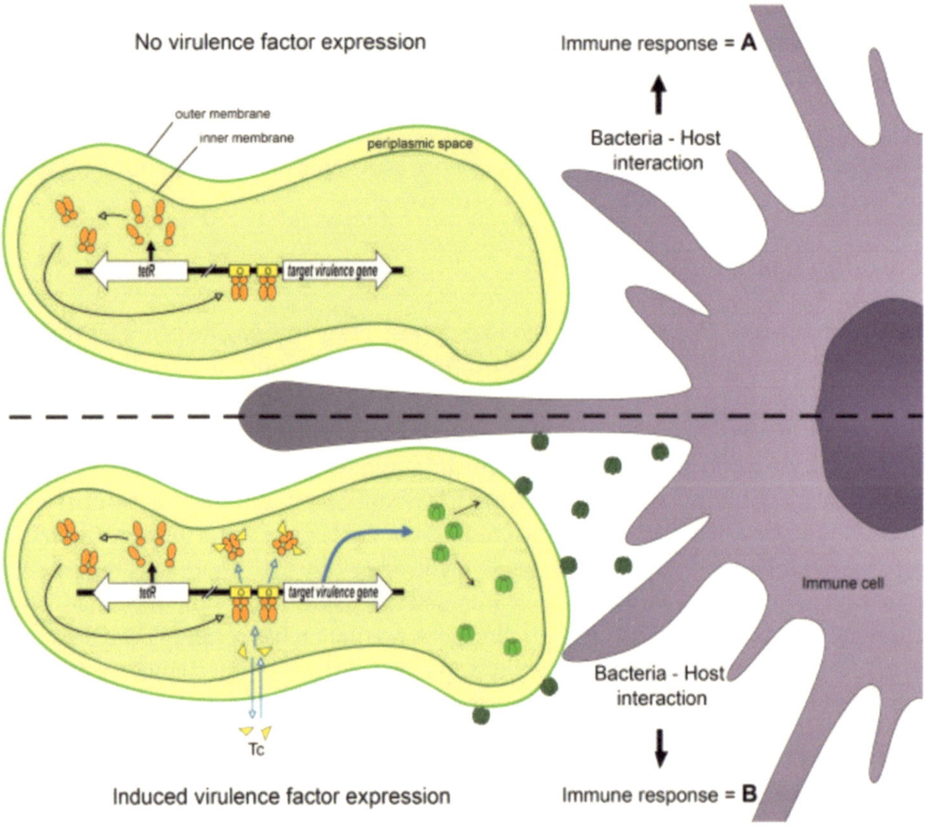

Figure 5. Using conditional mutants to study the role of genes in persistence. In the top panel the conditional *H. pylori* mutant constitutively expresses the *tet* repressor (orange circles), encoded by *tetR*, which binds to the tandem *tet* operators, *tetO*, preventing transcription of the target virulence gene. The host immune cells encounter bacteria lacking a virulence factor and produce a particular measurable response (immune response A). In the bottom panel, the molecular inducer of TetR, Tetracycline (Tc), indicated by filled yellow triangles, is administered to the system. Tc diffuses into the bacterial cell, binds to the repressor-operator complex and triggers a conformational change in TetR resulting in rapid dissociation of TetR from the DNA and a burst of target gene expression. The host immune cells encounter bacteria which express the target virulence factor and in turn produce a different response (immune response B).

a high degree of diversity in terms of insertions and deletions. There are 1406 genes shared by both strains, but 86 open reading frames are absent from strain 26695. Both strains contain a complete *cag* pathogenicity island that codes for a type IV secretion system to deliver the CagA cytotoxin protein. Comparison of the two genomes revealed between 6 to 7% of the genes were specific to each strain, with almost half of these genes being clustered in a single hyper-variable region or plasticity zone. The presence of a variable gene pool is indicative of horizontal gene transfer. Because strain-specific genes could be involved in gastric adaptation during co-evolution, this flexible gene pool was extensively investigated in many strains worldwide. *In silico* analysis of the two *H. pylori* genomes revealed that both housekeeping genes and virulence genes are transferred between *H. pylori* strains [278, 279].

Next generation sequencing has enabled the study of unrelated *H. pylori* strains isolated from unrelated individuals and further studies have focused on evolution of *H. pylori* within the same host. Commonly, isolates have been derived from chronically infected individuals that have been exposed to *H. pylori* for decades, such as 26695 and J99. More recently, analysis of the genetic relationships between strains of *H. pylori* that had been sequentially isolated from the same host at different times also showed high mutation rates and genetic diversity.

Inter-strain diversity is represented by variations in the number and contents of genes, chromosomal rearrangements and allelic diversities, and is not unique to *H. pylori* [280]. For *H. pylori*, each strain contains many strain-specific genes. It has been proposed that a particular bacterial species contains a core set of genes and auxiliary genes. The core genome contains genes that are present in all or nearly all of the strains. It determines the properties that are characteristic for the species. The auxiliary genes are present in some strains, and are determinants of the biological properties unique to each strain.

6.1. Chronic infection

The first studies of genetic diversity and evolution amongst *H. pylori* strains were performed using isolates derived from chronically infected individuals. Early studies of genetic change during *H. pylori* chronic infection were restricted to selected housekeeping genes within a bacterial population in single and mixed infected hosts.

Molecular fingerprinting studies using RAPD [281] and amplified fragment length polymorphisms (AFLP) [282] first showed that strains isolated from single patients were closely related, but were subtly different. Strains isolated at the same time or months and years apart also showed similar divergence [281-285]. Thus, while populations diverge within the host, divergence appears to occur slowly.

Newer technologies allowed for more accurate comparisons of *H. pylori* genomes. Salama *et. al.* reported genetic diversity amongst 15 unrelated *H. pylori* strains from different geographical locations and identified strain-specific genes based on whole genome *H. pylori* DNA microarray. Analysis of the genomic content of *H. pylori* strains from chronically infected patients found that 22% of *H. pylori* genes were dispensable and defined a minimal core genome of 1,281 *H. pylori* genes [286]. Of these, more than 300 genes were not homogeneously distributed and many of the dispensable genes were located in plasticity zones and in the *cag* pathogenicity island. Core genes encoded mostly metabolic and cellular processes, while strain-specific genes included genes unique to *H. pylori*, restriction modification genes, transposases and genes encoding cell surface proteins.

Gressmann *et al.* used a collection of 56 globally representative *H. pylori* strains that included examples from all known populations and subpopulations in comparative genome hybridizations with a microarray representing the genes of the combined genomes of 26695 and J99. The study found 1, 150 genes were conserved between the 56 strains and estimated that the core genome conserved in all *H. pylori* strains is ~1, 111 genes. The remaining 400 genes that each *H. pylori* genome contains come from a pool of genes that are strain-specific and located within the *cag* pathogenicity island [287], consistent with the findings of the previous study.

Other studies also identified the *cag* pathogenicity island and plasticity zones as regions of genetic diversity and DNA exchange. Israel *et. al.* examined the gene content of two *H. pylori* strains that had similar virulence genotypes (*cagA*$^+$ *vacA* s1a *iceA1*), but were phenotypically different and showed by *H. pylori* whole genome microarray analysis that the gene content within the *cag* island differed substantially [288]. Occhialini *et. al.* examined the composition of the plasticity zone in a collection of 43 *H. pylori* strains from diverse clinical origins and showed that the plasticity zone is highly mosaic and represents a large fragment of foreign DNA integrated into the genome [194].

Genetic variation can be generated in a bacterial population by mutation and/or recombination between different strains. The studies described so far focus on unrelated clinical isolates from unrelated infected individuals. However, to address the question of mutation and recombination rates of *H. pylori* during chronic infection, a comparison of *H. pylori* isolates from the same host must be made.

One of the first such studies compared the genome of J99, originally isolated in 1994, with multiple strains that had been isolated from the same patient six years later [289]. All follow-up strains differed from the original isolate by one or multiple gene losses or gains. Randomly amplified polymorphic DNA PCR and DNA sequencing of four unlinked loci revealed that these isolates were closely related to the original strain. In contrast, microarray analysis revealed differences in genetic content among all of the isolates that were not detected by randomly amplified polymorphic DNA PCR or sequence analysis [289]. Whole-genome microarray revealed a difference in genomic composition in 3% of J99 loci as well as the relatedness of these isolates to each other when compared with *H. pylori* isolates from other individuals.

Subsequent studies observed sequentially isolated *H. pylori* strains from the same host. One of the early reports examined the sequences of ten gene fragments (encoding house-keeping enzymes and virulence associated proteins) of paired sequential isolates from 26 patients in two geographical areas at between 3 month and 48 month intervals (average 1.8 year interval) and found that point mutations occur in the stomach of a single host and that mostly small DNA segments (median size of 417 base pairs) are exchanged with other bacteria in the stomach [175]. A Bayesian model was used to calculate mutation rate, import size and the frequency of recombination. On average, pairs of bacteria differed by ~100 DNA imports, corresponding to three percent of the genome or 50 kb. A mutation rate of 4.1×10^{-5} per year and base pair was estimated. Recombination occurred at a rate of 60 imports spanning 25, 000 base pair per genome per year. Authors concluded that recombination is so frequent that appreciable fractions of the entire genome are exchanged during the colonization of a single human, resulting in a highly flexible genome content and frequent shuffling of sequence polymorphisms throughout the local gene pool [175].

Kraft *et al.* examined paired strains of *H. pylori* with respect to their genomic contents using the DNA microarray method and also reported evolutionary changes in the *H. pylori* genome. Isolates were obtained from the same patients at intervals of 3 to 36 months. Of the 21 pairs of strains examined, 4 pairs showed differences in their genomic contents, suggesting the occurrence of evolutionary recombination events. These included a complete deletion and a partial loss of the *cag* pathogenicity island, a replacement of an open reading frame of unknown function, an acquisition of 14 genes in the plasticity zone, a duplication of the *ceuE* genes (HP1561/HP1562) and a truncation of tandem arranged *ackA* and *pta* genes resulting in the formation of pseudo-genes [290].

A more recent study estimated the short-term mutation and recombination rates of *H. pylori* by sequencing an average of 39, 300 base pairs in 78 gene fragments from 97 isolates [291]. These isolates included 34 pairs of sequential samples at intervals of 3 months to 10.2 years. They also included single isolates from 29 individuals from 10 families. The accumulation of sequence diversity increased with time of separation in a clock-like manner in the sequential isolates. Approximate Bayesian Computation was used to estimate the mutation and recombination rates, mean length of recombination tracts, and average diversity in those tracts. The short-term mutation rate is estimated to be 1.461026 (serial isolates) to 4.561026 (family isolates) per nucleotide per year and that three times as many substitutions are introduced by recombination as by mutation. Comparisons with the recent literature show that short-term mutation rates vary dramatically and can span a range of several orders of magnitude.

The above studies analysed the genetic relationships between strains of *H. pylori* sequentially isolated from the same patient. The studies are based mainly on multi-locus sequence analysis of mostly house-keeping genes and have limitations. Bayesian inference was used to estimate recombination and mutation but the multi-locus approach did not allow conclusions about the chromosomal distribution of import events or about the relative frequencies of imports in different categories of genes.

More recently, mutation and recombination rates have been estimated by a genome-wide analysis using pyro-sequencing technology. Kennemann *et al.* analysed the genomes of five sets of sequential isolates of *H. pylori,* including four pairs of isolates from the earlier studies (with isolation intervals of 3 years) and recent follow-up isolates for two of the pairs that were obtained 16 years after the first isolates. The genome comparisons of the four sets of isolates confirmed previous estimates of the length of imported fragments and reported an average length of 394 base pairs, which is in agreement with the previous estimate of 417 base pairs. The 16-year isolates differed from the initial isolates by far more SNPs and CNPs than the 3-year isolates, indicating that diversity caused by mutation and recombination had accumulated over time. The average genome-wide mutation rate for the four 3-year pairs of sequential isolates from chronically infected individuals was found to be 2.5×10^{-5} (range = $0.5–6.5 \times 10^{-5}$) per year per site. This rate is ~18-fold faster than the mutation rate previously calculated for serial *H. pylori* isolates based on analysis of housekeeping genes. The rate of recombination was 5.5×10^{-5} recombination events per initiation site and year, similar to what was previously estimated [92], but 122-fold higher than the rate of 4.4×10^{-7} calculated from housekeeping genes. These differences can be attributed to multiple factors. Faster rates can be expected for a genome-wide analysis, because housekeeping genes are likely to be under strong purifying selection, whereas the genome-wide analysis comprises noncoding DNA as well as genes under diversifying selection. In addition, the rates of mutation and recombination varied strongly between different infected individuals in both studies, which could be because of strain properties, the extent of mixed infections that determines the availability of exogenous

DNA, or varying selective forces in infected hosts. This study of *H. pylori* genomic evolution during human infection shows genome-wide recombination in *H. pylori* colonizing humans in a high-prevalence area with a high rate of mixed infections. Genome-wide analyses of the length of individual import events were in good agreement with earlier estimates, but two important findings have emerged: 1) imports were often clustered and 2) imports frequently affected genes coding for outer membrane proteins of the Hop family.

Taken together, these provide evidence of genetic variability and DNA exchange among *H. pylori* strains and demonstrate that gene contents of *H. pylori* isolates from the same and different individuals displays between 3% and 22% variability, respectively. Data indicate that within an apparently homogeneous population, remarkable genetic differences exist among single-colony isolates of *H. pylori* and provide direct evidence that this bacterium has the capacity to lose and possibly acquire exogenous DNA and is consistent with the theory of continuous microevolution within a cognate host.

H. pylori are naturally competent for transformation [151] and non-random distributed repetitive sequences are found in the genome, which leads to frequent recombination events [92]. Calculations of mutation and recombination frequencies with respect to insert sizes revealed that genetic diversity displayed by the panmictic population structure is a result of continuous DNA exchange between parental strains and daughter strains, which have accumulated mutations. This was supported by gene content analysis of isolates taken from single patients at different time points, which demonstrated that the great majority of genetic changes were caused by homologous recombination, indicating that adaptation of *H. pylori* to the host individual is more frequently mediated by sequence changes acquired by recombination events rather than loss or gain of genes [290].

The comparative studies of the *H. pylori* genome reveal the genomic changes during the cycle of invasion, colonization and transmission to a new host. Invasion into a new host seems to have little effect on the gene composition of *H. pylori*, suggesting that the current genome of *H. pylori* has sufficient capacities for permitting bacterial invasion into a human host. Once the infection is established, the bacterium has to cope with the dynamic changes of the physiological environment during the long-term coexistence with the host. Genomic diversifications, or gain and/or loss of genes, occur in response to these changes. The diversifications involve genes that are mainly those strain-specific genes observed from comparative studies of unrelated strains of *H. pylori*. Intra-host evolution of *H. pylori*, thus, results in the creation of a unique and strain-specific combination of genes enabling persistence in individual hosts.

6.2. Acute infection and human challenge studies

Most studies of *H. pylori* adaptation to the human host have relied on samples from adults who had most likely been infected since childhood thus showing changes only after a long adaption of the bacterium to the individual host. It is also of interest to understand the evolution of the *H. pylori* genome in the first weeks and months after infection to reflect the selective pressure occurring during adaptation to a new host.

A limited number of *H. pylori* challenge studies in humans have been performed over the past 2 decades, mainly to support the development of anti-Helicobacter vaccines. These studies have provided valuable samples for the study of intra-host adaptation of *H. pylori* during the acute phase of *H. pylori* infection.

The first human challenge study was documented by Graham *et al.* to develop a reliable challenge model to evaluate *H. pylori* vaccine candidates [292]. Healthy human volunteers were infected with the *H. pylori* strain BCS 100 and *H. pylori* clones were re-isolated from stomach biopsies 3 months after challenge. The Baylor challenge strain (BCS 100) is *cag* pathogenicity island negative, and positive for *vacA s1c-m1*.

Another challenge study using the same BCS 100 strain study was reported for the development of a vaccine against *H. pylori* [293]. Performed in Germany at the Paul Ehrlich Institute, a live vaccine against *H. py*lori was tested in human volunteers sero-negative for, and without evidence of, active *H. pylori* infection. Volunteers (n=58) were immunised orally with *Salmonella enterica* serovar Typhi Ty21a expressing *H. pylori* urease or HP0231, or solely with Ty21a, and then challenged with *H. pylori*. Gastric biopsies were taken before and after vaccination and pre- and post-challenge.

A third unpublished acute human challenge study using a CagA positive *H. pylori* strain was reported by Malfertheiner *et al.* at the AGA Annual Meeting 2011 (AGA abstract #432, S-86). In brief, 34 healthy subjects that tested negative for *H. pylori* infection received an experimental vaccine or placebo prior to subsequent challenge with *H. pylori* isolate at a dose of $5x10^6$ CFU. The isolate was susceptible to all current antibiotics used in *H. pylori* therapy. Subjects were evaluated at 2, 4 and 12 weeks after challenge and the published data revealed changes in pepsinogen I and II and gastrin-17 levels. Authors concluded that challenge with a CagA positive *H. pylori* strain induced moderate dyspeptic symptoms that resolve within a few days and profoundly affected gastric physiology with a distinct reactive pattern of serum pepsinogen I and II and gastrin-17.

With the challenge strain BCS 100 and the reisolate 8A3, the analysis of a pair of isolates for which the time elapsed between the infection and reisolation was exactly known, allowed the rate of genetic changes occurring in the early phase of *H. pylori* infection to be addressed. The genomes of the challenge strain (BCS 100) of the vaccine trial and a reisolate (8A3) from a volunteer (non-vaccinated control group) who had been infected with BCS 100 for 3 months [293] were sequenced. Whole-genome sequence comparison revealed very few differences between the two isolates [157]. Three point mutations were identified and confirmed by Sanger sequencing. All three were nonsynonymous mutations, leading to predicted single amino acid changes in the proteins δ-1-pyrroline-5-carboxylate dehydrogenase (PutA; HP0056), pyridoxal phosphate biosynthetic protein J (PdxJ; HP1582), and HP1181 (a predicted multidrug efflux transporter). In addition to point mutations, noted were repeat length differences (RLDs) in two different dinucleotide repeat sequences and one repeat consisting of multiple copies of an 8-basepair motif.

In striking contrast to the pairs from the earlier study of isolates from chronically infected individuals, no single recombination event was detected. This is most likely due to the lack of co-infection, more commonly observed in chronic infection. *H. pylori* prevalence has fallen in most Western countries, including Germany where the study was conducted, reducing the risk of acquiring multiple strains. A recent study of two pairs of sequential *H. pylori* isolates from Sweden also did not detect any evidence of recombination during chronic infection [294]. Likewise, there was no evidence of recombination during 3 months of infection of a volunteer in Germany, providing evidence that *H. pylori* can establish chronic infection after infection with a single strain and that its genome can be stable in the absence of mixed infection.

In addition, *H. pylori* isolates from four healthy adults (patients 101, 103, 104, and 105) who participated in the BCS 100 human challenge study [292] collected 15 days or 90 days post-infection were examined. Adult volunteers were not related to each other and were not related to the patient from which the challenge strain was obtained. Therefore, if host-specific differences select for genetic changes in the bacteria, such conditions would be present during this human challenge experiment. Comparative genome array analysis with single colony isolates demonstrated that their genomic contents were identical to the challenge strain. No rapid changes in gene content or sequence divergence up to 3 months after transmission was observed [295].

To date, no data has been published on the infectivity and colonisation rate of vaccinated and non-vaccinated subjects challenged with the CagA positive strain, or the genetic sequence of isolates collected at post-challenge time-points compared to the original challenge strain. This type of genome sequence analysis would provide new information on the adaptation of *H. pylori* during the acute phase of infection in the host and would allow comparison of genetic events occurring in the presence or absence of virulence genes such as CagA.

A fourth *H. pylori* human challenge study has recently been performed by investigators at Ondek Pty. Ltd. for the development of mucosal delivery technology based on live *H. pylori* (Benghezal *et al.* unpublished data). Five genotypically different strains of *H. pylori*, including CagA positive strains, were used to challenge healthy human volunteers in a Phase I study (clinical trial reference: SCGH HREC #2009-062). Briefly, 36 *H. pylori* sero-negative subjects were screened and randomised into 6 groups to receive either one of the 5 *H. pylori* strains or placebo. Subjects were monitored for the duration of the 12 week study and stomach biopsies were collected at 2 and 12 weeks post challenge, time points that depict an acute and start of the chronic phase of infection, respectively. Single colony isolates collected at the 2 and 12 week time points represent a unique resource for the investigation of *H. pylori* adaptation in humans based on a multi-strain, multi-person experimental study. Indeed, humans differ in physiologic and immunologic traits, and these traits change with age and in response to *H. pylori* infection. Such host diversity should select for adaptive changes in *H. pylori* genes important for host interaction. Yet the types of adaptive changes that *H. pylori* undergo during colonisation, the underlying mechanisms and functional significance and the resulting changes in the host response remain largely unknown. Thus a sweeping characterization of *H. pylori* adaptation is now made possible by the unique opportunity to access strains from the Ondek-sponsored clinical trial in which 6 subjects per group were each challenged with one of several *H. pylori* strains. *H. pylori* recovered during the acute (2 week) and chronic (12 week) phases of infection will be compared with input strains by genome sequencing to gain new perspectives on bacterial adaptation to different human traits. Of note, comparative genomic analysis of the input/output strains of *H. pylori* will provide insight into the genome plasticity and stability of a live bacterial vector after human challenge for further development of a novel mucosal delivery technology.

7. Perspectives

7.1. Insight into bacterial pathogenesis and microbial evolution

7.1.1. Genomic diversity

The sequencing of *H. pylori* host isolates has revealed the nature and extent of recombination arising from inter-strain horizontal transfer *in vivo*. Generation of genetic diversity by recombination likely relies on the presence of co-infection with multiple strains. Individuals who are already colonised are able to be infected with new additional strains [296]. A study of 127 individuals from three regions in Venezuela found evidence of mixed colonization in 55% of subjects [297]. Genome sequencing of sequential *H. pylori* isolates from chronically infected individuals in Columbia revealed high rates of recombination attributable to uptake of DNA from unrelated strains during co-infection [157]. Thus co-infection with multiple strains is likely to be common, at least in areas with endemic *H. pylori* infection [172, 298], as was the case through most of human history. Where recombination occurs between strains it has been found to introduce 100-fold more genetic alterations than mutation [172] and occurs genome-wide [157].

However, co-infection may be less pervasive in most Western countries where *H. pylori* prevalence is low. In the absence of mixed infection recombination has little effect on genetic diversity [172]. No evidence of recombination was found in a German individual experimentally infected with a single strain [157] or in sequential *H. pylori* isolates from Sweden [294]. The genome sequencing of *H. pylori* isolates from 52 members of two South African families found both high and low rates of recombination which the authors attributed to the presence of co-infection with multiple strains or infection with only a single strain, respectively [172]. Thus it is hypothesized that in instances of co-infection recombination can introduce genomic diversity but that a single strain of *H. pylori* can still establish a robust colonization and stably maintain its genome in the absence of recombination of DNA between strains, suggesting that intra-strain genetic diversity is a sufficient driver to adapt to the changing host. However, lack of opportunity for horizontal transfer between strains in mixed infections in developed countries may be accelerating the disappearance of *H. pylori* in these regions [176]. Indeed transient and self-clearing infections do occur [299] suggesting, in these instances, an inability of the bacterium to adapt to the host or a role of multiple infections in *H. pylori* transmission.

The competence of *H. pylori* likely confers evolutionary advantages. Competence has been found to confer a fitness advantage over non-competent strains *in vitro* [164]. Wild-type G27 was able to adapt to laboratory conditions more rapidly than a competence null *comH* mutant. Although competence is not required for gastric colonization in the gerbil model

[300], competence may be important for host adaptation. Natural transformation generates diversity by the introduction of new alleles and mosaic alleles in recipient strains. Greater genetic diversity amongst strains acts to increase the pool of variants available from which selection can act to confer an advantage on those who are fitter in the changing environment of the host or in different individuals. In the presence of co-infection recombination occurs throughout the time-course of infection. The continued requirement for host-adaptation results in the *in vivo* selection for genes that have undergone recombination that favour persistence [157, 172, 284, 301]. Evidence for recombination is often found in genes related to virulence and persistence.

Analysis of a mixed infection from a Lithuanian patient found that recombination between strains resulted in the loss of the *cag* pathogenicity island and changes in alleles encoding VacA and outer membrane proteins [301]. Genome sequencing of *H. pylori* strains isolated sequentially from chronically infected individuals demonstrated that the number of clustered nucleotide polymorphisms (CNPs), attributable to genetic recombination with DNA from different strains during co-infection, was much greater in strains isolated later in infection (16 years) than in those isolated earlier (3 years), demonstrating that recombination continues through the time-course of infection. CNPs occurred more regularly in some gene families than others; most notably in genes encoding outer membrane proteins, particularly those of the *hop* family [157] whose proteins are known to play key roles in adhesion [24]. This indicates that diversifying selection acts *in vivo* on recombined genes [157]. Indeed, genetic evidence of low effective population sizes in isolates from South Africa may reflect population bottlenecks arising from selection pressures imposed by the host immune system [172].

Horizontal gene transfer by natural transformation in the presence of multiple strains is a key driver in the genetic diversity of *H. pylori*. Evidence has emerged that this generation of genetic diversity plays a role in the ability of Helicobacter to continually adapt to the host throughout prolonged infection. Recombination has the advantage of allowing multiple beneficial mutations to be combined within the same genetic background by horizontal transfer rather than by sequential mutation. This would allow more rapid fixation of beneficial alleles [164]. Indeed, evidence is also emerging that *H. pylori* experiences selective pressure for fitter variants by the host immune system.

7.1.2. Epigenetic diversity

Recently, SMRT sequencing has been utilized to sequence the methylomes of *H. pylori* 26695 and J99. Analysis of the methylome following genetic manipulation of candidate methylases has allowed characterisation of a number of methyltransferases in *H. pylori*. Interestingly, a methyltransferase (HP1353) has been identified that contains two phase-variable repeat sequences. One phase variable repeat appears to function canonically to regulate expression of the methyltransferase. Phase variation of the second repeat appears to switch the protein between two forms that vary in their methylation recognition sequence. The protein thus has three different phase-variable states; off, methylation of recognition sequence 1, and methylation of recognition sequence 2 [302]. It is tempting to speculate that this represents an additional layer of complexity to the phasevarion. Should this methyltransferase regulate the transcription of other genes, it could, as a single methyltransferase, function to regulate two separate phasevarions.

Phase-variable methyltransferases have been identified in *H. pylori* and the investigation of their corresponding phasevarions has been initiated. The coordinated reversible switching of many genes within a phasevarion is postulated to play a role in host adaptation, immune evasion and pathogenicity. However, given the potential significance of the phasevarion, experimental evidence is lacking regarding the role of the phasevarion *in vivo* in host colonization, persistence, and disease pathology. In one study investigating the significance of methylation by the *iceA-hpyIM* R-M system, expression levels of *hpyIM* as determined from RT-PCR and/or RNA slot-blot analysis of RNA isolated from gastric biopsy specimens could not be correlated with *iceA* expression, disease sequelae, colonization density, or mucosal IL-8 levels. However, this methyltransferase has not been identified as having the potential to phase-vary and appears to be a stationary growth phase regulator [303].

Phase variation of individual genes and phasevarions impart to the bacterium an ability to rapidly and reversibly switch between a vast array of different phenotypes. It is postulated that for pathogenic bacteria, there is significant pressure to constantly avoid detection by the immune system. The ability to generate epigenetic and phenotypic variation in this way may enable a bacterial population to play a lottery against the human immune system in which at least the phenotype of one individual imparts sufficient fitness within a changing environment to allow persistence. Thus, both the continued characterisation of phasevarions and their *in vivo* relevance for host adaptation and virulence is of importance in our understanding of *H. pylori* persistence and pathogenesis.

7.1.3. H. pylori regulation of genetic diversity and evolution constraints?

The ability of *H. pylori* to generate genetic diversity is likely to be regulated so as to achieve a subtle balance between the generation of genetic diversity and maintaining the integrity of its small genome to establish persistent infection. The different mutation rates reported to date are in line with regulation of generation of genetic diversity in *H. pylori*. Phase variation of DNA glycosylase MutY, an enzyme of the base excision repair process, represents further evidence for regulation of genetic diversity [66, 67]. Alternatively, a constitutive high mutation rate (named the mutator phenotype in *E. coli*) could be counterbalanced by efficient mechanisms to maintain genome integrity, such as homologous recombination using DNA template from neighbouring cells by natural competence. This possibility has gained some support due to recent reports describing an increase of DNA uptake and RecA homologous recombination upon DNA damage [169] and poor persistence of the *dprA* mutant deficient in natural competence, although the initial colonization level was comparable to wild-type [246].

The ability of *H. pylori* to genetically adapt to the human host is remarkable based on adaptation to human subpopulations with 6 ancestral populations of *H. pylori* named ancestral European 1, ancestral European 2, ancestral East Asia, ancestral Africa1, ancestral Africa2 [2], and ancestral Sahul [1]. As described above, *H. pylori* genetic plasticity is the result of several mechanisms ranging from poor replication fidelity, lack of DNA repair genes and horizontal gene transfer promoted by natural competence, bacteriophage transduction, conjugation of

TnPZs and plasmid transfer. An extreme example of *H. pylori's* adaptive ability is exemplified by the host jump from humans to large felines, predicted to have occurred some 200, 000 years ago that resulted in a new species; *Helicobacter acinonychis*. This particular host jump was accompanied by relative conservation of the core genome, inactivation by different mechanisms of genes encoding surface proteins and acquisition of genes involved in sialyation of the bacterial surface to evade immune responses in the new host [210].

Altogether *H. pylori* micro-evolution within the human host and the above host jump conserved the core genome with changes affecting mainly hotspots and accessory genes. This suggests that constraints in the genome architecture and gene repertoire exist and these limit the evolutionary trajectories of *H. pylori*. Recent advances in evolutionary biology suggest a plurality of constraints on evolution, including the sequence type (coding sequence, structural RNAs, micro RNA and else) and genome architecture and gene repertoire underlying the sum of all phenotypic traits of the organism or phenome [304]. Thus to make sense of *H. pylori's* high mutation and recombination rates and investigate the role of genetic diversity in phenotypic adaptation to the human host, it is important to investigate the constraints, their networks and interactions limiting *H. pylori* evolvability.

7.1.4. Robustness and evolvability

Robustness of systems is the resistance to change under perturbation. Robustness, either mutational, or phenotypic, has been proposed to make biological systems more evolvable [305-308]. Studying *H. pylori* mutational and phenotypic robustness is a highly attractive approach to understand its adaptation to, and persistence in, the human host based on the latest findings and concepts of evolutionary biology.

The evolvability, or capacity of biological systems for adaptive evolution, was proposed to depend on their genotype-phenotype maps [309]. Evolutionary change takes place in a population with each population member having some genotype defining a collection of genotypes in the genotype space [308]. Through mutations, members of the population can change their location in the genotype space. In the population some individuals have a phenotype either superior, or inferior to the existing well-adapted phenotype. Natural selection, while eliminating poorly adapted individuals, preserves the well-adapted ones and selects superior ones. The genotype space reconciles the key problem of evolutionary adaptation of finding the rare superior genotype while preserving the population of well-adapted ones. A first characteristic of the genotype space is the existence of a set of genotypes with the same phenotype or connected genotype networks. The second characteristic of the genotype space is the number of genotypes that can be derived from any one genotype via mutation. The set of these genotypes is named neighbourhood genotype and its size is a simple measure of phenotypic variability of a genotype in response to mutation. In summary, the first feature of the genotype space allow individuals in a population to preserve their phenotype while changing their genotype and the neighbourhood genotype allows exploration of novel superior phenotypes in the population. Thus robustness is beneficial to both the individual and the population. As a consequence, robustness in the presence of genetic mutation/

recombination allows cryptic genetic diversity to accumulate (in the sense of a capacitor) and promotes evolutionary adaptation through greater phenotypic variability in the population.

Robustness as a variability principle in the context of the mutator phenotype of *H. pylori* (due to its high mutation and recombination rates) would reconcile the interest of the single cell and the cell population and may underlie *H. pylori* persistence in the gastric niche. A robust cell phenotype during persistent colonization of the gastric mucosa would not easily be disturbed by mutations, would be beneficial to single cells and would allow greater phenotypic variability to be achieved at the cell population level on a (micro-) evolutionary time scale by accumulation of cryptic genotypic diversity.

The presence of phasevarions in *H. pylori* raises the possibility to influence robustness by dramatically increasing phenotypic variability of the neighbourhood genotype by simple mutation. Greater robustness of *H. pylori* would enhance adaptation and persistence in the changing human gastric niche. Other interesting questions related to evolutionary dynamics are the size of the *H. pylori* population and its mutation rate and how these parameters influence robustness and adaptation to the host. For example, one could hypothesize that the lack of inter-strain recombination weakens the robustness of *H. pylori* leading to its disappearance in Western countries where multiple infections are rare.

To conclude, the investigation of *H. pylori* robustness to better understand the adaptation of this bacterium to the human host will require both computational modelling and experimental data on genotype-phenotype maps of *H. pylori* populations made accessible by the latest sequencing and high-content technologies.

7.1.5. Refining H. pylori persistence mathematical model

H. pylori apparently lacks active and costly sensory machinery gene regulation and its small genome suggests alternative adaptive mechanisms including small RNA regulation [52], automatic random genetic switches for generating diverse adaptive phenotypes [47, 50, 51, 53], and the numerous duplicate and divergent outer membrane genes, which could be part of a more general gene regulation network so far unidentified. Introducing random fluctuations for stochastic phenotype transitions in the *H. pylori* mathematical model of persistence published by Blaser and Kirshner [44] is highly relevant to the robustness principle of biological systems and their evolvability. Thus further refinement of this model by introducing random fluctuations for stochastic phenotype transitions in the spirit of Kussell and Leibler [310], could help to further our understanding of how *H. pylori* establishes the optimal balance between sensing changes and random phenotype switching to adapt to its niche. Model predictions could be tested experimentally in animal models, using the power of molecular-bacterial genetics, including tetracycline-based gene regulation [275, 277], to validate or invalidate aspects of the model and gain insight into the dynamics of *H. pylori* populations.

7.2. Therapeutic potential of targeting persistence mechanisms

H. pylori chronic infection remains a significant health burden, a long regimen of triple or quadruple antibiotic therapy is currently the only available treatment and antibiotic resistance is emerging [311]. Since no prophylactic or therapeutic vaccine has been successfully developed to date, new target ideas are needed for the development of innovative drug therapies to achieve *H. pylori* eradication. Targeting *H. pylori* persistence mechanisms is one such strategy that could encompass immune evasion, micro RNA regulation (of urease for example [52]), genetic and phenotypic diversity generation underlying host adaptation and robustness of biological systems. In this regard, phasevarions, recombination (XerH for example [312]), DNA repair, replication (low fidelity Polymerase I for example [48]) and competence would represent target pathways of choice. Also a drug targeting discrete sites on the urease complex surface shown to be required for infection [247] would have several advantages over eliciting site-specific urease antibodies to inhibit *H. pylori* persistence; e.g. better bioavailability in the mucus layer and a higher concentration that is more likely to achieve inhibition of the large amount of urease produced by *H. pylori*. Other potential targets are the UreI channel (whose structure is available for drug design [313]) that is required for buffering the periplasm during colonization [255-257], the gamma-gltutamyltransferase required for immune modulation and bacterial metabolism to maintain colonization [36], *H. pylori* LPS biosynthetic proteins contributing to gastric adaptation, adhesion and modulation of the host immune response by changing antigen expression in the same human host over time [314]. Compounds targeting the biosynthesis of glycolipids that *H. pylori* uses for immune evasion showed promising inhibition *in vitro* and further work is required to assess their potential [315]. With the recent adaptation of the tetracycline-based gene regulation system in *H. pylori* and its functionality *in vivo* [275, 277], potential targets can now be validated in animal models using tetracycline-based conditional knockouts. Furthermore, conditional knockouts will be instrumental in testing the rate of emergence of resistance for target candidates to select targets less prone to genetic adaptation before embarking on a long and costly drug discovery and development path. *H. pylori*-specific drugs targeting persistence mechanisms would have the advantage of leaving the gastrointestinal microbiota intact, avoiding side effects such as diarrhoea and increased patient compliance. Based on the use of triple and quadruple antibiotic therapies and the genetic plasticity of *H. pylori*, it is likely that more than one *H. pylori*-specific drug targeting persistence will be required to avoid emergence of resistance and achieve high eradication rate.

Acknowledgements

This work was supported by a NHMRC Sir McFarlane Burnett Fellowship grant (572723) to BJM, NHMRC Project Grant (634465) to BJM and MB and NHMRC Early Career Fellowship grant to AWD (1073250). We thank the team at Transittranslations who proofread the manuscript.

Author details

Mohammed Benghezal*, Jonathan C. Gauntlett, Aleksandra W. Debowski, Alma Fulurija, Hans-Olof Nilsson and Barry James Marshall

*Address all correspondence to: mohammed.benghezal@uwa.edu.au

Ondek Pty Ltd. and *Helicobacter pylori* Research Laboratory, Marshall Centre for Infectious Disease Research and Training, The University of Western Australia, School of Pathology & Laboratory Medicine, UWA Discipline of Microbiology & Immunology, Crawley WA, Australia

References

[1] Moodley Y, Linz B, Yamaoka Y, Windsor HM, Breurec S, et al. (2009) The peopling of the Pacific from a bacterial perspective. Science 323: 527-530.

[2] Falush D, Wirth T, Linz B, Pritchard JK, Stephens M, et al. (2003) Traces of human migrations in Helicobacter pylori populations. Science 299: 1582-1585.

[3] Dunn BE, Vakil NB, Schneider BG, Miller MM, Zitzer JB, et al. (1997) Localization of Helicobacter pylori urease and heat shock protein in human gastric biopsies. Infect Immun 65: 1181-1188.

[4] Suerbaum S, Michetti P (2002) Helicobacter pylori infection. N Engl J Med 347: 1175-1186.

[5] Blaser MJ, Atherton JC (2004) Helicobacter pylori persistence: biology and disease. J Clin Invest 113: 321-333.

[6] Monack DM, Mueller A, Falkow S (2004) Persistent bacterial infections: the interface of the pathogen and the host immune system. Nat Rev Microbiol 2: 747-765.

[7] Algood HM, Cover TL (2006) Helicobacter pylori persistence: an overview of interactions between H. pylori and host immune defenses. Clin Microbiol Rev 19: 597-613.

[8] Fischer W, Prassl S, Haas R (2009) Virulence mechanisms and persistence strategies of the human gastric pathogen Helicobacter pylori. Curr Top Microbiol Immunol 337: 129-171.

[9] Muller A, Solnick JV (2011) Inflammation, immunity, and vaccine development for Helicobacter pylori. Helicobacter 16 Suppl 1: 26-32.

[10] Ricci V, Romano M, Boquet P (2011) Molecular cross-talk between Helicobacter pylori and human gastric mucosa. World J Gastroenterol 17: 1383-1399.

[11] Kabir S (2011) The role of interleukin-17 in the Helicobacter pylori induced infection and immunity. Helicobacter 16: 1-8.

[12] Sundquist M, Quiding-Jarbrink M (2010) Helicobacter pylori and its effect on innate and adaptive immunity: new insights and vaccination strategies. Expert Rev Gastroenterol Hepatol 4: 733-744.

[13] Molnar B, Galamb O, Sipos F, Leiszter K, Tulassay Z (2010) Molecular pathogenesis of Helicobacter pylori infection: the role of bacterial virulence factors. Dig Dis 28: 604-608.

[14] Allison CC, Ferrero RL (2010) Role of virulence factors and host cell signaling in the recognition of Helicobacter pylori and the generation of immune responses. Future Microbiol 5: 1233-1255.

[15] Peek RM, Jr., Fiske C, Wilson KT (2010) Role of innate immunity in Helicobacter pylori-induced gastric malignancy. Physiol Rev 90: 831-858.

[16] Watanabe T, Asano N, Kitani A, Fuss IJ, Chiba T, et al. (2011) Activation of type I IFN signaling by NOD1 mediates mucosal host defense against Helicobacter pylori infection. Gut Microbes 2: 61-65.

[17] Atherton JC, Blaser MJ (2009) Coadaptation of Helicobacter pylori and humans: ancient history, modern implications. J Clin Invest 119: 2475-2487.

[18] Kobayashi M, Lee H, Nakayama J, Fukuda M (2009) Roles of gastric mucin-type O-glycans in the pathogenesis of Helicobacter pylori infection. Glycobiology 19: 453-461.

[19] O'Keeffe J, Moran AP (2008) Conventional, regulatory, and unconventional T cells in the immunologic response to Helicobacter pylori. Helicobacter 13: 1-19.

[20] D'Elios MM, Andersen LP (2007) Helicobacter pylori inflammation, immunity, and vaccines. Helicobacter 12 Suppl 1: 15-19.

[21] Robinson K, Argent RH, Atherton JC (2007) The inflammatory and immune response to Helicobacter pylori infection. Best Pract Res Clin Gastroenterol 21: 237-259.

[22] Suarez G, Reyes VE, Beswick EJ (2006) Immune response to H. pylori. World J Gastroenterol 12: 5593-5598.

[23] Velin D, Michetti P (2006) Immunology of Helicobacter pylori infection. Digestion 73: 116-123.

[24] Salama NR, Hartung ML, Muller A (2013) Life in the human stomach: persistence strategies of the bacterial pathogen Helicobacter pylori. Nat Rev Microbiol 11: 385-399.

[25] Yokota S, Okabayashi T, Rehli M, Fujii N, Amano K (2010) Helicobacter pylori lipopolysaccharides upregulate toll-like receptor 4 expression and proliferation of gastric

epithelial cells via the MEK1/2-ERK1/2 mitogen-activated protein kinase pathway. Infect Immun 78: 468-476.

[26] Cullen TW, Giles DK, Wolf LN, Ecobichon C, Boneca IG, et al. (2011) Helicobacter pylori versus the host: remodeling of the bacterial outer membrane is required for survival in the gastric mucosa. PLoS Pathog 7: e1002454.

[27] Gringhuis SI, den Dunnen J, Litjens M, van der Vlist M, Geijtenbeek TB (2009) Carbohydrate-specific signaling through the DC-SIGN signalosome tailors immunity to Mycobacterium tuberculosis, HIV-1 and Helicobacter pylori. Nat Immunol 10: 1081-1088.

[28] Necchi V, Manca R, Ricci V, Solcia E (2009) Evidence for transepithelial dendritic cells in human H. pylori active gastritis. Helicobacter 14: 208-222.

[29] Bergman MP, Engering A, Smits HH, van Vliet SJ, van Bodegraven AA, et al. (2004) Helicobacter pylori modulates the T helper cell 1/T helper cell 2 balance through phase-variable interaction between lipopolysaccharide and DC-SIGN. J Exp Med 200: 979-990.

[30] Appelmelk BJ, van Die I, van Vliet SJ, Vandenbroucke-Grauls CM, Geijtenbeek TB, et al. (2003) Cutting edge: carbohydrate profiling identifies new pathogens that interact with dendritic cell-specific ICAM-3-grabbing nonintegrin on dendritic cells. J Immunol 170: 1635-1639.

[31] Moran AP (2008) Relevance of fucosylation and Lewis antigen expression in the bacterial gastroduodenal pathogen Helicobacter pylori. Carbohydr Res 343: 1952-1965.

[32] Aspinall GO, Monteiro MA, Pang H, Walsh EJ, Moran AP (1994) O Antigen chains in the lipopolysaccharide of H.pylori NCTC 11637. O Antigen chains in the lipopolysaccharide of Hpylori NCTC 11637 1: 151-156.

[33] Andersen-Nissen E, Smith KD, Strobe KL, Barrett SL, Cookson BT, et al. (2005) Evasion of Toll-like receptor 5 by flagellated bacteria. Proc Natl Acad Sci U S A 102: 9247-9252.

[34] Gewirtz AT, Yu Y, Krishna US, Israel DA, Lyons SL, et al. (2004) Helicobacter pylori flagellin evades toll-like receptor 5-mediated innate immunity. J Infect Dis 189: 1914-1920.

[35] Lee SK, Stack A, Katzowitsch E, Aizawa SI, Suerbaum S, et al. (2003) Helicobacter pylori flagellins have very low intrinsic activity to stimulate human gastric epithelial cells via TLR5. Microbes Infect 5: 1345-1356.

[36] Schmees C, Prinz C, Treptau T, Rad R, Hengst L, et al. (2007) Inhibition of T-cell proliferation by Helicobacter pylori gamma-glutamyl transpeptidase. Gastroenterology 132: 1820-1833.

[37] Gebert B, Fischer W, Weiss E, Hoffmann R, Haas R (2003) Helicobacter pylori vacuolating cytotoxin inhibits T lymphocyte activation. Science 301: 1099-1102.

[38] Wunder C, Churin Y, Winau F, Warnecke D, Vieth M, et al. (2006) Cholesterol glucosylation promotes immune evasion by Helicobacter pylori. Nat Med 12: 1030-1038.

[39] Hitzler I, Sayi A, Kohler E, Engler DB, Koch KN, et al. (2012) Caspase-1 Has Both Pro-Inflammatory and Regulatory Properties in Helicobacter Infections, Which Are Differentially Mediated by Its Substrates IL-1beta and IL-18. J Immunol.

[40] Takashima M, Furuta T, Hanai H, Sugimura H, Kaneko E (2001) Effects of Helicobacter pylori infection on gastric acid secretion and serum gastrin levels in Mongolian gerbils. Gut 48: 765-773.

[41] Troost E, Hold GL, Smith MG, Chow WH, Rabkin CS, et al. (2003) The role of interleukin-1beta and other potential genetic markers as indicators of gastric cancer risk. Can J Gastroenterol 17 Suppl B: 8B-12B.

[42] El-Omar EM, Rabkin CS, Gammon MD, Vaughan TL, Risch HA, et al. (2003) Increased risk of noncardia gastric cancer associated with proinflammatory cytokine gene polymorphisms. Gastroenterology 124: 1193-1201.

[43] El-Omar EM, Carrington M, Chow WH, McColl KE, Bream JH, et al. (2000) Interleukin-1 polymorphisms associated with increased risk of gastric cancer. Nature 404: 398-402.

[44] Blaser MJ, Kirschner D (2007) The equilibria that allow bacterial persistence in human hosts. Nature 449: 843-849.

[45] Bjorkholm B, Sjolund M, Falk PG, Berg OG, Engstrand L, et al. (2001) Mutation frequency and biological cost of antibiotic resistance in Helicobacter pylori. Proc Natl Acad Sci U S A 98: 14607-14612.

[46] Kang J, Blaser MJ (2006) Bacterial populations as perfect gases: genomic integrity and diversification tensions in Helicobacter pylori. Nat Rev Microbiol 4: 826-836.

[47] Salaun L, Linz B, Suerbaum S, Saunders NJ (2004) The diversity within an expanded and redefined repertoire of phase-variable genes in Helicobacter pylori. Microbiology 150: 817-830.

[48] Garcia-Ortiz MV, Marsin S, Arana ME, Gasparutto D, Guerois R, et al. (2011) Unexpected role for Helicobacter pylori DNA polymerase I as a source of genetic variability. PLoS Genet 7: e1002152.

[49] Moccia C, Krebes J, Kulick S, Didelot X, Kraft C, et al. (2012) The nucleotide excision repair (NER) system of Helicobacter pylori: role in mutation prevention and chromosomal import patterns after natural transformation. BMC Microbiol 12: 67.

[50] Srikhanta YN, Gorrell RJ, Steen JA, Gawthorne JA, Kwok T, et al. (2011) Phasevarion mediated epigenetic gene regulation in Helicobacter pylori. PLoS One 6: e27569.

[51] Srikhanta YN, Maguire TL, Stacey KJ, Grimmond SM, Jennings MP (2005) The phasevarion: a genetic system controlling coordinated, random switching of expression of multiple genes. Proc Natl Acad Sci U S A 102: 5547-5551.

[52] Wen Y, Feng J, Sachs G (2013) Helicobacter pylori 5'ureB-sRNA, a cis-encoded antisense small RNA, negatively regulates ureAB expression by transcription termination. J Bacteriol 195: 444-452.

[53] Palmer ME, Lipsitch M, Moxon ER, Bayliss CD (2013) Broad conditions favor the evolution of phase-variable loci. MBio 4: e00430-00412.

[54] Ambur OH, Davidsen T, Frye SA, Balasingham SV, Lagesen K, et al. (2009) Genome dynamics in major bacterial pathogens. FEMS Microbiol Rev 33: 453-470.

[55] McCready SJ, Osman F, Yasui A (2000) Repair of UV damage in the fission yeast Schizosaccharomyces pombe. Mutat Res 451: 197-210.

[56] Alm RA, Trust TJ (1999) Analysis of the genetic diversity of Helicobacter pylori: the tale of two genomes. J Mol Med (Berl) 77: 834-846.

[57] Tomb JF, White O, Kerlavage AR, Clayton RA, Sutton GG, et al. (1997) The complete genome sequence of the gastric pathogen Helicobacter pylori. Nature 388: 539-547.

[58] Eisen JA (1998) A phylogenomic study of the MutS family of proteins. Nucleic Acids Res 26: 4291-4300.

[59] Wang G, Alamuri P, Humayun MZ, Taylor DE, Maier RJ (2005) The Helicobacter pylori MutS protein confers protection from oxidative DNA damage. Mol Microbiol 58: 166-176.

[60] LeClerc JE, Li B, Payne WL, Cebula TA (1996) High mutation frequencies among Escherichia coli and Salmonella pathogens. Science 274: 1208-1211.

[61] Oliver A, Canton R, Campo P, Baquero F, Blazquez J (2000) High frequency of hypermutable Pseudomonas aeruginosa in cystic fibrosis lung infection. Science 288: 1251-1254.

[62] Richardson AR, Yu Z, Popovic T, Stojiljkovic I (2002) Mutator clones of Neisseria meningitidis in epidemic serogroup A disease. Proc Natl Acad Sci U S A 99: 6103-6107.

[63] Dorer MS, Sessler TH, Salama NR (2011) Recombination and DNA repair in Helicobacter pylori. Annu Rev Microbiol 65: 329-348.

[64] Eutsey R, Wang G, Maier RJ (2007) Role of a MutY DNA glycosylase in combating oxidative DNA damage in Helicobacter pylori. DNA Repair (Amst) 6: 19-26.

[65] Huang S, Kang J, Blaser MJ (2006) Antimutator role of the DNA glycosylase mutY gene in Helicobacter pylori. J Bacteriol 188: 6224-6234.

[66] Kulick S, Moccia C, Kraft C, Suerbaum S (2008) The Helicobacter pylori mutY homologue HP0142 is an antimutator gene that prevents specific C to A transversions. Arch Microbiol 189: 263-270.

[67] Mathieu A, O'Rourke EJ, Radicella JP (2006) Helicobacter pylori genes involved in avoidance of mutations induced by 8-oxoguanine. J Bacteriol 188: 7464-7469.

[68] Eichman BF, O'Rourke EJ, Radicella JP, Ellenberger T (2003) Crystal structures of 3-methyladenine DNA glycosylase MagIII and the recognition of alkylated bases. EMBO J 22: 4898-4909.

[69] O'Rourke EJ, Chevalier C, Boiteux S, Labigne A, Ielpi L, et al. (2000) A novel 3-methyladenine DNA glycosylase from Helicobacter pylori defines a new class within the endonuclease III family of base excision repair glycosylases. J Biol Chem 275: 20077-20083.

[70] Baldwin DN, Shepherd B, Kraemer P, Hall MK, Sycuro LK, et al. (2007) Identification of Helicobacter pylori genes that contribute to stomach colonization. Infect Immun 75: 1005-1016.

[71] O'Rourke EJ, Chevalier C, Pinto AV, Thiberge JM, Ielpi L, et al. (2003) Pathogen DNA as target for host-generated oxidative stress: role for repair of bacterial DNA damage in Helicobacter pylori colonization. Proc Natl Acad Sci U S A 100: 2789-2794.

[72] Thompson SA, Latch RL, Blaser JM (1998) Molecular characterization of the Helicobacter pylori uvr B gene. Gene 209: 113-122.

[73] Kang J, Blaser MJ (2006) UvrD helicase suppresses recombination and DNA damage-induced deletions. J Bacteriol 188: 5450-5459.

[74] Lee GH, Jeong JY, Chung JW, Nam WH, Lee SM, et al. (2009) The Helicobacter pylori Mfd protein is important for antibiotic resistance and DNA repair. Diagn Microbiol Infect Dis 65: 454-456.

[75] Solnick JV, Hansen LM, Salama NR, Boonjakuakul JK, Syvanen M (2004) Modification of Helicobacter pylori outer membrane protein expression during experimental infection of rhesus macaques. Proc Natl Acad Sci U S A 101: 2106-2111.

[76] Amundsen SK, Fero J, Hansen LM, Cromie GA, Solnick JV, et al. (2008) Helicobacter pylori AddAB helicase-nuclease and RecA promote recombination-related DNA repair and survival during stomach colonization. Mol Microbiol 69: 994-1007.

[77] Oleastro M, Cordeiro R, Menard A, Gomes JP (2010) Allelic diversity among Helicobacter pylori outer membrane protein genes homB and homA generated by recombination. J Bacteriol 192: 3961-3968.

[78] Pohl MA, Kienesberger S, Blaser MJ (2012) Novel functions for glycosyltransferases Jhp0562 and GalT in Lewis antigen synthesis and variation in Helicobacter pylori. Infect Immun 80: 1593-1605.

[79] Talarico S, Whitefield SE, Fero J, Haas R, Salama NR (2012) Regulation of Helicobacter pylori adherence by gene conversion. Mol Microbiol 84: 1050-1061.

[80] Schmitt W, Odenbreit S, Heuermann D, Haas R (1995) Cloning of the Helicobacter pylori recA gene and functional characterization of its product. Mol Gen Genet 248: 563-572.

[81] Thompson SA, Blaser MJ (1995) Isolation of the Helicobacter pylori recA gene and involvement of the recA region in resistance to low pH. Infect Immun 63: 2185-2193.

[82] Amundsen SK, Fero J, Salama NR, Smith GR (2009) Dual nuclease and helicase activities of Helicobacter pylori AddAB are required for DNA repair, recombination, and mouse infectivity. J Biol Chem 284: 16759-16766.

[83] Marsin S, Mathieu A, Kortulewski T, Guerois R, Radicella JP (2008) Unveiling novel RecO distant orthologues involved in homologous recombination. PLoS Genet 4: e1000146.

[84] Marsin S, Lopes A, Mathieu A, Dizet E, Orillard E, et al. (2010) Genetic dissection of Helicobacter pylori AddAB role in homologous recombination. FEMS Microbiol Lett 311: 44-50.

[85] Wang G, Maier RJ (2008) Critical role of RecN in recombinational DNA repair and survival of Helicobacter pylori. Infect Immun 76: 153-160.

[86] Kang J, Blaser MJ (2008) Repair and antirepair DNA helicases in Helicobacter pylori. J Bacteriol 190: 4218-4224.

[87] Debowski AW, Carnoy C, Verbrugghe P, Nilsson H, Gauntlett JC, et al. (2012) Xer Recombinase and Genome Integrity in Helicobacter pylori, a Pathogen without Topoisomerase IV. PLoS One in press.

[88] Robinson K, Loughlin MF, Potter R, Jenks PJ (2005) Host adaptation and immune modulation are mediated by homologous recombination in Helicobacter pylori. J Infect Dis 191: 579-587.

[89] Fukui K, Nakagawa N, Kitamura Y, Nishida Y, Masui R, et al. (2008) Crystal structure of MutS2 endonuclease domain and the mechanism of homologous recombination suppression. J Biol Chem 283: 33417-33427.

[90] Pinto AV, Mathieu A, Marsin S, Veaute X, Ielpi L, et al. (2005) Suppression of homologous and homeologous recombination by the bacterial MutS2 protein. Mol Cell 17: 113-120.

[91] Kuempel PL, Henson JM, Dircks L, Tecklenburg M, Lim DF (1991) dif, a recA-independent recombination site in the terminus region of the chromosome of Escherichia coli. New Biol 3: 799-811.

[92] Aras RA, Fischer W, Perez-Perez GI, Crosatti M, Ando T, et al. (2003) Plasticity of repetitive DNA sequences within a bacterial (Type IV) secretion system component. J Exp Med 198: 1349-1360.

[93] Barrozo RM, Cooke CL, Hansen LM, Lam AM, Gaddy JA, et al. (2013) Functional plasticity in the type IV secretion system of Helicobacter pylori. PLoS Pathog 9: e1003189.

[94] van der Woude MW, Baumler AJ (2004) Phase and antigenic variation in bacteria. Clin Microbiol Rev 17: 581-611, table of contents.

[95] Salaun L, Snyder LA, Saunders NJ (2003) Adaptation by phase variation in pathogenic bacteria. Adv Appl Microbiol 52: 263-301.

[96] Guo X, Mrazek J (2008) Long simple sequence repeats in host-adapted pathogens localize near genes encoding antigens, housekeeping genes, and pseudogenes. J Mol Evol 67: 497-509.

[97] Alm RA, Ling LS, Moir DT, King BL, Brown ED, et al. (1999) Genomic-sequence comparison of two unrelated isolates of the human gastric pathogen Helicobacter pylori. Nature 397: 176-180.

[98] Saunders NJ, Peden JF, Hood DW, Moxon ER (1998) Simple sequence repeats in the Helicobacter pylori genome. Mol Microbiol 27: 1091-1098.

[99] Salaun L, Linz B, Suerbaum S, Saunders NJ (2004) The diversity within an expanded and redefined repertoire of phase-variable genes in Helicobacter pylori. Microbiology-Sgm 150: 817-830.

[100] Salaun L, Saunders NJ (2006) Population-associated differences between the phase variable LPS biosynthetic genes of Helicobacter pylori. BMC Microbiol 6: 79.

[101] Moran AP (1996) Helicobacter pylori expresses Lewis X. Helicobacter 1: 190-191.

[102] Appelmelk BJ, Shiberu B, Trinks C, Tapsi N, Zheng PY, et al. (1998) Phase variation in Helicobacter pylori lipopolysaccharide. Infect Immun 66: 70-76.

[103] Appelmelk BJ, Martin SL, Monteiro MA, Clayton CA, McColm AA, et al. (1999) Phase variation in Helicobacter pylori lipopolysaccharide due to changes in the lengths of poly(C) tracts in alpha3-fucosyltransferase genes. Infect Immun 67: 5361-5366.

[104] Nilsson C, Skoglund A, Moran AP, Annuk H, Engstrand L, et al. (2008) Lipopolysaccharide diversity evolving in Helicobacter pylori communities through genetic modifications in fucosyltransferases. PLoS One 3: e3811.

[105] Appelmelk BJ, Martino MC, Veenhof E, Monteiro MA, Maaskant JJ, et al. (2000) Phase variation in H type I and Lewis a epitopes of Helicobacter pylori lipopolysaccharide. Infect Immun 68: 5928-5932.

[106] Langdon R, Craig JE, Goldrick M, Houldsworth R, High NJ (2005) Analysis of the role of HP0208, a phase-variable open reading frame, and its homologues HP1416 and HP0159 in the biosynthesis of Helicobacter pylori lipopolysaccharide. J Med Microbiol 54: 697-706.

[107] Sanabria-Valentin E, Colbert MT, Blaser MJ (2007) Role of futC slipped strand mispairing in Helicobacter pylori Lewisy phase variation. Microbes Infect 9: 1553-1560.

[108] Wirth HP, Yang M, Peek RM, Jr., Hook-Nikanne J, Fried M, et al. (1999) Phenotypic diversity in Lewis expression of Helicobacter pylori isolates from the same host. J Lab Clin Med 133: 488-500.

[109] Linden S, Boren T, Dubois A, Carlstedt I (2004) Rhesus monkey gastric mucins: oligomeric structure, glycoforms and Helicobacter pylori binding. Biochem J 379: 765-775.

[110] Goodwin AC, Weinberger DM, Ford CB, Nelson JC, Snider JD, et al. (2008) Expression of the Helicobacter pylori adhesin SabA is controlled via phase variation and the ArsRS signal transduction system. Microbiology 154: 2231-2240.

[111] Peck B, Ortkamp M, Diehl KD, Hundt E, Knapp B (1999) Conservation, localization and expression of HopZ, a protein involved in adhesion of Helicobacter pylori. Nucleic Acids Res 27: 3325-3333.

[112] Kennemann L, Brenneke B, Andres S, Engstrand L, Meyer TF, et al. (2012) In vivo sequence variation in HopZ, a phase-variable outer membrane protein of Helicobacter pylori. Infect Immun 80: 4364-4373.

[113] Ilver D, Arnqvist A, Ogren J, Frick IM, Kersulyte D, et al. (1998) Helicobacter pylori adhesin binding fucosylated histo-blood group antigens revealed by retagging. Science 279: 373-377.

[114] Dossumbekova A, Prinz C, Mages J, Lang R, Kusters JG, et al. (2006) Helicobacter pylori HopH (OipA) and bacterial pathogenicity: genetic and functional genomic analysis of hopH gene polymorphisms. J Infect Dis 194: 1346-1355.

[115] Yamaoka Y, Kita M, Kodama T, Imamura S, Ohno T, et al. (2002) Helicobacter pylori infection in mice: Role of outer membrane proteins in colonization and inflammation. Gastroenterology 123: 1992-2004.

[116] Yamaoka Y, Kikuchi S, el-Zimaity HM, Gutierrez O, Osato MS, et al. (2002) Importance of Helicobacter pylori oipA in clinical presentation, gastric inflammation, and mucosal interleukin 8 production. Gastroenterology 123: 414-424.

[117] Tannaes T, Dekker N, Bukholm G, Bijlsma JJ, Appelmelk BJ (2001) Phase variation in the Helicobacter pylori phospholipase A gene and its role in acid adaptation. Infect Immun 69: 7334-7340.

[118] Moran AP, Knirel YA, Senchenkova SN, Widmalm G, Hynes SO, et al. (2002) Phenotypic variation in molecular mimicry between Helicobacter pylori lipopolysaccharides and human gastric epithelial cell surface glycoforms. Acid-induced phase

variation in Lewis(x) and Lewis(y) expression by H. Pylori lipopolysaccharides. J Biol Chem 277: 5785-5795.

[119] Dumrese C, Slomianka L, Ziegler U, Choi SS, Kalia A, et al. (2009) The secreted Helicobacter cysteine-rich protein A causes adherence of human monocytes and differentiation into a macrophage-like phenotype. FEBS Lett 583: 1637-1643.

[120] Khamri W, Moran AP, Worku ML, Karim QN, Walker MM, et al. (2005) Variations in Helicobacter pylori lipopolysaccharide to evade the innate immune component surfactant protein D. Infect Immun 73: 7677-7686.

[121] Bergman M, Del Prete G, van Kooyk Y, Appelmelk B (2006) Helicobacter pylori phase variation, immune modulation and gastric autoimmunity. Nat Rev Microbiol 4: 151-159.

[122] Salaun L, Ayraud S, Saunders NJ (2005) Phase variation mediated niche adaptation during prolonged experimental murine infection with Helicobacter pylori. Microbiology 151: 917-923.

[123] Styer CM, Hansen LM, Cooke CL, Gundersen AM, Choi SS, et al. (2010) Expression of the BabA adhesin during experimental infection with Helicobacter pylori. Infect Immun 78: 1593-1600.

[124] Weiser JN, Maskell DJ, Butler PD, Lindberg AA, Moxon ER (1990) Characterization of repetitive sequences controlling phase variation of Haemophilus influenzae lipopolysaccharide. J Bacteriol 172: 3304-3309.

[125] Boyer HW (1971) DNA restriction and modification mechanisms in bacteria. Annu Rev Microbiol 25: 153-176.

[126] Wilson GG, Murray NE (1991) Restriction and modification systems. Annu Rev Genet 25: 585-627.

[127] Low DA, Weyand NJ, Mahan MJ (2001) Roles of DNA adenine methylation in regulating bacterial gene expression and virulence. Infect Immun 69: 7197-7204.

[128] Srikhanta YN, Fox KL, Jennings MP (2010) The phasevarion: phase variation of type III DNA methyltransferases controls coordinated switching in multiple genes. Nat Rev Microbiol 8: 196-206.

[129] Srikhanta YN, Dowideit SJ, Edwards JL, Falsetta ML, Wu HJ, et al. (2009) Phasevarions mediate random switching of gene expression in pathogenic Neisseria. PLoS Pathog 5: e1000400.

[130] Fox KL, Srikhanta YN, Jennings MP (2007) Phase variable type III restriction-modification systems of host-adapted bacterial pathogens. Mol Microbiol 65: 1375-1379.

[131] Akopyants NS, Fradkov A, Diatchenko L, Hill JE, Siebert PD, et al. (1998) PCR-based subtractive hybridization and differences in gene content among strains of Helicobacter pylori. Proc Natl Acad Sci U S A 95: 13108-13113.

[132] Lin LF, Posfai J, Roberts RJ, Kong H (2001) Comparative genomics of the restriction-modification systems in Helicobacter pylori. Proc Natl Acad Sci U S A 98: 2740-2745.

[133] Furuta Y, Kobayashi I (2012) Mobility of DNA sequence recognition domains in DNA methyltransferases suggests epigenetics-driven adaptive evolution. Mob Genet Elements 2: 292-296.

[134] Gawthorne JA, Beatson SA, Srikhanta YN, Fox KL, Jennings MP (2012) Origin of the diversity in DNA recognition domains in phasevarion associated modA genes of pathogenic Neisseria and Haemophilus influenzae. PLoS One 7: e32337.

[135] Kong H, Lin LF, Porter N, Stickel S, Byrd D, et al. (2000) Functional analysis of putative restriction-modification system genes in the Helicobacter pylori J99 genome. Nucleic Acids Res 28: 3216-3223.

[136] de Vries N, Duinsbergen D, Kuipers EJ, Pot RG, Wiesenekker P, et al. (2002) Transcriptional phase variation of a type III restriction-modification system in Helicobacter pylori. J Bacteriol 184: 6615-6623.

[137] Skoglund A, Bjorkholm B, Nilsson C, Andersson AF, Jernberg C, et al. (2007) Functional analysis of the M.HpyAIV DNA methyltransferase of Helicobacter pylori. J Bacteriol 189: 8914-8921.

[138] Kumar R, Mukhopadhyay AK, Ghosh P, Rao DN (2012) Comparative transcriptomics of H. pylori strains AM5, SS1 and their hpyAVIBM deletion mutants: possible roles of cytosine methylation. PLoS One 7: e42303.

[139] Nedenskov-Sørensen P, Bukholm G, Bøvre K (1990) Natural competence for genetic transformation in Campylobacter pylori. J Infect Dis 161: 365-366.

[140] Bakkali M (2013) Could DNA uptake be a side effect of bacterial adhesion and twitching motility? Arch Microbiol 195: 279-289.

[141] Seitz P, Blokesch M (2013) Cues and regulatory pathways involved in natural competence and transformation in pathogenic and environmental Gram-negative bacteria. FEMS Microbiol Rev 37: 336-363.

[142] Hofreuter D, Odenbreit S, Haas R (2001) Natural transformation competence in Helicobacter pylori is mediated by the basic components of a type IV secretion system. Mol Microbiol 41: 379-391.

[143] Stingl K, Muller S, Scheidgen-Kleyboldt G, Clausen M, Maier B (2010) Composite system mediates two-step DNA uptake into Helicobacter pylori. Proc Natl Acad Sci U S A 107: 1184-1189.

[144] Yeh YC, Lin TL, Chang KC, Wang JT (2003) Characterization of a ComE3 homologue essential for DNA transformation in Helicobacter pylori. Infect Immun 71: 5427-5431.

[145] Humbert O, Dorer MS, Salama NR (2011) Characterization of Helicobacter pylori factors that control transformation frequency and integration length during inter-strain DNA recombination. Mol Microbiol 79: 387-401.

[146] Mortier-Barrière I, Velten M, Dupaigne P, Mirouze N, Piètrement O, et al. (2007) A key presynaptic role in transformation for a widespread bacterial protein: DprA conveys incoming ssDNA to RecA. Cell 130: 824-836.

[147] Kang J, Huang S, Blaser MJ (2005) Structural and functional divergence of MutS2 from bacterial MutS1 and eukaryotic MSH4-MSH5 homologs. J Bacteriol 187: 3528-3537.

[148] Zhang XS, Blaser MJ (2012) DprB facilitates inter- and intragenomic recombination in Helicobacter pylori. J Bacteriol 194: 3891-3903.

[149] Smeets LC, Kusters JG (2002) Natural transformation in Helicobacter pylori: DNA transport in an unexpected way. Trends Microbiol 10: 159-162; discussion 162.

[150] Hofreuter D, Odenbreit S, Henke G, Haas R (1998) Natural competence for DNA transformation in Helicobacter pylori: identification and genetic characterization of the comB locus. Mol Microbiol 28: 1027-1038.

[151] Karnholz A, Hoefler C, Odenbreit S, Fischer W, Hofreuter D, et al. (2006) Functional and topological characterization of novel components of the comB DNA transformation competence system in Helicobacter pylori. J Bacteriol 188: 882-893.

[152] Lin TL, Shun CT, Chang KC, Wang JT (2006) Isolation and characterization of a competence operon associated with transformation and adhesion in Helicobacter pylori. Microbes Infect 8: 2756-2765.

[153] Hofreuter D, Karnholz A, Haas R (2003) Topology and membrane interaction of Helicobacter pylori ComB proteins involved in natural transformation competence. Int J Med Microbiol 293: 153-165.

[154] Aras RA, Takata T, Ando T, van der Ende A, Blaser MJ (2001) Regulation of the HpyII restriction-modification system of Helicobacter pylori by gene deletion and horizontal reconstitution. Mol Microbiol 42: 369-382.

[155] Levine SM, Lin EA, Emara W, Kang J, DiBenedetto M, et al. (2007) Plastic cells and populations: DNA substrate characteristics in Helicobacter pylori transformation define a flexible but conservative system for genomic variation. FASEB J 21: 3458-3467.

[156] Zhang XS, Blaser MJ (2012) Natural transformation of an engineered Helicobacter pylori strain deficient in type II restriction endonucleases. J Bacteriol 194: 3407-3416.

[157] Kennemann L, Didelot X, Aebischer T, Kuhn S, Drescher B, et al. (2011) Helicobacter pylori genome evolution during human infection. Proc Natl Acad Sci U S A 108: 5033-5038.

[158] Ando T, Israel DA, Kusugami K, Blaser MJ (1999) HP0333, a member of the dprA family, is involved in natural transformation in Helicobacter pylori. J Bacteriol 181: 5572-5580.

[159] Smeets LC, Bijlsma JJ, Kuipers EJ, Vandenbroucke-Grauls CM, Kusters JG (2000) The dprA gene is required for natural transformation of Helicobacter pylori. FEMS Immunol Med Microbiol 27: 99-102.

[160] Dwivedi GR, Sharma E, Rao DN (2013) Helicobacter pylori DprA alleviates restriction barrier for incoming DNA. Nucleic Acids Res 41: 3274-3288.

[161] Kang J, Tavakoli D, Tschumi A, Aras RA, Blaser MJ (2004) Effect of host species on recG phenotypes in Helicobacter pylori and Escherichia coli. J Bacteriol 186: 7704-7713.

[162] Loughlin MF, Barnard FM, Jenkins D, Sharples GJ, Jenks PJ (2003) Helicobacter pylori mutants defective in RuvC Holliday junction resolvase display reduced macrophage survival and spontaneous clearance from the murine gastric mucosa. Infect Immun 71: 2022-2031.

[163] Smeets LC, Bijlsma JJ, Boomkens SY, Vandenbroucke-Grauls CM, Kusters JG (2000) comH, a novel gene essential for natural transformation of Helicobacter pylori. J Bacteriol 182: 3948-3954.

[164] Baltrus DA, Guillemin K, Phillips PC (2008) Natural transformation increases the rate of adaptation in the human pathogen Helicobacter pylori. Evolution 62: 39-49.

[165] Kostidis K, Thackray P, Bardhan KD, Potter CW, Sayers JR ComH: isolation, purification and characterisation of a unique H. pylori protein. Gut 56: A166.

[166] O'Rourke EJ, Pinto AV, Petroni EA, Tolmasky ME, Ielpi L (2004) Evidence for the active role of a novel nuclease from Helicobacter pylori in the horizontal transfer of genetic information. J Bacteriol 186: 2586-2593.

[167] Liechti GW, Goldberg JB (2013) Helicobacter pylori Salvages Purines from Extracellular Host Cell DNA Utilizing the Outer Membrane-Associated Nuclease NucT. J Bacteriol 195: 4387-4398.

[168] Baltrus DA, Guillemin K (2006) Multiple phases of competence occur during the Helicobacter pylori growth cycle. FEMS Microbiol Lett 255: 148-155.

[169] Dorer MS, Fero J, Salama NR (2010) DNA damage triggers genetic exchange in Helicobacter pylori. PLoS Pathog 6: e1001026.

[170] Kulick S, Moccia C, Didelot X, Falush D, Kraft C, et al. (2008) Mosaic DNA imports with interspersions of recipient sequence after natural transformation of Helicobacter pylori. PLoS One 3: e3797.

[171] Lin EA, Zhang XS, Levine SM, Gill SR, Falush D, et al. (2009) Natural transformation of helicobacter pylori involves the integration of short DNA fragments interrupted by gaps of variable size. PLoS Pathog 5: e1000337.

[172] Didelot X, Nell S, Yang I, Woltemate S, van der Merwe S, et al. (2013) Genomic evolution and transmission of Helicobacter pylori in two South African families. Proc Natl Acad Sci U S A 110: 13880-13885.

[173] Israel DA, Lou AS, Blaser MJ (2000) Characteristics of Helicobacter pylori natural transformation. FEMS Microbiol Lett 186: 275-280.

[174] Suerbaum S, Smith JM, Bapumia K, Morelli G, Smith NH, et al. (1998) Free recombination within Helicobacter pylori. Proc Natl Acad Sci U S A 95: 12619-12624.

[175] Falush D, Kraft C, Taylor NS, Correa P, Fox JG, et al. (2001) Recombination and mutation during long-term gastric colonization by Helicobacter pylori: estimates of clock rates, recombination size, and minimal age. Proc Natl Acad Sci U S A 98: 15056-15061.

[176] Suerbaum S, Josenhans C (2007) Helicobacter pylori evolution and phenotypic diversification in a changing host. Nat Rev Microbiol 5: 441-452.

[177] Schröder G, Lanka E (2005) The mating pair formation system of conjugative plasmids-A versatile secretion machinery for transfer of proteins and DNA. Plasmid 54: 1-25.

[178] Penfold SS, Lastovica AJ, Elisha BG (1988) Demonstration of plasmids in Campylobacter pylori. J Infect Dis 157: 850-851.

[179] Höfler C, Fischer W, Hofreuter D, Haas R (2004) Cryptic plasmids in Helicobacter pylori: putative functions in conjugative transfer and microcin production. Int J Med Microbiol 294: 141-148.

[180] Hofreuter D, Haas R (2002) Characterization of two cryptic Helicobacter pylori plasmids: a putative source for horizontal gene transfer and gene shuffling. J Bacteriol 184: 2755-2766.

[181] De Ungria MC, Kolesnikow T, Cox PT, Lee A (1999) Molecular characterization and interstrain variability of pHPS1, a plasmid isolated from the Sydney strain (SS1) of Helicobacter pylori. Plasmid 41: 97-109.

[182] Heuermann D, Haas R (1995) Genetic organization of a small cryptic plasmid of Helicobacter pylori. Gene 165: 17-24.

[183] Joo JS, Song JY, Baik SC, Lee WK, Cho MJ, et al. (2012) Genetic organization and conjugal plasmid DNA transfer of pHP69, a plasmid from a Korean isolate of Helicobacter pylori. J Microbiol 50: 955-961.

[184] Kleanthous H, Clayton CL, Tabaqchali S (1991) Characterization of a plasmid from Helicobacter pylori encoding a replication protein common to plasmids in gram-positive bacteria. Mol Microbiol 5: 2377-2389.

[185] Minnis JA, Taylor TE, Knesek JE, Peterson WL, McIntire SA (1995) Characterization of a 3.5-kbp plasmid from Helicobacter pylori. Plasmid 34: 22-36.

[186] Backert S, Kwok T, König W (2005) Conjugative plasmid DNA transfer in Helicobacter pylori mediated by chromosomally encoded relaxase and TraG-like proteins. Microbiology 151: 3493-3503.

[187] Rohrer S, Holsten L, Weiss E, Benghezal M, Fischer W, et al. (2012) Multiple pathways of plasmid DNA transfer in Helicobacter pylori. PLoS One 7: e45623.

[188] Quiñones M, Knesek JE, McIntire SA (2001) Sequence and gene expression analyses of plasmid pHPM8 from Helicobacter pylori reveal the presence of two operons with putative roles in plasmid replication and antibiotic activity. Plasmid 46: 223-228.

[189] Kuipers EJ, Israel DA, Kusters JG, Blaser MJ (1998) Evidence for a conjugation-like mechanism of DNA transfer in Helicobacter pylori. J Bacteriol 180: 2901-2905.

[190] Oyarzabal OA, Rad R, Backert S (2007) Conjugative transfer of chromosomally encoded antibiotic resistance from Helicobacter pylori to Campylobacter jejuni. J Clin Microbiol 45: 402-408.

[191] Fischer W, Windhager L, Rohrer S, Zeiller M, Karnholz A, et al. (2010) Strain-specific genes of Helicobacter pylori: genome evolution driven by a novel type IV secretion system and genomic island transfer. Nucleic Acids Res 38: 6089-6101.

[192] Kersulyte D, Velapatino B, Mukhopadhyay AK, Cahuayme L, Bussalleu A, et al. (2003) Cluster of type IV secretion genes in Helicobacter pylori's plasticity zone. J Bacteriol 185: 3764-3772.

[193] Kersulyte D, Lee W, Subramaniam D, Anant S, Herrera P, et al. (2009) Helicobacter Pylori's plasticity zones are novel transposable elements. PLoS One 4: e6859.

[194] Occhialini A, Marais A, Alm R, Garcia F, Sierra R, et al. (2000) Distribution of open reading frames of plasticity region of strain J99 in Helicobacter pylori strains isolated from gastric carcinoma and gastritis patients in Costa Rica. Infect Immun 68: 6240-6249.

[195] Romo-Gonzalez C, Salama NR, Burgeno-Ferreira J, Ponce-Castaneda V, Lazcano-Ponce E, et al. (2009) Differences in genome content among Helicobacter pylori isolates from patients with gastritis, duodenal ulcer, or gastric cancer reveal novel disease-associated genes. Infect Immun 77: 2201-2211.

[196] de Jonge R, Kuipers EJ, Langeveld SC, Loffeld RJ, Stoof J, et al. (2004) The Helicobacter pylori plasticity region locus jhp0947-jhp0949 is associated with duodenal ulcer

disease and interleukin-12 production in monocyte cells. FEMS Immunol Med Microbiol 41: 161-167.

[197] Lehours P, Dupouy S, Bergey B, Ruskone-Foumestraux A, Delchier JC, et al. (2004) Identification of a genetic marker of Helicobacter pylori strains involved in gastric extranodal marginal zone B cell lymphoma of the MALT-type. Gut 53: 931-937.

[198] Proenca Modena JL, Lopes Sales AI, Olszanski Acrani G, Russo R, Vilela Ribeiro MA, et al. (2007) Association between Helicobacter pylori genotypes and gastric disorders in relation to the cag pathogenicity island. Diagn Microbiol Infect Dis 59: 7-16.

[199] Rhead JL, Letley DP, Mohammadi M, Hussein N, Mohagheghi MA, et al. (2007) A new Helicobacter pylori vacuolating cytotoxin determinant, the intermediate region, is associated with gastric cancer. Gastroenterology 133: 926-936.

[200] Rizwan M, Alvi A, Ahmed N (2008) Novel protein antigen (JHP940) from the genomic plasticity region of Helicobacter pylori induces tumor necrosis factor alpha and interleukin-8 secretion by human macrophages. J Bacteriol 190: 1146-1151.

[201] Santos A, Queiroz DM, Menard A, Marais A, Rocha GA, et al. (2003) New pathogenicity marker found in the plasticity region of the Helicobacter pylori genome. J Clin Microbiol 41: 1651-1655.

[202] Sugimoto M, Watada M, Jung SW, Graham DY, Yamaoka Y (2012) Role of Helicobacter pylori plasticity region genes in development of gastroduodenal diseases. J Clin Microbiol 50: 441-448.

[203] Wozniak RA, Waldor MK (2010) Integrative and conjugative elements: mosaic mobile genetic elements enabling dynamic lateral gene flow. Nat Rev Microbiol 8: 552-563.

[204] Brüssow H, Canchaya C, Hardt WD (2004) Phages and the evolution of bacterial pathogens: from genomic rearrangements to lysogenic conversion. Microbiol Mol Biol Rev 68: 560-602, table of contents.

[205] Marshall BJ, Armstrong JA, Francis GJ, Nokes NT, Wee SH (1987) Antibacterial action of bismuth in relation to Campylobacter pyloridis colonization and gastritis. Digestion 37 Suppl 2: 16-30.

[206] Schmid EN, von Recklinghausen G, Ansorg R (1990) Bacteriophages in Helicobacter (Campylobacter) pylori. J Med Microbiol 32: 101-104.

[207] Heintschel von Heinegg E, Nalik HP, Schmid EN (1993) Characterisation of a Helicobacter pylori phage (HP1). J Med Microbiol 38: 245-249.

[208] Vale FF, Matos APA, Carvalho P, Vítor JMB (2008) Helicobacter pylori phage screening. Microsc Microanal 14.

[209] Lehours P, Vale FF, Bjursell MK, Melefors O, Advani R, et al. (2011) Genome sequencing reveals a phage in Helicobacter pylori. MBio 2.

[210] Eppinger M, Baar C, Linz B, Raddatz G, Lanz C, et al. (2006) Who ate whom? Adaptive Helicobacter genomic changes that accompanied a host jump from early humans to large felines. PLoS Genet 2: e120.

[211] Luo CH, Chiou PY, Yang CY, Lin NT (2012) Genome, integration, and transduction of a novel temperate phage of Helicobacter pylori. J Virol 86: 8781-8792.

[212] Uchiyama J, Takeuchi H, Kato S, Takemura-Uchiyama I, Ujihara T, et al. (2012) Complete genome sequences of two Helicobacter pylori bacteriophages isolated from Japanese patients. J Virol 86: 11400-11401.

[213] Uchiyama J, Takeuchi H, Kato S, Gamoh K, Takemura-Uchiyama I, et al. (2013) Characterization of Helicobacter pylori bacteriophage KHP30. Appl Environ Microbiol 79: 3176-3184.

[214] Chen J, Novick RP (2009) Phage-mediated intergeneric transfer of toxin genes. Science 323: 139-141.

[215] Sharma CM, Hoffmann S, Darfeuille F, Reignier J, Findeiss S, et al. (2010) The primary transcriptome of the major human pathogen Helicobacter pylori. Nature 464: 250-255.

[216] Gottesman S, Storz G (2011) Bacterial small RNA regulators: versatile roles and rapidly evolving variations. Cold Spring Harb Perspect Biol 3.

[217] Storz G, Vogel J, Wassarman KM (2011) Regulation by small RNAs in bacteria: expanding frontiers. Mol Cell 43: 880-891.

[218] Geissmann T, Possedko M, Huntzinger E, Fechter P, Ehresmann C, et al. (2006) Regulatory RNAs as mediators of virulence gene expression in bacteria. Handb Exp Pharmacol: 9-43.

[219] Romby P, Vandenesch F, Wagner EG (2006) The role of RNAs in the regulation of virulence-gene expression. Curr Opin Microbiol 9: 229-236.

[220] Waters LS, Storz G (2009) Regulatory RNAs in bacteria. Cell 136: 615-628.

[221] Babitzke P, Romeo T (2007) CsrB sRNA family: sequestration of RNA-binding regulatory proteins. Curr Opin Microbiol 10: 156-163.

[222] Wassarman KM (2007) 6S RNA: a regulator of transcription. Mol Microbiol 65: 1425-1431.

[223] Henkin TM (2008) Riboswitch RNAs: using RNA to sense cellular metabolism. Genes Dev 22: 3383-3390.

[224] Zhang J, Lau MW, Ferre-D'Amare AR (2010) Ribozymes and riboswitches: modulation of RNA function by small molecules. Biochemistry 49: 9123-9131.

[225] Brennan RG, Link TM (2007) Hfq structure, function and ligand binding. Curr Opin Microbiol 10: 125-133.

[226] Gorke B, Vogel J (2008) Noncoding RNA control of the making and breaking of sugars. Genes Dev 22: 2914-2925.

[227] Storz G, Altuvia S, Wassarman KM (2005) An abundance of RNA regulators. Annu Rev Biochem 74: 199-217.

[228] Vanderpool CK, Balasubramanian D, Lloyd CR (2011) Dual-function RNA regulators in bacteria. Biochimie 93: 1943-1949.

[229] Pernitzsch SR, Sharma CM (2012) Transcriptome complexity and riboregulation in the human pathogen Helicobacter pylori. Front Cell Infect Microbiol 2: 14.

[230] Parkhill J, Wren BW, Mungall K, Ketley JM, Churcher C, et al. (2000) The genome sequence of the food-borne pathogen Campylobacter jejuni reveals hypervariable sequences. Nature 403: 665-668.

[231] Lasa I, Toledo-Arana A, Dobin A, Villanueva M, de los Mozos IR, et al. (2011) Genome-wide antisense transcription drives mRNA processing in bacteria. Proc Natl Acad Sci U S A 108: 20172-20177.

[232] Thibonnier M, Thiberge JM, De Reuse H (2008) Trans-translation in Helicobacter pylori: essentiality of ribosome rescue and requirement of protein tagging for stress resistance and competence. PLoS One 3: e3810.

[233] Wassarman KM, Storz G (2000) 6S RNA regulates E. coli RNA polymerase activity. Cell 101: 613-623.

[234] Barrick JE, Sudarsan N, Weinberg Z, Ruzzo WL, Breaker RR (2005) 6S RNA is a widespread regulator of eubacterial RNA polymerase that resembles an open promoter. RNA 11: 774-784.

[235] Faucher SP, Friedlander G, Livny J, Margalit H, Shuman HA (2010) Legionella pneumophila 6S RNA optimizes intracellular multiplication. Proc Natl Acad Sci U S A 107: 7533-7538.

[236] Wen Y, Feng J, Scott DR, Marcus EA, Sachs G (2011) A cis-encoded antisense small RNA regulated by the HP0165-HP0166 two-component system controls expression of ureB in Helicobacter pylori. J Bacteriol 193: 40-51.

[237] Williams SM, Chen YT, Andermann TM, Carter JE, McGee DJ, et al. (2007) Helicobacter pylori chemotaxis modulates inflammation and bacterium-gastric epithelium interactions in infected mice. Infect Immun 75: 3747-3757.

[238] McGee DJ, Langford ML, Watson EL, Carter JE, Chen YT, et al. (2005) Colonization and inflammation deficiencies in Mongolian gerbils infected by Helicobacter pylori chemotaxis mutants. Infect Immun 73: 1820-1827.

[239] Croxen MA, Sisson G, Melano R, Hoffman PS (2006) The Helicobacter pylori chemotaxis receptor TlpB (HP0103) is required for pH taxis and for colonization of the gastric mucosa. J Bacteriol 188: 2656-2665.

[240] Schreiber S, Konradt M, Groll C, Scheid P, Hanauer G, et al. (2004) The spatial orientation of Helicobacter pylori in the gastric mucus. Proc Natl Acad Sci U S A 101: 5024-5029.

[241] Shimomura H, Hayashi S, Yokota K, Oguma K, Hirai Y (2004) Alteration in the composition of cholesteryl glucosides and other lipids in Helicobacter pylori undergoing morphological change from spiral to coccoid form. FEMS Microbiol Lett 237: 407-413.

[242] Chaput C, Ecobichon C, Cayet N, Girardin SE, Werts C, et al. (2006) Role of AmiA in the morphological transition of Helicobacter pylori and in immune escape. PLoS Pathog 2: e97.

[243] Nagai S, Mimuro H, Yamada T, Baba Y, Moro K, et al. (2007) Role of Peyer's patches in the induction of Helicobacter pylori-induced gastritis. Proc Natl Acad Sci U S A 104: 8971-8976.

[244] Wang G, Maier SE, Lo LF, Maier G, Dosi S, et al. (2010) Peptidoglycan deacetylation in Helicobacter pylori contributes to bacterial survival by mitigating host immune responses. Infect Immun 78: 4660-4666.

[245] Harris AG, Wilson JE, Danon SJ, Dixon MF, Donegan K, et al. (2003) Catalase (KatA) and KatA-associated protein (KapA) are essential to persistent colonization in the Helicobacter pylori SS1 mouse model. Microbiology 149: 665-672.

[246] Dorer MS, Cohen IE, Sessler TH, Fero J, Salama NR (2013) Natural competence promotes Helicobacter pylori chronic infection. Infect Immun 81: 209-215.

[247] Schoep TD, Fulurija A, Good F, Lu W, Himbeck RP, et al. (2010) Surface properties of Helicobacter pylori urease complex are essential for persistence. PLoS One 5: e15042.

[248] Ha NC, Oh ST, Sung JY, Cha KA, Lee MH, et al. (2001) Supramolecular assembly and acid resistance of Helicobacter pylori urease. Nat Struct Biol 8: 505-509.

[249] Pinkse MW, Maier CS, Kim JI, Oh BH, Heck AJ (2003) Macromolecular assembly of Helicobacter pylori urease investigated by mass spectrometry. J Mass Spectrom 38: 315-320.

[250] Marcus EA, Scott DR (2001) Cell lysis is responsible for the appearance of extracellular urease in Helicobacter pylori. Helicobacter 6: 93-99.

[251] Hu LT, Mobley HL (1990) Purification and N-terminal analysis of urease from Helicobacter pylori. Infect Immun 58: 992-998.

[252] Marshall BJ, Barrett LJ, Prakash C, McCallum RW, Guerrant RL (1990) Urea protects Helicobacter (Campylobacter) pylori from the bactericidal effect of acid. Gastroenterology 99: 697-702.

[253] Cao P, McClain MS, Forsyth MH, Cover TL (1998) Extracellular release of antigenic proteins by Helicobacter pylori. Infect Immun 66: 2984-2986.

[254] Voland P, Weeks DL, Marcus EA, Prinz C, Sachs G, et al. (2003) Interactions among the seven Helicobacter pylori proteins encoded by the urease gene cluster. Am J Physiol Gastrointest Liver Physiol 284: G96-G106.

[255] Scott DR, Marcus EA, Weeks DL, Lee A, Melchers K, et al. (2000) Expression of the Helicobacter pylori ureI gene is required for acidic pH activation of cytoplasmic urease. Infect Immun 68: 470-477.

[256] Weeks DL, Eskandari S, Scott DR, Sachs G (2000) A H+-gated urea channel: the link between Helicobacter pylori urease and gastric colonization. Science 287: 482-485.

[257] Weeks DL, Gushansky G, Scott DR, Sachs G (2004) Mechanism of proton gating of a urea channel. J Biol Chem 279: 9944-9950.

[258] Scott DR, Marcus EA, Wen Y, Singh S, Feng J, et al. (2010) Cytoplasmic histidine kinase (HP0244)-regulated assembly of urease with UreI, a channel for urea and its metabolites, CO2, NH3, and NH4(+), is necessary for acid survival of Helicobacter pylori. J Bacteriol 192: 94-103.

[259] Eaton KA, Krakowka S (1994) Effect of gastric pH on urease-dependent colonization of gnotobiotic piglets by Helicobacter pylori. Infect Immun 62: 3604-3607.

[260] Williams CL, Preston T, Hossack M, Slater C, McColl KEL (1996) Helicobacter pylori utilises urease for amino acid synthesis. FEMS Immunol Med Microbiol 13: 87-94.

[261] Kuwahara H, Miyamoto Y, Akaike T, Kubota T, Sawa T, et al. (2000) Helicobacter pylori urease suppresses bactericidal activity of peroxynitrite via carbon dioxide production. Infect Immun 68: 4378-4383.

[262] Schwartz JT, Allen LA (2006) Role of urease in megasome formation and Helicobacter pylori survival in macrophages. J Leukoc Biol 79: 1214-1225.

[263] Makristathis A, Rokita E, Labigne A, Willinger B, Rotter ML, et al. (1998) Highly significant role of Helicobacter pylori urease in phagocytosis and production of oxygen metabolites by human granulocytes. J Infect Dis 177: 803-806.

[264] Rokita E, Makristathis A, Presterl E, Rotter ML, Hirschl AM (1998) Helicobacter pylori urease significantly reduces opsonization by human complement. J Infect Dis 178: 1521-1525.

[265] Celli JP, Turner BS, Afdhal NH, Keates S, Ghiran I, et al. (2009) Helicobacter pylori moves through mucus by reducing mucin viscoelasticity. Proc Natl Acad Sci U S A 106: 14321-14326.

[266] Harris PR, Ernst PB, Kawabata S, Kiyono H, Graham MF, et al. (1998) Recombinant Helicobacter pylori urease activates primary mucosal macrophages. J Infect Dis 178: 1516-1520.

[267] Harris PR, Mobley HL, Perez-Perez GI, Blaser MJ, Smith PD (1996) Helicobacter pylori urease is a potent stimulus of mononuclear phagocyte activation and inflammatory cytokine production. Gastroenterology 111: 419-425.

[268] Wroblewski LE, Shen L, Ogden S, Romero-Gallo J, Lapierre LA, et al. (2009) Helicobacter pylori dysregulation of gastric epithelial tight junctions by urease-mediated myosin II activation. Gastroenterology 136: 236-246.

[269] Tanahashi T, Kita M, Kodama T, Yamaoka Y, Sawai N, et al. (2000) Cytokine expression and production by purified Helicobacter pylori urease in human gastric epithelial cells. Infect Immun 68: 664-671.

[270] Fan X, Gunasena H, Cheng Z, Espejo R, Crowe SE, et al. (2000) Helicobacter pylori urease binds to class II MHC on gastric epithelial cells and induces their apoptosis. J Immunol 165: 1918-1924.

[271] Boneca IG, Ecobichon C, Chaput C, Mathieu A, Guadagnini S, et al. (2008) Development of inducible systems to engineer conditional mutants of essential genes of Helicobacter pylori. Appl Environ Microbiol 74: 2095-2102.

[272] Zawilak-Pawlik A, Kois A, Stingl K, Boneca IG, Skrobuk P, et al. (2007) HobA--a novel protein involved in initiation of chromosomal replication in Helicobacter pylori. Mol Microbiol 65: 979-994.

[273] Bertram R, Hillen W (2008) The application of Tet repressor in prokaryotic gene regulation and expression. Microb Biotechnol 1: 2-16.

[274] Sun Y, Chen X, Xiao D (2007) Tetracycline-inducible expression systems: new strategies and practices in the transgenic mouse modeling. Acta Biochim Biophys Sin (Shanghai) 39: 235-246.

[275] Debowski AW, Verbrugghe P, Sehnal M, Marshall BJ, Benghezal M (2013) Development of a Tetracycline-Inducible Gene Expression System for the Study of Helicobacter pylori Pathogenesis. Appl Environ Microbiol 79: 7351-7359.

[276] McClain MS, Duncan SS, Gaddy JA, Cover TL (2013) Control of gene expression in Helicobacter pylori using the Tet repressor. J Microbiol Methods 95: 336-341.

[277] Debowski AW, Himbeck R, Middelton M, Camilleri T, Sehnal M, et al. (2011) A tetracycline-based conditional knockout demonstrates the role of urease in colonization and maintenance of Helicobacter pylori infection. CHRO A114.

[278] Garcia-Vallve S, Janssen PJ, Ouzounis CA (2002) Genetic variation between Helicobacter pylori strains: gene acquisition or loss? Trends Microbiol 10: 445-447.

[279] Saunders NJ, Boonmee P, Peden JF, Jarvis SA (2005) Inter-species horizontal transfer resulting in core-genome and niche-adaptive variation within Helicobacter pylori. BMC Genomics 6: 9.

[280] Pupo E, Padron A, Santana E, Sotolongo J, Quintana D, et al. (2005) Preparation of plasmid DNA-containing liposomes using a high-pressure homogenization--extrusion technique. J Control Release 104: 379-396.

[281] Wong BC, Yin Y, Berg DE, Xia HH, Zhang JZ, et al. (2001) Distribution of distinct vacA, cagA and iceA alleles in Helicobacter pylori in Hong Kong. Helicobacter 6: 317-324.

[282] Owen RJ, Ferrus M, Gibson J (2001) Amplified fragment length polymorphism genotyping of metronidazole-resistant Helicobacter pylori infecting dyspeptics in England. Clin Microbiol Infect 7: 244-253.

[283] Carroll IM, Ahmed N, Beesley SM, Khan AA, Ghousunnissa S, et al. (2004) Microevolution between paired antral and paired antrum and corpus Helicobacter pylori isolates recovered from individual patients. J Med Microbiol 53: 669-677.

[284] Kuipers EJ, Israel DA, Kusters JG, Gerrits MM, Weel J, et al. (2000) Quasispecies development of Helicobacter pylori observed in paired isolates obtained years apart from the same host. J Infect Dis 181: 273-282.

[285] Smeets LC, Arents NL, van Zwet AA, Vandenbroucke-Grauls CM, Verboom T, et al. (2003) Molecular patchwork: Chromosomal recombination between two Helicobacter pylori strains during natural colonization. Infect Immun 71: 2907-2910.

[286] Salama N, Guillemin K, McDaniel TK, Sherlock G, Tompkins L, et al. (2000) A whole-genome microarray reveals genetic diversity among Helicobacter pylori strains. Proc Natl Acad Sci U S A 97: 14668-14673.

[287] Gressmann H, Linz B, Ghai R, Pleissner KP, Schlapbach R, et al. (2005) Gain and loss of multiple genes during the evolution of Helicobacter pylori. PLoS Genet 1: e43.

[288] Israel DA, Salama N, Arnold CN, Moss SF, Ando T, et al. (2001) Helicobacter pylori strain-specific differences in genetic content, identified by microarray, influence host inflammatory responses. J Clin Invest 107: 611-620.

[289] Israel DA, Salama N, Krishna U, Rieger UM, Atherton JC, et al. (2001) Helicobacter pylori genetic diversity within the gastric niche of a single human host. Proc Natl Acad Sci U S A 98: 14625-14630.

[290] Kraft C, Stack A, Josenhans C, Niehus E, Dietrich G, et al. (2006) Genomic changes during chronic Helicobacter pylori infection. J Bacteriol 188: 249-254.

[291] Morelli G, Didelot X, Kusecek B, Schwarz S, Bahlawane C, et al. (2010) Microevolution of Helicobacter pylori during prolonged infection of single hosts and within families. PLoS Genet 6: e1001036.

[292] Graham DY, Opekun AR, Osato MS, El-Zimaity HM, Lee CK, et al. (2004) Challenge model for Helicobacter pylori infection in human volunteers. Gut 53: 1235-1243.

[293] Aebischer T, Bumann D, Epple HJ, Metzger W, Schneider T, et al. (2008) Correlation of T cell response and bacterial clearance in human volunteers challenged with Heli-

cobacter pylori revealed by randomised controlled vaccination with Ty21a-based Salmonella vaccines. Gut 57: 1065-1072.

[294] Lundin A, Bjorkholm B, Kupershmidt I, Unemo M, Nilsson P, et al. (2005) Slow genetic divergence of Helicobacter pylori strains during long-term colonization. Infect Immun 73: 4818-4822.

[295] Salama NR, Gonzalez-Valencia G, Deatherage B, Aviles-Jimenez F, Atherton JC, et al. (2007) Genetic analysis of Helicobacter pylori strain populations colonizing the stomach at different times postinfection. J Bacteriol 189: 3834-3845.

[296] Beji A, Vincent P, Darchis I, Husson MO, Cortot A, et al. (1989) Evidence of gastritis with several Helicobacter pylori strains. Lancet 2: 1402-1403.

[297] Ghose C, Perez-Perez GI, van Doorn LJ, Dominguez-Bello MG, Blaser MJ (2005) High frequency of gastric colonization with multiple Helicobacter pylori strains in Venezuelan subjects. J Clin Microbiol 43: 2635-2641.

[298] Patra R, Chattopadhyay S, De R, Ghosh P, Ganguly M, et al. (2012) Multiple infection and microdiversity among Helicobacter pylori isolates in a single host in India. PLoS One 7: e43370.

[299] Marshall BJ, Armstrong JA, McGechie DB, Glancy RJ (1985) Attempt to fulfil Koch's postulates for pyloric Campylobacter. Med J Aust 142: 436-439.

[300] Kavermann H, Burns BP, Angermuller K, Odenbreit S, Fischer W, et al. (2003) Identification and characterization of Helicobacter pylori genes essential for gastric colonization. J Exp Med 197: 813-822.

[301] Kersulyte D, Chalkauskas H, Berg DE (1999) Emergence of recombinant strains of Helicobacter pylori during human infection. Mol Microbiol 31: 31-43.

[302] Krebes J, Bunk B, Spröer C, Luong K, Morgan RD, et al. (2013) Comprehensive methylome analysis of the human gastric pathogen, Helicobacter pylori. 17th International Workshop on Campylobacter, Helicobacter and Related Organisms Abstract O57a.

[303] Takeuchi H, Israel DA, Miller GG, Donahue JP, Krishna U, et al. (2002) Characterization of expression of a functionally conserved Helicobacter pylori methyltransferase-encoding gene within inflamed mucosa and during in vitro growth. J Infect Dis 186: 1186-1189.

[304] Koonin EV, Wolf YI (2010) Constraints and plasticity in genome and molecular-phenome evolution. Nat Rev Genet 11: 487-498.

[305] Levy SF, Siegal ML (2012) The robustness continuum. Adv Exp Med Biol 751: 431-452.

[306] Masel J, Siegal ML (2009) Robustness: mechanisms and consequences. Trends Genet 25: 395-403.

[307] Masel J, Trotter MV (2010) Robustness and evolvability. Trends Genet 26: 406-414.

[308] Wagner A (2012) The role of robustness in phenotypic adaptation and innovation. Proc Biol Sci 279: 1249-1258.

[309] Wagner GP, Altenberg L (1996) Perspective: Complex Adaptations and the Evolution of Evolvability. Evolution 50: 967-976.

[310] Kussell E, Leibler S (2005) Phenotypic diversity, population growth, and information in fluctuating environments. Science 309: 2075-2078.

[311] Vakil N, Vaira D (2013) Treatment for H. pylori infection: new challenges with antimicrobial resistance. J Clin Gastroenterol 47: 383-388.

[312] Debowski AW, Carnoy C, Verbrugghe P, Nilsson HO, Gauntlett JC, et al. (2012) Xer recombinase and genome integrity in Helicobacter pylori, a pathogen without topoisomerase IV. PLoS One 7: e33310.

[313] Strugatsky D, McNulty R, Munson K, Chen CK, Soltis SM, et al. (2013) Structure of the proton-gated urea channel from the gastric pathogen Helicobacter pylori. Nature 493: 255-258.

[314] Nilsson C, Skoglund A, Moran AP, Annuk H, Engstrand L, et al. (2006) An enzymatic ruler modulates Lewis antigen glycosylation of Helicobacter pylori LPS during persistent infection. Proc Natl Acad Sci U S A 103: 2863-2868.

[315] Gunasekara S, Vrielink A, Stubbs KA (2010) Preliminary studies into the inhibition of the cholesterol alpha-glucosyltransferase from Helicobacter pylori using azasugars. Carbohydr Res 345: 960-964.

[316] Thomson N, Sebaihia M, Cerdeno-Tarraga A, Bentley S, Crossman L, et al. (2003) The value of comparison. Nat Rev Microbiol 1: 11-12.

Chapter 2

Immune Response to *Helicobacter pylori*

Batool Mutar Mahdi

Additional information is available at the end of the chapter

http://dx.doi.org/10.5772/57480

1. Introduction

Helicobacter pylori (H. pylori) is a Gram-negative microaerophilic spiral bacterium previously known Campylobacterpylori. It has a significant attention since its isolation and characterisation in 1983 [1]. It colonizes the gastrointestinal mucosa of its host in spite of a strong persistent humoral and cellular immune response to *H. pylori* at the local and systemic level, the organism persists for the lifetime of its host.

It is a pathogen, playing an important role in the aetiology of gastritis (especially active antral gastritis). Gastritis is a histopathologic term characterized by chronic inflammation of the stomach mucosa. It is classification based on the underlying cause (eg, *H. pylori,* that cause atrophic gastritis, bile reflux, nonsteroidal anti-inflammatory drugs [NSAIDs], autoimmunity, or allergic response) [2]. Gastritis is also classified as erosive or nonerosive based on the severity of mucosal injury by endoscopy. Other classification is according to the site of involvement (cardia, body, antrum). Histological classification is acute or chronic based on the inflammatory cell type. Acute gastritis is characterized by PMN infiltration of the mucosa of the antrum and body. Chronic gastritis implies some degree of atrophy or metaplasia. It predominantly involves the antrum with subsequent loss of G cells and decreased gastrin secretion or the corpus with loss of oxyntic glands, leading to reduced acid, pepsin, and intrinsic factor [3, 4, 5].

H. pylori causes more than half of peptic ulcers worldwide. The bacterium causes peptic ulcers by damaging the mucous membrane of the stomach and duodenum. Damage to the mucous membrane causing stomach acid to get through to the sensitive lining layer. Together, the stomach acid and *H. pylori* irritate the lining of the stomach or duodenum and cause an ulcer [6].Ulcers in the stomach and duodenum result when the consequences of inflammation allow stomach acid and the digestive enzyme pepsin to overwhelm the mechanisms that protect the stomach and duodenal mucous membranes. The location of colonization of *H. pylori,* which affects the location of the ulcer, depends on the acidity of the stomach [7].The majority of patients with duodenal ulcer (DU) are infected with *H. pylori* [8].

H. pylori infection is a major cause of gastric adenocarcinoma, specifically non-cardia gastric cancer. H. pylori infection also causes gastric mucosa-associated lymphoid tissue (MALT) lymphoma [9]. Some *H. pylori* bacteria had a toxin produced by a gene called cytotoxin-associated gene A (*cagA*) injected into the junctions where cells of the stomach lining. This toxin (known as CagA) alters the structure of stomach cells and allows the bacteria to attach to them more easily. Long-term exposure to the toxin causes chronic inflammation [10]. Other type of cancer is gastric MALT lymphoma is a rare type of non-Hodgkin lymphoma that is characterized by the slow multiplication of B lymphocytes. Normally, the lining of the stomach lacks lymphoid tissue, but growth of this tissue is often stimulated in response to colonization of *H. pylori* [11]. Nearly all patients with gastric MALT lymphoma show signs of *H. pylori* infection, and the risk of developing this tumor is more than six times higher in infected people than in uninfected people [12]

The prevalence of gastric cancers among *H. pylori*-infected patients varies between individuals, countries, and geographic areas, *H. pylori* disease-related outcomes are believed to be determined by interaction between host factors, bacterial factors, and their *interaction* with the *environment* [13] produces different diseases in different persons. High and low acid secretion rates probably contribute to duodenal ulceration and gastric carcinogenesis, respectively. *H. pylori*products and certain cytokines released in gastritis release gastrin from G-cells but inhibit parietal cells. Also tumour necrosis *factor* alpha inhibits somatostatin-cells and interleukin 1 beta inhibits enterochromaffin-like cells. The net result is that antral gastritis tends to increase, whilst corpus gastritis tends to decrease acid secretion. Corpus atrophy further lowers acid through loss of parietal cells. Factors postulated to increase corpus gastritis include: *host* genetics, early acquisition of bacteria, more aggressive strains, poor general health and diets high in salt or lacking in antioxidant vitamins [14]. *Other factor is environmental* factors that play an important role in the manifestation, course, and prognosis of diseases of *H. pylori*-induced gastritis. This disease is the outcome of allelic group of a *host* and the microbial (microflora) and physical environments. *Host* alleles predisposing to a disease in one genomic and/or *environmental* surroundings may not be deleterious in other group, in addition to that microbes can have different effects in different hosts and under different *environmental* conditions [15]. *H. pylori* eradication may not eliminate the risk of gastric cancer. Therapy of this bacteria may be used in high-risk populations to reduce gastric cancer incidence. It can reverse many biochemical, genetic, and epigenetic changes that *H. pylori* infection induces in the stomach [16]. The major factors playing a pathogenic role in *H. pylori*-related non-cancer diseases are host polymorphisms in genes involved in inflammation and protection against oxidative damage, host exposure to dietary genotoxic agents, and bacterial genetic polymorphisms [17]. The study of *host*-bacterial *interaction* is key to detection the molecular and cellular pathways involved and will lead to developing preventive and therapeutic modules against this pathogen [18].

http://dx.doi.org/10.5772/57480

Gastric inflammation nearly always precedes the development of peptic ulceration, and is a critical component in initiating the multi-step progression towards gastric carcinogenesis due to this interaction between these three factors [19].

H. pylori is spread from person to person by two routes, oral-oral and faecal-oral route [20].Food prepared under less ideal conditions or exposed to contaminated water or soil may increase the risk. Inadequate sanitation practices, low social class, and crowded or high-density living conditions seem to be related to a higher prevalence of *H. pylori* infection. Therefore poor hygiene and crowded conditions may facilitate transmission of infection among family members Understanding the route of *H. pylori* transmission is important if public health measures to prevent its spread. Iatrogenic transmission of *H. pylori* following endoscopy is the only proven mode. The person-to-person mode of transmission is supported by the higher incidence of infection among institutionalized children and adults and detection of *H. pylori* DNA in vomitus, saliva, dental plaque, gastric juice, and feces. Waterborne transmission, probably due to fecal contamination or contaminated well water, may be an important source of infection, especially in parts of the world in which untreated water is common. *H. pylori* has been isolated in domestic cats, housefly. However, evidence is lacking that H. *pylori* can be transmitted to humans from flies that have been in contact with *H. pylori*-infected feces. Mode of transmission of *H. pylori* is important to prevent its spread and identifying high-risk populations [21, 22].

The pathogenesity of this bacterium depend on the production of several virulence factors. The most important ones are CagA (cytotoxic associated gene A) and VacA (vacuolizating cytotoxin A). The immunodominant CagA protein is encoded by genes called the cagA-PAI (pathogenicity island), a 40 kb genomic fragment containing ORFs (open reading frames) encoding approximately 31 genes that forms a type IV secretion system, which is found in 60–70% of *H pylori* strains and can be divided into two regions, cag I and cag II, according to a novel insertion sequence [23] This secretion system (T4SS) forms a pilus that delivers CagA, an oncoprotein, into the cytosol of gastric epithelial cells through a rigid needle structure covered by CagY, a VirB10-homologous protein and CagT, a Virb7-homologous protein, at the base [24]. This is accomplished by a specialized adhesin of the pilus surface, the CagL protein, which binds to and activates host cell integrins for subsequent delivery of CagA across the host cell membrane. Injected CagA becomes tyrosine-phosphorylated by Src and Abl family kinases and mimics a host cell protein in binding and activation of multiple signalling factors. After the induction of membrane dynamics, actin cytoskeletal rearrangements and the disruption of cell-to-cell junctions as well as proliferative, pro-inflammatory and anti-apoptotic nuclear responses. All these signalling cascades contribute in *H. pylori* pathogenesis [25]. Therefore, CagA remains the only identified effector mechanism that is translocated by the T4SS of *H. pylori* into gastric epithelial cells where it induces host cell kinases that phosphorylate tyrosine residues in CagA adjacent to the site of bacterial adhesion on the host gastric epithelial cells, which in turn activate eukaryotic signal transduction pathways and cytoskeletal plasticity [26]. Wild-type *H pylori* (not phosphorylation-resistant CagA)induced a growth factor-like response in gastric epithelial cells. CagA formed a physical complex with the SRC homology 2 domain (SH2)-containing tyrosine phosphatase SHP-2 in a phosphorylation-dependent manner and stimulated the phosphatase activity. On the other hand, the CagA effect on cells was reproduced by constitutively active SHP-2. Thus, upon translocation, CagA perturbs cellular functions by deregulating SHP-2 [27]. Injected CagA associates with the epithelial tight-junction scaffolding protein ZO-1 and the transmembrane protein junctional adhesion molecule, causing an ectopic assembly of tight-junction components at sites of bacterial attachment, and altering the composition and function of the apical-junctional complex. Long-term CagA delivery to polarized epithelia caused a disruption of the epithelial barrier function and dysplastic alterations in epithelial cell morphology [28].

Regarding VacA, there is a significant polymorphism in this gene (vacA s, vacA i and vacA m). There are two types of the s (s1 and s2), i (i1 and i2), and m (m1 and m2) regions of *vacA* [29]. Three polymorphic subtypes, namely m1T, m1Tm2 and m2. The s1a/i1/m1Tm2 genotype had a higher frequency of lymphoid follicle formation in the corpus than the s1a/i1/m1T and s1a/i1/m2 strains while *vacA* s1/m1 strains are most closely associated with gastric carcinoma [30]. The method PCR- genotyping from gastric biopsy had advantages over routine diagnostic tools such as histological *H. pylori* detection, which has high interobserver variation, very much depending on the experience of the pathologist, and over *H. pylori* culture, which is more time-consuming, requires expertise, and is not always successful. In general, PCR-based techniques show high sensitivity for *H. pylori* detection and permit further characterization of bacteria virulence-associated genotypes. In archive materials, the genotyping of the *vacA* i region allows the analysis of the *H. pylori* strains in the same biopsy specimen that can also be used for histopathological evaluation, conferring a more reliable measurement of the effects of local infecting strains. Another advantage of the use of archive materials is that it permits retrospective studies to be performed without the need of *H. pylori* isolation from fresh biopsy specimens [31].

In most cases, the infection is asymptomatic and clinical manifestation appears in only 10-15% of infected individuals. This is due to virulence of *H. pylori* strains and host immune response to this bacterium [32]. The different clinical outcomes may be explained by bacterial factors and the host immune responses. *H. pylori* induce a strong immune response with infiltration of neutrophils, B- and T-cells into the gastroduodenal mucosa that fails to clear the infection. Several virulence factors have been associated with the development of gastroduodenal disease, e.g. the cytotoxin-associated gene A (CagA) and a vacuolating toxin [33] individuals infected with strains lacking these genetic markers may still develop peptic ulcers, and that many individuals infected with bacterial strains bearing these genotypes do not develop any symptoms [34]. On other hand, the lower epithelial cytokine responses may be of importance for the pathogenesis of *H. pylori*-induced ulcers, most likely can be explained by host factors, i.e. mainly a decreased ability of the epithelium to produce cytokines, but possibly partly also down-regulation by regulatory T cells [35]. *H. pylori*infection induces strong antibody responses in the human gastric mucosa, both in asymptomatic carriers and in ulcer patients [36].

This will shed a light on the immune response to *H. pylori* colonization and its effect on clinical outcomes.

http://dx.doi.org/10.5772/57480

2. Host immune response to *H. pylori*

The immune response towards bacterial pathogens can be divided into an innate and an adaptive response.

2.1. Innate immune response to *H. pylori*

Recognition of bacterial antigenic molecules is mediated by TLRs (Toll-like receptors) that are expressed by distinct cell types throughout the gastrointestinal tract, and play an important role in regulation of the innate immune response especially TLR4 It is expressed on antigen-presenting cells such as monocytes and dendritic cells. Bacterial contact with monocytes and other APCs leads to the secretion of proinflammatory cytokines such as TNF-α (tumour necrosis factor-α), IL (interleukin)-1β and IL-8. *H. pylori* infection has been shown to be associated with increased levels of these cytokines which, in turn, act as local chemoattractants, inducing granulocytic infiltration [37]. The gastric epithelia of children respond to *H. pylori* infection by increasing the expression of TLR2, TLR4, TLR5, TLR9 and the cytokines IL-8, IL-10 and TNF-α that participate actively in innate immune responses [38]. Their role in the progression of gastric lesions leading to cancer is associated with decreasing levels of TLRs inhibitors and elevated TLRs levels throughout all the spectrum of lesions [39].

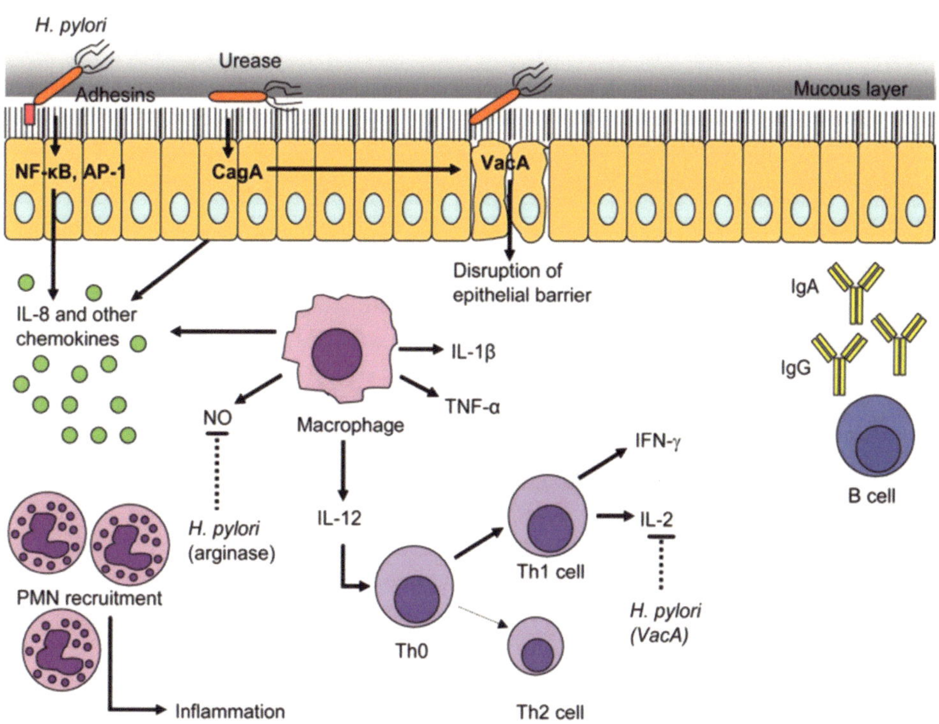

Figure 1. *H. pylori* pathogenesis, the inflammatory immune response and some of escape mechanisms [54].

2.2. Adaptive immunity: cellular immune response and humoral response

2.2.1. Cellular immune response

Adaptive immune responses towards *H. pylori* infection have been developed after failure of innate immune response to eliminate the pathogen. The immune response to *Helicobacter pylori* is a versatile group of mechanisms involving responses that are both protective and damaging to the host. The innate and the adaptive immune responses lead to damaging inflammatory responses allowing for persistence of many infections [40]. *H. pylori* associated inflammatory reaction is characterized by a mucosal infiltration of different cells like polymorphonuclear leukocytes (PMN), T cells, macrophages, and plasma cells [41] in addition to that *H. pylori* adheres to the cells of gastric mucosa and secretes different molecules that can change gastric epithelial cell function [42]. Chronic active gastritis is associated with an increased CD4/CD8 T-cell ratio within the gastric mucosa and accumulation of CD4+ T-helper lymphocytes in the lamina propia of the gastric mucosa. *H. pylori* infection results in a Th1-predominant host immune response in the gastric mucosa and induction of IFN-γ (interferon-γ) and IFN-γ -related genes. A Th1-predominant immune response is associated with elevated levels of the pro-inflammatory cytokines IL-12, IL-18 and TNF-α([43]. Other cell that infiltrates the gastric mucosa was Th17 which are $CD4^+$ T cells associated with infections and inflammation. Th17 are induced during both *H. pylori* infection and gastric cancer in the inflammatory process of gastric stroma and may be an important link between inflammation and carcinogenesis [44]. The host genetic milieu contributes to the inflammatory response to *H. pylori* infection is IL-1B. The *IL-1B* gene encodes the expression of IL-1β, a potent pro-inflammatory cytokine and powerful inhibitor of gastric acid secretion that had a most important responsibility in initiating and amplifying the inflammatory response to *H. pylori* infection [45]. It had been that IL-1 polymorphism had an effect on IL-1 production in gastric mucosa infected with *H. pylori* [46]. This indicate that individual genetic polymorphism had an effect on disease expression.

Yuceyar etal 2002 [47] found that there is no alteration in total T and B lymphocytes and CD4+ T, CD8+ T lymphocytes and natural killer cells of both duodenal ulcer and chronic antral gastritis patients compared to normal persons. Although there was a slight increase in the proportion of active T lymphocytes in duodenal ulcer and chronic antral gastritis groups comparing to healthy subjects the difference was not statistically significant. This indicate that there is no systemic alteration in the specific immune system in response to *H. pylori* in patients with duodenal ulcer and chronic antral gastritis. Other study confirmed the systemic immune response to helicobacters at the cellular level in patients with *Helicobacter pylori* infection by leukocyte migration inhibition test was performed and a highly significant inhibitory effect on leukocyte migration was found in patients with *Helicobacter pylori* infection [48].

2.2.2. Humoral immune response

H. pylori induce a strong specific systemic and local antibody response and infected individual had antibodies against whole bacteria or part of it [49]and increase in plasma cells in gastric mucosa which produce IgA [50]. Other important antibody was IgG that binds to *H. pylori* and enhance phagocytosis [51].This antibodies lead to complement activation by either classical or alternative pathways [52]. In addition to that, the role of the secretory IgA is important in neutralizing urease and VacA as well as inhibiting adherence of *H. pylori* to gastric mucosa [53].The immune response to *H. pylori* can be summarized by figure -1- [54]. There is high seroprevalence of *H. pylori* antibodies undervalue of past infection, the relation of the *H. pylori* cytotoxin to gastric precancerous lesions is warranted. There is a strong mucosal IgA response to *H. pylori* in non-neoplastic antral mucosa of gastric cancer patients irrespective of the biopsy urease results [55].

2.2.2.1. Evasion of immune response by H. pylori

Helicobacter pylori is a gastric bacterial pathogen that evades host immune responses in vivo by different mechanisms like inducing apoptosis of macrophages in association with alterations in the mitochondrial pathway [56].

Elimination of this key immunomodulatory cell may represent a *mechanism* employed by the bacterium to evade host immune responses. It can survive intracellularly within macrophages by interfering with lysosomal proteins, similar to *Mycobacterium tuberculosis* [57]. *H. pylori* like many other pathogen escape the immune system by production an enzyme arginase that prevent nitrous oxide production [58].

Vacuolating cytotoxin secreted by *H. pylori* has turned out to be a potent immunomodulatory toxin. VacA-deficient *H. pylori* induced significantly higher expression of integrin-linked kinase (ILK) and endothelial nitric oxygen synthase (eNOS), and significantly more production of reactive oxygen species (ROS) in monocyte/macrophage-like U937 cells, as compared with isogenic vacA+ *H. pylori*. Thus, vacA-deficient *H. pylori* appears to upregulate ILK expression, which modulates the expression of eNOS and as a result, stimulates the production of ROS. It is VacA that prevents such a process by inhibiting ILK expression, helping *H. pylori escape* host immunoreaction and persist in gastric mucosa [59].

In addition to that, *H. pylori* LPS exhibits a reduced endotoxic potency in terms of pyrogenicity, lethality, toxicity, mitogenicity and the lower immune response elicited by *H. pylori* LPS in comparison with other enterobacterial LPS may represent an *escape mechanism* from the host [60]. *H. pylori*, possess flagellin molecules that cannot be recognized by TLR5 that is important for its survival [61]. *H. pylori* infection could alter cellular gene expression processes that evade host immune mechanism by activating NF-κB and Wnt/β-catenin signaling pathway, disturb metal ion homeostasis, and induce carcinogenesis [62].

VacA of *H pylori* act as an immunomodulator by interfering with the IL-2 signalling pathway in T-cells by blocking Ca2+ mobilization and the activity of the Ca2+/calmodulin-dependent phosphatase calcineurin [63]. It also interferes with antigen presentation mediated by MHC class II [64]. VacA by itself act as immunosuppressive by a direct action on T-cells rather than APCs [65]. *VacA* is a crucial element for *H. pylori* to *escape* from host immune defense by means of differentially regulating the expression of some related genes by altering their mRNA expression at different times [66].

2.2.2.2. *Vaccination against H. pylori infection*

Helicobacter pylori can persist in the gastric mucosa of infected individuals for life, in the face of chronic inflammation and low pH. Efforts to develop vaccines have largely failed and, in the wake of emerging antibiotic resistance, novel therapeutic approaches have developed [67].

There is a consent that vaccines are essential to limit the severity of this infection. Great development has been made since its detection 25 years ago the virulence factors and several aspects of the pathogenesis of the *H. pylori* gastric diseases. Several key bacterial factors have been identified: urease, vacuolating cytotoxin, cytotoxin-associated antigen, the pathogenicity island, neutrophil-activating protein, and among others. These proteins, in their native or recombinant forms, have been shown to confer protection against infectious challenge with *H. pylori* in animal models. However, a quantity of clinical trials in healthy volunteers have been conducted using urease given orally as a soluble protein or expressed in bacterial vectors with limited results or a mixture of *H. pylori* antigens was reported to be highly immunogenic in *H. pylori*-negative volunteers following intramuscular administration of the vaccine with aluminium hydroxide as an adjuvant [69].

H. pylori is a mucosa-associated organism, it was initially thought that an IgA type anti-*Helicobacter* antibody response would be essential for protective immunity [69]. An adjuvant is an important component of any oral/mucosal vaccine as it is responsible for stimulating immune system, but due to toxicities associated with these agents, there are currently no suitable and safe adjuvants available for use in humans. Another important limitation to effective oral immunization is that it requires multiple doses and a large amount of antigen administration. These studies showed that mucosal immunity can be induced by oral or intranasal routes of immunization. The intranasal route of immunization is similar to the oral route in that it also requires the administration of bacterial antigen in conjunction with an adjuvant multiple times [70].

Considering the side effects of oral adjuvants, researches have focused attention on making oral immunization safe and effective for human usage. Thus, *E. coli LT* heat-labile toxin that was used as an oral adjuvant in humans did show a significant decrease in gastric *H. pylori* density but was associated with cramping and diarrhea [71]. Another approach is to use other mucosal routes such as the nasal mucosa and the rectal mucosa for effective immunization. When mice were immunized orally, rectally and intranasally in combination with *E. coli* heat-labile toxin (LT) and subsequently challenged with purified *H. pylori* antigen, mice immunized by either of the routes were found to be protected against this challenge compared with controls. These studies showed that mucosal immunity can be induced by oral or intranasal routes of immunization. The intranasal route of immunization is similar to the oral route in that it also requires the administration of bacterial antigen in conjunction with an adjuvant multiple times [72].

Although the intransal route of immunization seems the most efficient and effective route of mucosal immunization, it still has some disadvantages histologic inflammation in the olfactory bulb and cause paralysis of facial nerves [72]. Intranasal route could also result in oral ingestion thus exposing the subject to various side effects and toxicities. Eriksson et al. [73] found that

CTA1-DD adjuvant was to be safe for intranasal administration without any accumulation in the nervous tissue.

Other modalities of administering vaccines such as the intraperitoneal (i.p.) and subcutaneous (s.c.) routes are also being done. Mice were vaccinated i.p. using *H. pylori* antigen in combination with aluminum hydroxide and upon rechallenge with *H. pylori* were found to confer protection that was shown by absence of bacteria, both histologically and in culture of gastric biopsy tissues. This immunity was noted to be antibody independent and achieved by IL-5-secreting T cells [74]. The results of these experiments suggest that until a safe, effective, and inexpensive mucosal (oral/nasal) vaccine becomes available, systemic immunizations should be a consideration.

Urease is important as a vaccine antigen has been confirmed by numerous studies in mice, ferrets, and non-human primates [75]. Urease conferred protection against helicobacter infection when delivered either as a native protein or as an enzymatically inactive recombinant protein [76]. Therapeutic immunisation with urease has recently been reported in ferrets naturally infected with *H. mustelae*. [77]. Infection with *H. mustelae*occurs in ferrets soon after weaning, persists for life, induces active chronic gastritis, and is associated with the development of ulceration in a subgroup of infected animals [78]. Thus, therapeutic immunisation is possible in a natural setting of helicobacter infection, confirming that the inability of the natural immune response to clear helicobacter infection can be overcome.

Other method of delivery of the antigen used in mice by immunisation with genetically engineered bacteria expressing *H. pylori* antigens elicits a protective immune response against gastric helicobacter infections. Immunisation with live bacterial vaccines usually requires only one or two doses, does not depend on the addition of extra mucosal adjuvant, and the vaccine can be produced at very low cost. Additional improvements to the vaccine should result from a better understanding of the natural immune responses to helicobacter infection and of the mechanisms by which vaccination restores protection [79].

Zhang etal, 2013 [80] used recombinant technology, Lactococcus lactis (L. lactis) could serve as an antigen-delivering vehicle for the development of edible *vaccine*. They produced edible UreB (urease B) *vaccine* derived from L. lactis against H. *pylori*. The UreB subunit is the most effective and common immunogen of all strains of H. *pylori*. The UreB was produced as a chimeric protein fused with IL-2 (human interleukin 2) as the mucosal adjuvant. Mucosal immunization of mice with recombinant L. lactis NZ9000 containing the UreB-IL-2 protein elicited more anti-UreB antibody that specifically bounded to the purified bacterial UreB protein and more cytokines such as IFN-γ, IL-4, and IL-17, and had a lower H. *pylori* burden and urease activity than control mice. These results suggest that the recombinant L. lactis expressing UreB-IL-2 can be potentially used as an edible *vaccine* for controlling H. *pylori* infection.

Altman etal, 2013 [81] demonstrated that synthetic glycoconjugates based on delipidated lipopolysaccharide (LPS) of *Helicobacter pylori* and containing an α(1-6)-glucan chain induced broadly cross-reactive functional antibodies in immunized animals. Thus, they prepared glycoconjugates based on dextrans produced by lactic acid bacteria Leuconostoc mesenteroides B512F and consisting of linear α(1-6)-glucan chains with limited branching. Three dextrans with averaged molecular masses of 5, 000 Da, 3, 500 Da and 1, 500 Da, respectively, were modified with a diamino group-containing linker and conjugated to a carrier protein, tetanus toxoid (TT) or diphtheria toxoid (DT. The conjugates were immunogenic in both rabbits and mice and induced specific IgG responses against α(1-6)- glucan -expressing H. *pylori* LPS. Studies performed with post-immune sera of mice and rabbits immunized with dextran-based conjugates demonstrated cross-reactivity with LPS from typeable and non-typeable strains of H. *pylori* and selected mutants. The post-immune sera from rabbits that received the conjugates exhibited functional activity against α(1-6)-glucan-positive strains of *H. pylori*. These data provide evidence that dextran-based conjugates may offer a simplified approach to the development of carbohydrate-based *vaccines* against *H. pylori*.

Helicobacter pylori neutrophil-activating protein (NAP) is a toll-like receptor 2 (TLR2) agonist and potent immunomodulator inducing Th1-type immune response. Iankov etal 2013 [82]studied the humoral immune response against NAP-tagged antigens, encoded by attenuated measles virus (MV) vector platform, in MV infection susceptible type I interferon receptor knockout and human CD46 transgenic (Ifnarko-CD46Ge) mice. Immunogenicity of MV expressing a full-length human immunoglobulin lambda light chain (MV-lambda) was compared to that of MV expressing lambda-NAP chimeric protein (MV-lambda-NAP). MV-lambda-NAP immunized Ifnarko-CD46Ge mice developed significantly higher (6-20-fold) anti-lambda ELISA titers as compared to the MV-lambda-immunized control animal group, indicating that covalently-linked NAP co-expression significantly enhanced lambda immunogenicity. In contrast, ELISA titers against MV antigens were not significantly different between the animals vaccinated with MV-lambda or MV-lambda-NAP. NAP-tagged antigen expression did not affect development of protective anti-measles immunity. Both MV-lambda and MV-lambda-NAP-immunized groups showed strong virus neutralization serum titers in plaque reduction microneutralization test. They concluded that MV-encoded lambda-NAP is highly immunogenic as compared to the unmodified full-length lambda chain. Boost of immune response to poor immunogens using live vectors expressing NAP-tagged chimeric antigens is an attractive approach with potential application in immunoprophylaxis of infectious diseases and cancer immunotherapy.

An important consideration in the development of subunit *vaccines* is the loss of activity caused by physical instability of the protein. CagL is a protein present in strains of *H. pylori*. It contributes to bacterial adherence via α5β1 integrin, thereby making it an attractive subunit *vaccine* candidate. Choudhari etal, 2013 [83] used CagL in different pH and temperature conditions using a variety of spectroscopic techniques. Stability was assessed in terms of transition temperature with the accumulated data, and then incorporated into an empirical phase diagram (EPD) that provided an overview of CagL physical stability. These analyses indicated maximum CagL stability at pH 4-6 up to 40°C in the absence of excipient. Using this EPD analysis, aggregation assays were developed to screen a panel of excipients with some found to inhibit CagL aggregation. These analyses will help in the formulation of a stable *vaccine* against H.*pylori*.

Helicobacter pylori is a major human pathogen that colonizes the stomach and is the lead etiological agent for several pathologies. Sutton P and Chionh YT 2013 [84] demonstrated that effective *vaccine* against these bacteria would be invaluable for protecting against gastric adenocarcinoma. However, the development of such a *vaccine* has stalled and the field has progressed little in the last decade. The key problems that are preventing the development of a *H. pylori vaccine*. Primarily, this involves the inability to produce a completely protective immune response. The knock-on effects of this include a loss of industry investment. Overcoming these problems will likely involve defeating the immune-evasion defenses of *H. pylori*, in particular the mechanism(s) by which it evades antibody-mediated attack.

Chronic *H. pylori* infection can be successfully eradicated by intragastric vaccination with *H. pylori* antigens such as recombinant VacA and CagA, which were administered together with a genetically detoxified mutant of the heat-labile enterotoxin of Escherichia coli (referred to as LTK63), in which the serine in position 63 was replaced by a lysine. The therapeutic vaccination confers efficacious protection against reinfection [85]. Vaccines against *Helicobacter pylori* could circumvent the problem of increasing antibiotic resistance. They would be particularly useful in developing countries, where re-infection rates are high following standard eradication regimes. The vaccine could be given orally with an *H. pylori* whole cell sonicate preparation and cholera toxin adjuvant. Protection was associated with increased serum *H. pylori* IgG antibodies. In this type of vaccine the levels of gastric IL-12p40 and IFN-gamma transcripts were significantly decreased. Gastric IL-10 and TGF-beta transcripts were found only at relatively low levels [86]. Other type of vaccines were used a recombinant antigen ureB138 (a segment of the beta-subunit of urease) against *Helicobacter pylori* infection [87]. Using mucosal vaccination with *H. pylori* antigens when given together with cholera toxin (CT) adjuvant, but not without adjuvant, can induce protective immune responses against *H. pylori* infection. However, the toxicity of CT prevents its use as a mucosal adjuvant in humans. The using a nontoxic double mutant Escherichia coli heat-labile toxin, LT(R192G/L211A) (dmLT), as a mucosal adjuvant in an experimental H. pylori vaccine and compared it to CT in promoting immune responses and protection against *H. pylori* infection. Immunization via the sublingual or intragastric route with *H. pylori* lysate antigens and dmLT resulted in a significant decrease in bacterial load after challenge. Cellular immune responses in the sublingually route resulting in enhanced *in vitro* proliferative and cytokine responses from spleen and mesenteric lymph node cells to *H. pylori* antigens. Thus, dmLT is an attractive adjuvant for inclusion in a mucosal vaccine against *H. pylori* infection [88].

3. Conclusions

Helicobacter infection is an important cause of cancer development. Immune response to this bacterial infection is playing an important role in gastric inflammation. The infection may be innocent or subclinical. Therefore, frequent patients screening for this bacteria and eradication of *Helicobacter* spp. is very crucial. Researches about these bacteria are very essential starting from laboratory animal to application of the researches from lab bench to clinic. Innate and adaptive immune responses of the host are seriously significant for the development of new plans to prevent the development of *H. pylori*-induced gastroduodenal disease and production a vaccine to eradicate this infection. It will be necessary to determine the feasibility of using different epitopes extracted from *H. pylori* in a vaccine design.

Author details

Batool Mutar Mahdi

Clinical Immunology, Department of Microbiology, HLA Research Unit, Al-Kindy College of Medicine, Baghdad University, Baghdad, Iraq

References

[1] Marshall BJ, Warren JR. Unidentified curved bacilli in the stomach of patients with gastritis and peptic ulceration. Lancet 1984; i: 1311-5.

[2] Gao L, Weck MN, Stegmaier C, Rothenbacher D, Brenner H. Alcohol consumption and chronic atrophic gastritis: Population-based study among 9, 444 older adults from Germany. *Int J Cancer*. Jun 2 2009;

[3] Weck MN, Gao L, Brenner H. Helicobacter pylori infection and chronic atrophic gastritis: associations according to severity of disease. *Epidemiology*. 2009;20(4):569-74.

[4] Dixon MF, Genta RM, Yardley JH, Correa P. Classification and grading of gastritis. The updated Sydney System. International Workshop on the Histopathology of Gastritis, Houston 1994. *Am J Surg Pathol*. 1996;20(10):1161-81.

[5] Blaser MJ, Atherton JC. "*Helicobacter pylori* persistence: biology and disease". *J. Clin. Invest.* 2004;113 (3): 321–33.

[6] *Helicobacter pylori* and peptic ulcer disease; economics of peptic ulcer disease and *H. pylori* infection. Centers for Disease Control and Prevention website. www.cdc.gov/ulcer/economic.htm.

[7] Dixon MF. "Patterns of inflammation linked to ulcer disease".Baillieres Best Pract Res Clin Gastroenterol.2000;14 (1): 27–40.

[8] Ciociola AA, McSorley DJ, Turner K, et al. *Helicobacter pylori* infection rates in duodenal ulcer patients in the United States may be lower than previously estimated. Am J Gastroenterol 1999; 94:1834.

[9] Parsonnet J, Friedman GD, Vandersteen DP et al. *Helicobacter pylori* infection and gastric lymphoma. N. Engl. J. Med. 1994;330, 1267–1271.

[10] Wen S, Moss SF. Helicobacter pylori virulence factors in gastric carcinogenesis. Cancer Letters2009; 282(1):1–8.

[11] Kusters JG, van Vliet AH, Kuipers EJ. Pathogenesis of Helicobacter pylori infection. *Clinical Microbiology Reviews* 2006; 19(3):449–490.

[12] Sagaert X, Van Cutsem E, De Hertogh G, Geboes K, Tousseyn T. Gastric MALT lymphoma: A model of chronic inflammation-induced tumor development. Nature Reviews Gastroenterology & Hepatology 2010; 7(6):336–346.

[13] Menaker RJ, Sharaf AA, Jones NL. *Helicobacter pylori* infection and gastric cancer: host, bug, environment, or all three? Curr Gastroenterol Rep. 2004 ;6(6):429-35.

[14] Calam J.Host mechanisms: are they the key to the various clinical outcomes of *Helicobacter pylori* infection? Ital J Gastroenterol Hepatol. 1997 ;29(4):375-82.

[15] Bleich A, Mahler M. Environment as a critical factor for the pathogenesis and outcome of gastrointestinal disease: experimental and human inflammatory bowel disease and helicobacter-induced gastritis. Pathobiology. 2005;72(6):293-307.

[16] Kabir S. Effect of *Helicobacter pylori* eradication on incidence of gastric cancer in human and animal models: underlying biochemical and molecular events. Helicobacter 2009; 14(3): 159-171.

[17] Izzotti A, Durando P, Ansaldi F, Gianiorio F, Pulliero A. Interaction between *Helicobacter pylori*, diet, and genetic polymorphisms as related to non-cancer diseases. Mutat Res. 2009 ; 10;667(1-2):142-57.

[18] McNamara D, El-Omar E.*Helicobacter pylori* infection and the pathogenesis of gastric cancer: a paradigm for host-bacterial interactions. Dig Liver Dis. 2008 ;40(7):504-9.

[19] Correa P. Human gastric carcinogenesis: a multistep and multifactorial process-First American Cancer Society Award Lecture on Cancer Epidemiology and Prevention. Cancer Res 1992; 52: 6735-6740.

[20] Brown LM. *Helicobacter pylori*: epidemiology and routes of transmission. Epidemiol. Rev. 2000;22, 283–297.

[21] Brown LM.*Helicobacter pylori*: epidemiology and routes of transmission. Epidemiol Rev. 2000;22(2):283-97.

[22] Mégraud F.Transmission of *Helicobacter pylori*: faecal-oral versus oral-oral route. Aliment Pharmacol Ther. 1995;9 Suppl 2:85-91.

[23] Mobley HL. Defining *Helicobacter pylori* as a pathogen: strain heterogeneity and virulence. Am. J. Med1996;100, 2S–9S, discussion 9S–11S.

[24] Rohde M, Puls J, Buhrdorf R, Fischer W, Haas R. A novel sheated surface organelle of the *Helicobacter pylori* cag type IV secretion system. Molecular Microbiology 2003; 49(1): 219-234.

[25] Backert S, Selbach M. Role of type IV secretion in *Helicobacter pylori* pathogenesis. Cellular Microbiology 2008; 10(8): 1573-1581.

[26] Odenbreit S, Puls J, Sedlmaier B, Gerland E, Fisher W, Haas R. Translocation of *Helicobacter pylori* CagA into gastric epithelial cells by type IV secretion. Science 2000; 287(5457): 1497-1500.

[27] Higashi H, Tsutsumi R, Muto S, Sugiyama T, Azuma T, Asaka M, Hatakeyama M. SHP-2 tyrosine phosphatase as na intracellular target of *Helicobacter pylori* CagA protein. Science 2002; 295: 683-686.

[28] Amieva MR, Vogelmann R, Covacci A, Tompkins LS, Nelson WJ, Falkow S. Disruption of the epithelial apical-junctional complex by *Helicobacter pylori* CagA. Science 2003; 300(5624): 1430-1434.

[29] Portal-Celhay C and Perez-Perez GI. Immune responses to *Helicobacter pylori* colonization: mechanisms and clinical outcomes. Clin. Sci. 2006;110, 305–314.

[30] Miehlke, S., Kirsch, C., Agha-Amiri, K. et al. The *Helicobacter pylori* vacA s1 m1 genotype and cagA is associated with gastric carcinoma in Germany. Int. J. Cancer.2000. 87, 322–327.

[31] Ferreira RM, Machado JC, Letley D, Atherton JC, Pardo ML, Gonzalez CA, Carneiro F, Figueiredo C. A novel method for genotyping the *Helicobacter pylori* vacA intermediate region directly in gastric biopsy specimens. J Clin Microbiol 2012, 50(12): 3893-9.

[32] Stromberg E, Edebo A, Svennerholm AM, Lindholm C.Decreased epithelial cytokine responses in the duodenal mucosa of *Helicobacter pylori*-infected duodenal ulcer patients. Clin Diagn Lab Immunol. 2003; 10:116-124.

[33] Hamlet A, Thoreson AC, Nilsson O, et al. Duodenal Helicobacter pylori infection differs in cagA genotype between asymptomatic subjects and patients with duodenal ulcers. *Gastroenterology*.1999;116:259–68.

[34] van Doorn LJ, Figueiredo C, Sanna R, et al. Clinical relevance of the cagA, vacA, and iceA status of Helicobacter pylori. *Gastroenterology*.1998;115:58–66.

[35] Stromberg E, Edebo A, Lundin S, Bergin P, Brisslert M, Svennerholm A and Lindholm C.Down-regulation of epithelial IL-8 responses in *Helicobacter pylori*-infected duodenal ulcer patients depends on host factors, rather than bacterial factors.Clin Exp Immunol. 2005 ; 140(1): 117–125.

[36] Mattsson A, Quiding-Jarbrink M, Lonroth H, Hamlet A and Ahlstedt I.Antibody-Secreting Cells in the Stomachs of Symptomatic and Asymptomatic *Helicobacter pylori*-Infected Subjects Infect. Immun. June 1998 vol. 66 no. 6 2705-2712

[37] Crabtree, J. E. Immune and inflammatory responses to *Helicobacter pylori* infection. Scand. J. Gastroenterol. 1996;215: 3S–10S.

[38] Lagunes-Servin H, Torres J, Maldonado-Bernal C, Pérez-Rodríguez M, Huerta-Yépez S, Madrazo de la Garza A, Muñoz-Pérez L, Flores-Luna L, Ramón-García G, Camorlinga-Ponce M. Toll-Like Receptors and Cytokines are Upregulated during *Helicobacter pylori* Infection in Children. Helicobacter. 2013 Jul 22. doi: 10.1111/hel.12067. [Epub ahead of print]

[39] Pimentel-Nunes P, Gonçalves N, Boal-Carvalho I, Afonso L, Lopes P, Roncon-Albuquerque R, Henrique R, Moreira-Dias L, Leite-Moreira A and Dinis-Ribeiro M.*Helicobacter pylori* Induces Increased Expression of Toll-Like Receptors and Decreased Toll-Interacting Protein in Gastric Mucosa that Persists Throughout Gastric Carcinogenesis.Helicobacter2013;18:22-32.

[40] Ihan A, Pinchuk IV, Beswick EJ. Inflammation, immunity, and vaccines for *Helicobacter pylori* infection.Helicobacter. 2012 Sep;17 Suppl 1:16-21.

[41] Avilés-Jiménez F, Reyes-Leon A, NietoPatlán E, Hansen LM, Burgueño J, Ramos IP et al. In vivo expression of *Helicobacter pylori* virulence genes in patients with gastritis, ulcer, and gastric cancer. Infect Immun 2012;80:594-601.

[42] Chatterjee A, Chatterjee S, Bandyopadhyay SK. *H pylori*-induced gastric ulcer: pathophysiology and herbal remedy. Int J Biol Med Res 2012;3:1461-5.

[43] Tummala, S., Keates, S. and Kelly, C. P. Update on the immunologic basis of *Helicobacter pylori* gastritis. Curr. Opin. Gastroenterol.2004; 20, 592–597.

[44] Irina V. Pinchuk, Katherine T. Morris, Robert A. Nofchissey, Rachel B. Earley, Jeng-Yih Wu, Thomas Y. Ma, and Ellen J. Beswick. Stromal Cells Induce Th17 during *Helicobacter pylori* Infection and in the Gastric Tumor Microenvironment.*PLoS One.* 2013; 8: e53798.

[45] Noach, L. A., Bosma, N. B., Jansen, J., Hoek, F. J., van Deventer, S. J. and Tygat, G. N. Mucosal tumor necrosis factor-α, interleukin-1β, and interleukin-8 production in patients with *Helicobacter pylori* infection. Scand. J. Gastroenterol. 1994;29, 425–429.

[46] Hwang, I. R., Kodama, T., Kikuchi, S. et al. (2002) Effect of interleukin 1 polymorphisms on gastric mucosal interleukin 1beta production in *Helicobacter pylori* infection. Gastroenterology 123, 1793–1803

[47] Yuceyar H, Saruc M, Kokuludag A, Terzioglu E, Goksel G, Isisag A. The systemic cellular immune response in the *Helicobacter pylori*-associated duodenal ulcer and chronic antral gastritis" Hepatogastroenterology 2002, 49(46): 1177-9.

[48] Fixa B, Komárková O, Krejsek J, Nozicka Z, Bures J. Specific cellular immune response in patients with *Helicobacter pylori* infection. Hepatogastroenterology 1990, 37(6):606-7.

[49] Nessa J, Chart H, Owen RJ and Drasar B. Human serum antibody response to *H pylori* whole cell antigen in an institutionalized Bangaladish population. J Appl microb. 2001;90:68-72.

[50] Mattsson A, Quiding-Jabrink M, Lonroth H, Hamlet A, Ahlstedt I and Svennerholm A. Antibody secreting cells in the stomach of symptomatic and asymptomatic *H pylori* infected subjects. 1998; 66:2705-2712.

[51] Tosi, M. F. and Czinn, S. J. Opsonic activity of specific human IgG against *Helicobacter pylori.* J. Infect. Dis.1990; 162, 156–162.

[52] Berstad, A. E, Holbjorn, K., Bukholm, G., Moran, A. P. and Brandtzaeg, P Complement activation directly induced by *Helicobacter pylori.* Gastroenterology;2001 120, 1108–1116.

[53] Cover TL. The vaculating cytotoxin of *H pylori*. Mol 241-246.

[54] Portal-Celhay C and Perez-Perez G. Immune responses to *Helicobacter pylori* colonization: mechanisms and clinical outcomes.Clinical Science.2006; 110: 305–314.

[55] Crabtree JE, Wyatt JI, Sobala GM.Systemic and mucosal humoral responses to *Helicobacter pylori* in gastric cancer.. Gut1993, 34:1339-43.

[56] Menaker RJ, Ceponis PJ, Jones NL. *Helicobacter pylori* induces apoptosis of macrophages in association with alterations in the mitochondrial pathway. Infect Immun. 2004 ;72:2889-98.

[57] Ramarao, N. and Meyer, T. F. *Helicobacter pylori* resists phagocytosis by macrophages: quantitative assessment by confocal microscopy and fluorescenceactivated cell sorting. Infect. Immun. 2001; 69, 2604–2611

[58] Gobert, A. P., McGee, D. J., Akhtar, M. et al. *Helicobacter pylori* arginase inhibits nitric oxide production by eukaryotic cells: a strategy for bacterial survival. Proc. Natl. Acad. Sci. 2001; 98:13844–13849.

[59] Yuan J, Li P, Tao J, Shi X, Hu B, Chen H, Guo X. H. pylori escape host immunoreaction through inhibiting ILK expression by VacA. Cell Mol Immunol. 2009;6:191-197.

[60] Perez-Perez, G. I., Shepherd, V. L., Morrow, J. D. and Blaser, M. J. Activation of human THP-1 cells and rat bone marrow-derived macrophages by *Helicobacter pylori* lipopolysaccharide. Infect. Immun. 1995;63, 1183–1187

[61] Andersen-Nissen, E., Smith, K. D., Strobe, K. L. et al. Evasion of Toll-like receptor 5 by flagellated bacteria. Proc. Natl. Acad. Sci.2005; 102:9247–9252.

[62] Yang ZM, Chen WW, Wang YF. Gene expression profiling in gastric mucosa from *Helicobacter pylori*-infected and uninfected patients undergoing chronic superficial gastritis. PLoS One. 2012;7:e33030.

[63] Boncristiano, M., Paccani, S. R., Barone, S. et al. The *Helicobacter pylori* vacuolating toxin inhibits T cell activation by two independent mechanisms. J. Exp. Med. 2003;198: 1887–1897.

[64] Molinari, M., Salio, M., Galli, C. et al. Selective inhibition of Ii-dependent antigen presentation by *Helicobacter pylori* toxin VacA. J. Exp. Med. 1998;187 :135–140

[65] Gebert, B., Fischer, W., Weiss, R., Hoffmann, R. andHaas, R. *Helicobacter pylori* vacuolating cytotoxin inhibits T-lymphocyte activation. Science.2003; 301: 1099–1102.

[66] Yuan JP, Li T, Li ZH, Yang GZ, Hu BY, Shi XD, Shi TL, Tong SQ, Guo XK. mRNA expression profiling reveals a role of *Helicobacter pylori* vacuolating toxin in escaping host defense. World J Gastroenterol. 2004 ;10:1528-32.

[67] Every AL. Key host-pathogen interactions for designing novel interventions against *Helicobacter pylori*. Trends Microbiol. 2013;21(5):253-9.

[68] Del Giudice G, Malfertheiner P, Rappuoli R. Development of vaccines against *Helicobacter pylori*. Expert Rev Vaccines. 2009 ;8(8):1037-49.

[69] Sutton P. Progress in vaccination against *Helicobacter pylori*. *Vaccine* 2001;19:2286–90.

[70] Kleanthous H, Myers GA, Georgakopoulos KM, et al. Rectal and intranasal immunizations with recombinant urease induce distinct local and serum immune responses in mice and protect against *Helicobacter pylori* infection. Infect Immun 1998;66:2879–86.

[71] Michetti P, Kreiss C, Kotloff KL, et al. Oral immunization with urease and *Escherichia coli* heat-labile enterotoxin is safe and immunogenic in*Helicobacter pylori*-infected adults. *Gastroenterology* 1999;116:804–12.

[72] Blanchard TG, Eisenberg JC, Matsumoto Y. Clearance of *Helicobacter pylori* infection through immunization: the site of T cell activation contributes to vaccine efficacy. Vaccine 2004;22:888–97.

[73] Eriksson AM, Schon KM, Lycke NY. The cholera toxin-derived CTA1-DD vaccine adjuvant administered intranasally does not cause inflammation or accumulate in the nervous tissues. J Immunol 2004;173:3310–9.

[74] Gottwein JM, Blanchard TG, Targoni OS, et al. Protective anti-Helicobacter immunity is induced with aluminum hydroxide or complete Freund's adjuvant by systemic immunization. J Infect Dis 2001;184:308–14.

[75] Stadtlander CTKH, Gangemi JD, Khanolvar SS, Kitsos CM, Farris HE, Fulton LK, et al. Immunogenicity and Safety of recombinant *Helicobacter pylori* urease in a nonhuman primate. Dig Dis Sci;1996 41:1853–1862.

[76] Michetti P, CorthésyTheulaz I, Davin C, Haas R, y AC, Heitz M, et al.Immunization of BALB/c mice against Helicobacter felis infection with H. pylori urease. Gastroenterology.1994;107:1002–1011.

[77] Cuenca R, Blanchard TG, Czinn SJ, Nedrud JG, Monath TP, Lee CK, et al. Therapeutic immunization against Helicobacter mustelae in naturally infected ferrets. Gastroenterology.1996; 110:1770–1775.

[78] Kreiss C, Buclin T, Cosma M, CorthésyTheulaz I, Michetti PSafety of oral immunization with recombinant urease in patients with *Helicobacter pylori* infection. Lancet. 1996; 347:1630–1631.

[79] Corthésy-Theulaz I, Bachmann D, Hopkins S, Kraehenbuhl J-P, Michetti P, Blum AL Mucosal immunization against *Helicobacter pylori* in mice via attenuated recombinant Salmonella. Gastroenterology.1997; 112:A953.

[80] Zhang HX, Qiu YY, Zhao YH, Liu M, Yu AL. Immunogenicity of oral vaccination with Lactococcus lactis derived vaccine candidate antigen (UreB) of*Helicobacter pylori* fused with the human interleukin 2 as adjuvant.Mol Cell Probes. 2013 Sep 13. pii: S0890-8508(13)00048-0. doi: 10.1016/j.mcp.2013.08.003. [Epub ahead of print]

[81] Altman E, Chandan V, Harrison B. The potential of dextran-based glycoconjugates for development of *Helicobacter pylori* vaccine.Glycoconj J. 2013 Aug 30. [Epub ahead of print].

[82] Iankov ID, Federspiel MJ, Galanis E. Measles virus expressed *Helicobacter pylori* neutrophil-activating protein significantly enhances the immunogenicity of poor immunogens.Vaccine. 2013;31(42):4795-801.

[83] Choudhari SP, Pendleton KP, Ramsey JD, Blanchard TG, Picking WD. A systematic approach toward stabilization of CagL, a protein antigen from *Helicobacter pylori* that is a candidate subunit vaccine. J Pharm Sci. 2013 ;102(8):2508-19.

[84] Sutton P, Chionh YT.Why can't we make an effective vaccine against *Helicobacter pylori*? Expert Rev Vaccines. 2013 ;12(4):433-41.

[85] Ghiara P, Rossi M, Marchetti M, Di Tommaso A, Vindigni C, Ciampolini F et al. Therapeutic intragastric vaccination against Heliconbacter pylori in mice eradicates an otherwise chronic infection and confers protection against reinfection. Infect Immun 1997, 65(12): 4996-5002.

[86] Jeremy AH, Du Y, Dixon MF, Robinson PA, Crabtree JE. Protection against *Helicobacter pylori* infection in the Mongolian gerbil after prophylatic vaccination.Microbes Infect 2006, 8(2):340-6.

[87] Morihara F, Fujii R, Hifurni E, Nishizono A, Uda T. Effects of vaccination by a recombinant antigen ureB138 (a segment of the beta-subunit of urease) against *Helicobacter pylori* infection. J Med Microbiol 2007, 56(6):847-53.

[88] Sjökvist Ottsjö L, Flach CF, Clements J, Holmgren J, Raghavan S. A double mutant heat-labile toxin from Escherichia coli, LT(R192G/L211A), is an effective mucosal adjuvant for vaccination against *Helicobacter pylori* infection. Infect Immun 2013, 81(5): 1532-40.

Section 2

Questions Concerning Possible Routes of H. pylori Transmission: Water

Chapter 3

Can Drinking Water Serve as a Potential Reservoir of *Helicobacter pylori*? Evidence for Water Contamination by *Helicobacter pylori*

Malgorzata Plonka, Aneta Targosz and
Tomasz Brzozowski

Additional information is available at the end of the chapter

http://dx.doi.org/10.5772/57568

1. Introduction

This review was designed to highlight the available evidence that suggests drinking water and possible survival in water as a probable transmission mode for *H. pylori*.

Although the natural niche for *H. pylori* is the human stomach, for widespread infection to occur the organism may need to survive in the external environment [1]. Documented evidence relating to the survival of *H.pylori* outside the gastric niche is extremely limited. However, there are no established culture methods for the detection of viable *H. pylori* in the environment, in particular drinking water supplies, preventing the development of true epidemiological and risk assessments [2]. A number of drinking water studies have identified *H. pylori* in water pre- and post-chlorination [3]. Baker and colleague [4] found that *H. pylori* were more resistant to low levels of free chlorine than E. coli or C. jejuni. Moreno and colleagues [5] have shown that *H. pylori* could survive disinfection procedures that are normally used in drinking water treatment when bacterium *H. pylori* was found in the viable but not-culturable (VBNC) state. However, they did find that culture of *H. pylori* was lost after 5 min in water despite free chlorine levels of 0.96 mg/2l of water. Children born into high-income families supplied with municipal water are considered 12 times more likely to become colonized with *H. pylori* than those supplied from community wells. This suggests that municipal water is a possible risk factor in the transmission and acquisition of *H. pylori*. It is plausible to suggest that breaks in municipal pipes allow for infiltration of contaminated surface water [6].

2. *Helicobacter pylori* — sources and pathways of transmission

2.1. A Brief history

It has been over a century since Walery Jaworski at Cracow University detected a spiral bacteria named *Vibrio rugula,* in the sediment after gastric washing from patients with gastric cancer and over a quarter of century since Marshall and Warren drew attention to the spiral bacteria, *H. pylori* as a pathogen in various gastric diseases. The Nobel Prize was awarded to Marshall and Warren in 2005 for the discovery of *H. pylori* within the gastric mucosa and its role in gastritis and peptic ulcer disease [7].

H. pylori infecting almost half of the world's population, has become the cause of one of the most common infections. It is a pathogen of constant interest among researchers still looking for the answers to many questions. One of them is the question: "How are *H. pylori* transmitted and what is its source?"

The answer to this question hangs within the realm of conjecture, because - so far - no dominant route of infection by *H. pylori* has been defined. The following routes of transmission are currently taken into consideration: oral - oral transmission, fecal - oral transmission, iatrogenic transmission and vector-borne transmission (Fig. 1). The most likely way in which the *H. pylori* infection is spread has been found to be by passing from person to person by oral- oral or fecal - oral transmission [8, 9]. All the scientists involved in research on the etiology of *H. pylori* infection are unanimous about the fact that this bacterium has to get invaded into the stomach through the mouth - this is a non-invasive micro-organism, and therefore cannot colonize the gastric mucosa in any other way.

2.2. Oral-oral transmission

Data for the confirmation of oral - oral transmission is based on various observations that are related to, among others, research on infection within the family. Research showed that if one person in the family was found to be infected with *H. pylori,* the probability of infecting the other family members was significantly higher [10, 11]. By studying the frequency of infected couples, Italian and German epidemiologists have shown the relationship between the prevalence of infection among uninfected spouses and the length of time in which they live with an infected partner [12, 13]. German studies [14, 15] have also demonstrated particularly strong dependence of the cross-infection between mother and child, with emphasis on the key role of the mother in this form of transmission. Evidence for the dominance of the oral- oral and fecal - oral transmissions was also provided by research conducted in closed institutions such as care facilities for the mentally and physically handicapped, nursing homes, preschools/ kindergartens and orphanages. Research conducted by Lambert and others [16], carried out on adult residents of a home for mentally and physically handicapped persons in Australia, reported a higher prevalence rate of *H. pylori* infection in the population of the institution, than in the general population, as well as the relationship between the prevalence of infection and the length of stay in such a care facility. Similar conclusions were reached by Dutch and Japanese researchers [17, 18]. Indeed, a higher degree of *H. pylori* infection was also detected

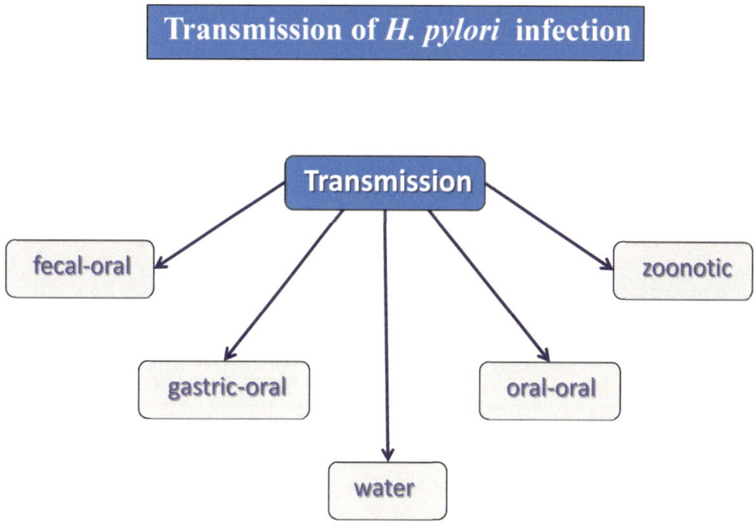

Lee A et al., 1999, Brown LM et al., 2000 Konturek PC et al. 2009

Figure 1. The different mode of transmission of *H.pylori* in humans.

in closed institutions: in England [19, 20], Russia [21], and France [22]. The oral - oral route of transmission is confirmed by the presence of bacteria in the saliva, the dental plate and dental pockets. Evidence that the bacterium *H. pylori* can be transmitted by saliva come from studies conducted by Mègraund`s [23], Pytko - Polonczyk et al [24] and Parsonnet et al [25]. Mègraund in the cited work [23] also reported an increased risk of transmission associated with the chewing of food by mothers in West Africa before the feeding it to their children. The transmission of bacteria through vomiting up the stomach contents into the mouth was confirmed in clinical trials by Parsonnet et al [25] who bred *H. pylori* from all samples collected from 16 vomiting seropositive asymptomatic patients.

2.3. Fecal -oral transmission

An important argument for transmission of *H. pylori* by the fecal - oral route was the isolation and growth of the bacteria from human faeces by Thomas et al [26]. Another proponent of the spreading of the *H. pylori* infection by the fecal - oral route is a David Graham, who demonstrated the transmission's similarity to other bacterial gastrointestinal infections transmitted in this way, in particular hepatitis A (HAV) [27].

An important factor in the acquisition of *H. pylori* infection by the fecal - oral route may be the contamination of water with faeces (Fig. 2). The active, spiral form of *H. pylori* can survive in river water for at least a week, and coccoid of the bacteria can survive for a year or more. Klein et al [28] also demonstrated that *H. pylori* can survive in water, and then penetrate into particular parts and organs of the gastrointestinal tract through the contaminated water. They found that the water resources in Lima (Peru) may be responsible for the bacterium *H. pylori* infection, especially if it is stored in tanks or extracted from urban scenes.

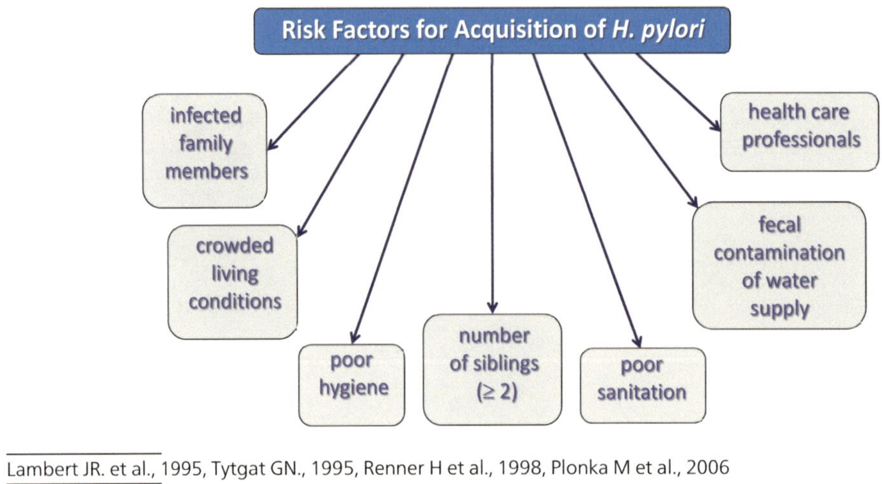

Figure 2. Major epidemiologic risk factors for acquisition of *H.pylori* in humans.

2.4. Iatrogenic and vector-borne transmission

In view of the widespread use of the gastroscopy as a means for diagnosing the upper gastro-intestinal tract disorders, the iatrogenic transmission of *H. pylori* could be a potential risk factor for infecting patients undergoing colonoscopies. Tytgat [29] proposed that the major cause of this phenomenon is the complex structure of gastroscope and the difficulties involved in its disinfection. It should be noted, however, that the risk of bug infection in this way is negligible. Lin et al [30, 31] believe that the medical staff performing endoscopic examinations are at greater risk of becoming infected with *H. pylori*, as opposed to dentists and dental nurses whose level of risk is negligible. This suggests that infected gastric mucosa may play a more important role in the spread of infection than infected saliva. Although the principal reservoir for *H. pylori* infection seems to be a human being, there may be other reservoirs of *H. pylori*, such as livestock. Handt et al [32] isolated *H. pylori* from cats and implied that this so called "pet transmission" may have public health implications. However, there is no convincing epidemiological data of *H. pylori* infection in cats, which is why the current risk of infection from cats is considered to be rather small. Other animal organisms that were found to be colonized with *H. pylori* are monkeys [33]. The monkey to human mode of transmission of *H. pylori* could be, however, unlikely due to limited human contact with monkeys. However, a much more likely vector in the transmission of *H. pylori* is a housefly. It was Grubel et al [34, 35] who found that houseflies infected with *H.pylori* in the laboratory may be a reservoir of living bacteria, found both in the gut and on the hairs covering the fly's body. The probability that flies can carry *H. pylori* from infected faeces to food or human mucosal surfaces is indirectly confirmed by numerous epidemiological studies conducted in countries with particularly difficult sanitary conditions such as Colombia, Peru and Japan (Fig. 3). However, there is no direct evidence that the flies which have been in contact, under natural conditions, with faeces infected by *H. pylori* are the source of infection or that this microorganism can be transferred from contaminated flies to food in an amount sufficient enough to infect humans [36]. Goodman et al [37] have found interesting results on the risk of *H. pylori* infection in children from the Colombian Andes, who played with sheep (Fig. 3). A study by Dore et al [38] revealed a significantly higher prevalence of *H. pylori* infection among Sardinian sheep herders, but not among members of their families. Papiez et al [39] and Plonka et al [40] detected an increased risk of *H. pylori* infection in both Polish sheepherders from the Tatra Mountains, as well as entire families in that region. Despite the significance of issue at hand, the epidemiology of the *H. pylori* infection still remains obscure. Studies often present conflicting results, especially when it comes to sources and modes of transmission of infection and associated risk factors. In world literature, authors of various studies emphasize the high volatility of risk, depending on environmental and geographical factors. They also emphasize the lack of a sufficient number of epidemiological studies in the countries of Central and Eastern Europe, including Poland.

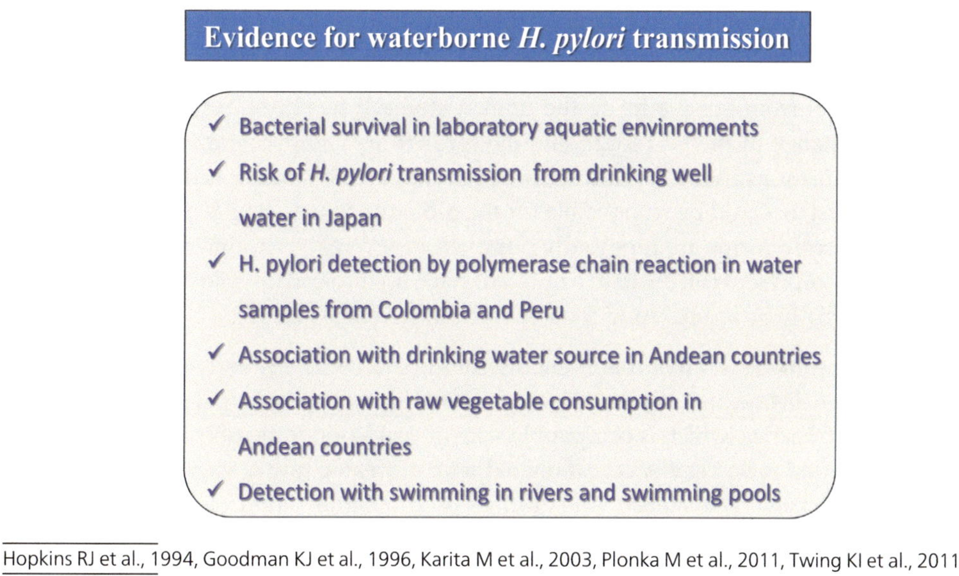

Figure 3. Literature evidence that water may serve as a potential source and reservoir of *H.pylori*.

2.5. Water serves as a potential reservoir of *H. pylori*

The breakthrough discovery that water can be a source and route of the *H. pylori* infection resulted in a flurry of research. The fact that water can be a source of *H. pylori* infection was reported in a study, conducted in the Colombian Andes, by Goodman and others [37]. They found that drinking water from streams, bathing and swimming in streams and pools significantly increases the risk of infection in children in Colombia (Fig. 3). Similar conclusions were reached by Klein et al [28] on the basis of the abovementioned studies conducted in Lima. However, Teh et al [41] of Taiwan and Hopkins et al [42] in Chile found no increased risk in subjects who acquired their drinking water from rivers, and even in those that swam near the polluted beaches in local rivers, irrigation canals or lakes. The problem of *H.pylori* contamination of water resources requires further studies with a proper way of assessment of bacteria in water environment.

3. Methods for the detection of waterborne *H. pylori*

The following methods are used in order to detect the presence of *H. pylori* in water samples taken from a variety of intakes:

1. Culturable methods – that utilize the specialized media bacterial growth, and
2. The methods of molecular assessment of *H. pylori* using the polymerase chain reaction (PCR).

3.1. Culturable methods in the culturing of *H. pylori*

H. pylori is a Gram-negative bacterium, measuring 2 to 4 μm in length and 0.5 to 1 μm in width. Culturing *H. pylori* from areas outside the human stomach has been difficult because of a morphological change in the bacterium and overgrowth by competing microorganisms. *H. pylori* rapidly transforms into a coccoid form which is in a viable but nonculturable (VNBC) state. The VBNC state could be responsible for the difficulty in isolating *H. pylori* from water samples [43]. Coccoid forms are repeatedly observed in several environments, but since it is not known if they represent cell death or a resistant state, their role in the transmission pathway of *H. pylori*, especially by animals and food, is still controversial [44, 45].

We found only a few studies that report successful isolation of *H. pylori* from environmental water samples [46]. In one case, the bacterium was isolated from a municipal wastewater canal on the US-Mexico border, which is compatible with a fecal – oral route of contamination [47]. This canal was found to be heavily contaminated with untreated raw sewage in an area know to have a high *H. pylori* prevalence. The authors used a combination of non standardized immunomagnetically separation (IMS) and culturing techniques. Following separation the bead-*H. pylori* conjugates were streaked onto Columbia blood agar plates and incubated for 3 to 5 days in microaerophilic condition at 37°C, the small, gray colonies were selected and stained with Gram stain to verify morphology. Colonies with Gram-negative rods or coccoid forms were tested by three diagnostic techniques: a rapid urea test, of cytochrome oxidase test and catalase test. In order to fully confirm detection of *H. pylori* one should remember that besides to be positive in all the three mentioned tests, *H. pylori* is a Gram-negative bacterium. A total of 37 out of 132 isolates from culture were selected as putative *H. pylori* and then 23 out of 37 isolates were confirmed to be *H. pylori* by 16S rRNA PCR (Fig. 4).

In the second case, *H. pylori was* isolated from a seawater sample [48]. Colonies were only obtained in residues on 200 μm filters but not in residues on 0.64 and 0.22 μm filters. *H. pylori* could only be isolated from fractionated seawater samples, containing large zooplankton organisms; without zooplankton, *H. pylori* cells could not be recovered from any other fractions by growth-dependent detection protocols [48, 49]. This suggests that bacterium *H. pylori* requires an organic or proteins matrix to remain culturable. This should be further investigated and other studies attempting to isolate *H. pylori* from water sources using similar approaches are needed.

In another study [50] drinking water samples (n= 600) were collected from ground-drilled water supplied by water and sanitation agencies in different localities within the Lahore metropolitan area, Pakistan, and were used within six hours for culturing of *H. pylori*. Water Samples with isolated bacteria was cultured on modified *H. pylori* medium and detected by biochemical tests. The culture-based method sometimes may lead to false negative results due to contamination of microbial species present in the environment that contain the combination of antibiotic resistant genes. In order to remove this discrepancy the grown bacterial cultures were rechecked on another *H. pylori* agar plate followed by urease and catalase tests and was also checked under a microscope to minimize the probability of mixed microbial growth. It was found that 225 out of 600 drinking water samples (37.5%) were positive for *H. pylori* on the *H. pylori* agar medium. The samples that were positive for *H. pylori* were selected on the basis of the formation of a discrete red color zone around the bacterial colony during incubation in 5% CO_2 at 37°C for 3-5 days. And then PCR analysis showed that 90 out of 225 *H. pylori* positive drinking water samples were confirmed 139 bp gene segment of 16S rRNA *H. pylori* strains from water in the Lahore metropolitan area were studied to find the presence of virulence genes and also to correlate with the global genetic structure and evolution of *H. pylori*. The presence of *H. pylori* in drinking water samples of Lahore metropolitan city was approximately 40%, which is an alarming situation. The presence of a high percentage of *H. pylori* contamination in different water sources may be due to low socioeconomic factors such as a lack of public health education, poverty, overcrowding, poor sanitation and unsafe water supplies (Fig. 2). The results for the presence of *H. pylori* in the test samples are in agreement with the results of other studies [51]. The epidemiological survey also suggests that water is the potential source for the transmission of *H. pylori* infection [52] suggesting that water is one of the vectors required for prevalence and transmission of *H. pylori*.

Survival studies in water samples demonstrate that *H. pylori* can be cultured for a limited period of time in a temperature dependent manner [53, 54]. Elevated temperature results in loss of cultivability [55]. The presence of *H. pylori* associated with biofilm from wells, rivers and water distribution systems has been reported recently [56, 57]. Biofilms are slimy films of bacteria, other microbes and organic materials that cover underwater surfaces, particularly inside plumbing. This makes them rather inaccessible and provides a matrix difficult to be reached by disinfectants. The detachment of biofims is the principal form of contamination of treated water [58, 59]. Aside from these studies, positive culture of *H pylori* from drinking water has not been successful, despite efforts to produce a culture-specific media sensitive and selective enough to isolate and grow this organism. A simple plating medium for the detection of *H. pylori* in the environment was investigated independently by Stoodley et al [59], however, the culturable methods employed were unsuccessful in the culturing of *H. pylori*.

3.2. The methods of molecular assessment of *H. pylori*

3.2.1. Fluorescent in situ hybridization (FISH)

Fluorescent in situ hybridization (FISH) with rRNA oligonucleotide probes has been used for detection and identification of VBNC forms of bacteria [62]. In addition to PCR, FISH was validated as a quick and sensitive method for detection of *H. pylori* in environmental samples [63].

In the United States, actively respiring *H. pylori* from surface and well water has been detected using fluorescent antibody - tetrazolium reduction (FACTC) microscopy [64] and confirmed using species-specific PCR [65]. Sen et al. [66] investigated the development of internal controls for PCR assays by spiking drinking water with 100 cells of *H. pylori* and demonstrated similar cycle thresholds to those of recombinant *Escherichia coli* during chlorine disinfection. In addition to PCR, FISH was validated as a quick and sensitive method for detection of *H. pylori* in environmental samples [63]. These findings suggest the presence of *H. pylori* in the natural environment and a possible waterborne route of transmission.

3.2.2. The determination of gene expression by PCR method in the biological material collected from humans and from water sources

This method allows the identification of DNA which is specific for *H. pylori* in biological material: gastric juice, saliva, feces and as shown, this method could be useful to detect the presence of *H. pylori* in water. The application of this technique to test for *H. pylori* has allowed the cloning and sequencing of important genes involved in colonization and pathogenesis, and for the development of simple patterns to determine a sequence of *H. pylori*-specific genes. It also allows for the detection of the protein CagA and VacA which are encoded by the pathogenic genes of cagA and vacA found in particular strains of *H. pylori* bacteria that cause serious gastric disorders including chronic gastritis, peptic gastric and duodenal diseases and /or even gastric cancer.

Despite the numerous research findings identifying *H. pylori* in water, it is important to consider the fact that the use of PCR and other molecular methods for the detection of pathogens in environmental samples has limitations. This is principally due to the inability of PCR to differentiate between naked DNA from dead and living cells. Consequently, to scientifically interpret data regarding the epidemiology of *H. pylori*, cultured bacteria from appropriate water sources are necessary (Fig. 4).

H. pylori rapidly transforms into VBNC state which is induced by low nutrient and hyperosmotic conditions [67 - 69]. Such stressed conditions are commonly found in water and the watery environment. Nayak and Rose [70] demonstrated that quantitative polymerase chain reaction (qPCR) could determine *H. pylori* concentrations in water. In this study real time qPCR was shown to be a specific, sensitive and rapid method to quantify *H. pylori* in sewage. Prior to these studies a two-stage *in vitro* method for detection of *H. pylori* in spiked water and fecal samples.

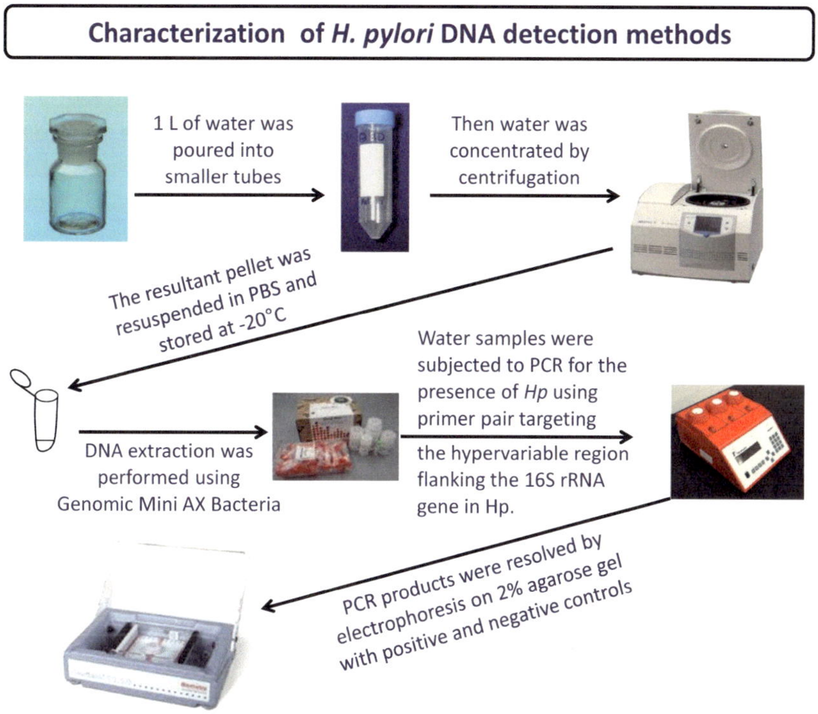

Figure 4. *H.pylori* detection by the assessment of *H.pylori* DNA and 16S rRNA by PCR technique. Proposed steps of detection of *H.pylori* in municipal water.

Janzon et al [71] developed tested and optimized two complementary *H. pylori* specific real-time PCR assays for quantification of *H. pylori* DNA in water. The minimum detection level of the assays including collection procedures and DNA extraction was shown to be approximately 250 *H. pylori* genomes per water sample. They analyzed samples of drinking and environmental water ($n = 75$) and natural water biofilms ($n = 21$) from a high-endemic area in Bangladesh. They could not identify *H. pylori* DNA in any of the samples, even though other pathogenic bacteria have been found previously in the same water samples by using the same methodology. A series of control experiments were performed to ensure that the negative results were not falsely caused by PCR inhibition, nonspecific assays, degradation of template DNA, or low detection sensitivity. Their results suggest that it is unlikely that the predominant transmission route of *H. pylori* in this area is waterborne.

3.2.2.1. H. pylori DNA is not detected in environmental and wastewater samples

Since *H. pylori* DNA was not detected in the household waters, the presence of *H. pylori* DNA in different environmental water sources in Dhaka was evaluated. A total of 15 water samples from ponds and lakes and 6 wastewater samples were collected in the larger Dhaka area between November 2005 and March 2006. The sample volumes ranged between 150 ml and 1,000 ml. Also, these samples were all negative for the presence of *H. pylori* DNA.

3.2.2.2. Determination of inhibitors in samples subjected for PCR.

To evaluate the possibility that the absence of *H. pylori* DNA in the water samples was caused by substances inhibiting the PCR process, two *H. pylori* strains, Hel513 and Hel703, were incubated at approximately 107 bacteria per ml in water samples from three drinking water sources and one pond in Dhaka and in PBS as a control and sampled after 1 and 21 days. The detection rates of less than 100% compared to the level for the control incubated in PBS indicated that PCR inhibitors were present in one of the drinking water sources and in the pond water. However, ten-fold dilution of the purified DNA was shown to remove the effect of the PCR inhibitors.

To further determine the presence of inhibitory factors in the field study water and biofilm samples from Dhaka, the real-time PCR analysis was repeated on all field samples but spiked with 1,000 genomes of *H. pylori* strain J99 in each PCR. Detection rates lower than 30% were found in 41% of the drinking water samples. However, 10-fold dilution of the DNA was shown to remove the inhibitory effect in 90% of samples, but still without positive results. These analyses showed that levels of *H. pylori* DNA were below 250 genome copies in 38% of the samples and below at least 2,500 genome copies in another 52% of the samples. Similar results were found in biofilm and environmental water samples. Interestingly, fewer than 10% of the wastewater samples showed presence of inhibitors, presumably because these were extracted using the Qiagen stool kit, which removes PCR inhibitors but decreases the DNA yield.

3.2.2.3. H. pylori DNA and RNA stability during long-term incubation in tap water and seawater

Possible degradation of *H. pylori* DNA in water was studied using two different *H. pylori* strains, Hel513 and Hel703. Because of the possible confounding effect of inhibitors in the water in Dhaka, water was taken from Gothenburg, Sweden, for this experiment. Morphology, culturability, *hpaA* and *glmM* gene numbers, and RNA integrity were analyzed at different time points. A majority of the initially spiral-shaped *H. pylori* bacteria converted into the coccoid shape within 24 h, and on day 7, no spiral-shaped bacteria were detected and no viable bacteria were recovered. Real-time PCR assays revealed that the copy numbers of both *H. pylori* genes were constant in tap water for up to 35 days, followed by small decreases at 100 days, whereas copy numbers in seawater decreased up to 50-fold after 100 days. However, gel electrophoresis of total RNA showed that RNA was degraded in tap water within 7 days, with no visible 23S or 16S fragments.

4. Evidence that biofilms in water distribution systems may harbor *H. pylori*

It is well known that waterborne bacteria can attach to surfaces by aggregating in a hydrated exopolymer known as a biofilm [72, 73]. The association of bacteria, particularly pathogens, with biofilm communities within a water distribution system may offer vulnerable and susceptible bacteria protection from disinfection and protozoan predation [74]. In fact microorganisms in drinking water are predominantly associated with biofilms rather than in the planktonic state [72, 73, 75]. There is evidence that biofilms in water distribution systems may harbor *H. pylori* [76-78]. In addition a study undertaken in Western Africa, utilizing 16S rDNA sequences, has shown evidence that *H. pylori* can be detected in natural biofilms [79]. A more recent study by Watson and colleagues [80] showed a close link between *Helicobacter* DNA in showerhead biofilm used in domestic households.

4.1. Cultivability of *H. pylori in* water and water-associated biofilms and implications for transmission

Adams et al. [81] have shown that in pure culture *H. pylori* cells remain cultivable longer at 15°C than at 20°C, but in their study it was not possible to recover cultivable *H. pylori* from water samples and biofilms. However, considering the shape of the cells detected by PNA-FISH (peptide nucleic acid fluorescence in situ hybridization) and considering that cultivable cells are spiral shaped, while coccoid cells are VBNC and therefore likely to be non-cultivable, the expectation is that there should be more cultivable *H. pylori* cells at 20°C. It is assumed demonstrating that the behavior of this pathogen in heterotrophic biofilms might be completely different than its behavior in pure culture. Additionally, the PNA probe used in this work targets sites on the 16S rRNA molecule, and it is known that the RNA content of a cell can be indicative of viability which suggests that the cells detected were still viable [82]. It has been shown that the concentration of all *H. pylori* cells in the biofilms formed in this work is either higher than or very similar to the concentrations found when pure-culture biofilms were formed [83]. In addition, the detection of *H. pylori* embedded in biofilms suggests that there is a close association with other bacteria present in the biofilms. These two factors, together with the persistence of a bright PNA-FISH signal, which is indicative of a high rRNA content, suggest that the heterotrophic bacteria present in the biofilms formed in this study were not a negative influence on *H. pylori* but only induced its transformation to the more robust coccoid morphology [84-86].

4.2. The existence of *H. pylori* in the drinking water

The evidence based medicine regarding *H. pylori* transmission is not convincing, making it difficult to avoid the notion that the burden/inconvenience accounts for this bacterial infection. The microbiological and epidemiological studies confirmed that in certain conditions the intake of water contaminated with *H. pylori* might be considered as potential source of human infection with this bug. The water could be considered as a reservoir of *H. pylori* [87].

In the U.S. the problem of drinking water pollution is handled by the Environmental Protection Agency (EPA). On the basis of a survey which was carried out, the Agency has developed and issued a list of microbiological contaminants of water, which are likely to significantly affect the public health of consumers of drinking water. The list includes three species of bacteria: *Aeromonas, Mycobacterium avium* and *H. pylori*.

The water contamination of bacteria was documented specially in suburban areas because the number of systems for discharging sewage to sewage treatment plants is inadequate. The reason of these bacterial contaminations is not fully understood but some mechanisms were already proposed. Moreover, many farms and households either have their own small wastewater treatment plants, which do not always function properly, or in worse cases, waste is disposed of by releasing pollutants into nearby rivers, streams or roadside ditches. Some farms have leaky septic tanks often built near wells from which they derive all their household water.

Recent advances in the role of the particular ionic concentrations and the possible correlation between the presence or absence of contamination of water samples tested for *H. pylori* may be an important contribution for tracing the presence of this microorganism in environmental conditions and attempting to define the role of microelements regarding the inhibition or stimulation of *H. pylori* proliferation in water environment.

Determining the concentrations of the suggested ions and the possible correlation between the presence and absence of contamination of water samples tested for *H. pylori* may be an important contribution for tracing the development of this organism in environmental conditions and to attempt to define the role of microelements on the inhibition or stimulation of *H. pylori* proliferation.

4.2.1. Sample preparation

The samples were collected, cooled and stored in polyethylene containers prior to analyses. Before quantitative elemental analysis, if appropriate the samples were filtered and diluted adequately to fit the analytical signal to the linear range of calibration curve.

4.2.2. Quantitative determination of metals

Quantitative determinations of sodium and potassium were made using flame photometry method in air acetylene flame in standard conditions (Perkin Elmer AAS spectrometer Model 3110, USA).

Determinations of Fe, Mg and Zn were performed by means of atomic absorption spectrometry, flame technique (air acetylene flame) using Perkin Elmer AAS spectrometer Model 3110, USA. In both methods, analyses were preceded by thorough optimization of measurement conditions (flame characteristic, burner position, and nebulizer performance). Spectral conditions are given in Table 1.

Element	Method	Lamp type	Wavelength (nm)	Slit (nm)
K	AES		766.5	0.7
Na	AES		589.0	0.2
Fe	F AAS	HCL	248.3	0.2
Mg	F AAS	HCL	285.2	0.7
Zn	F AAS	HCL	213.9	0.7

Table 1. Spectral conditions of elements determination.

All measurements were made using the calibration curve technique. In case of Mg measurements, the samples characterized by high Na concentration were quantified using the method of standard additions calibration. Measurements were made in triplicate.

4.2.3. The methods of molecular assessment of H. pylori

We have collected 150 water samples from different municipal water distribution systems (n=49), rivers (n=48), water reservoirs (n=39) and drinking water tanks and wells (n=14) and they were analyzed between June and December 2012. Samples of 1000 ml water were poured into smaller tubes water and were processed to remove organic matter by centrifugation at 121xg for 5 min. The supernatant was concentrated by centrifugation at 7740xg for 15 min. The resultant pellet was dissolve in 1 ml of PBS, followed by centrifugation at 10 000Xg for 5 min. Finally the pellet was stored at -20°C. Total DNA from concentrated samples for PCR was purified using Genomic Mini or Genomic Mini AX Bacteria (A & A Biotechnology, Gdynia, Poland). DNA was stored at -20°C. All PCR amplifications were performed using the GoTaq DNA Polymerase (Promega, WI, USA) in Thermo cycler T3 (Biometra, Gottingen, Germany).

A negative control with sterile water and positive control with *H. pylori* 43504 DNA were included.

PCR with primers specific for *Helicobacter spp.* and *H. pylori* (Table 2) were used to screen samples for potential presence of *H. pylori.*

First, samples were analyzed for *Helicobacter* species with phosphoglucosamine mutase gene and 23S rRNA *Helicobacter spp.* and then were further tested with primer specific for 16S rRNA hyper variable flanking region of *H. pylori.*

For DNA visualization, electrophoresis or PCR products was performed through 2% agarose gel containing ethidium bromide and gels were photographed under UV light. A 100 bp and 50 bp ladder were used as a molecular weight marker.

Primer	Target site	Sequence (5'→3')	Ref*
GlmM-forward	phosphoglucosamine mutase gene	AGG CTT TTA GGG GTG TTA GGG GTT T	[85]
GlmM-reverse		AAG CTT ACT TTC TAA CAC TAA CGC	
Cluster2	16S rRNA hyper variable flanking region of *H. pylori*	GGC GTT ATC AAC AGA ATG GC	[86]
B1J99		CTC AGT TCG GAT TGT AGG CTG C	
HelGen-forward	23S rRNA *Helicobacter spp.*	AAC GGG GCT AAG ATA GAC	[87]
HelGen-reverse		TCT CAT CTA CCT GTG TCG	

*References

Table 2. PCR primer used in this study.

5. Conclusions that arise in relation to the presented results

On the basis of a chemometric analysis that involved the use of multidimensional data analysis known as multivariate data analysis it was possible to distinguish water samples containing DNA *H. pylori* and from samples that did not contain the DNA (Fig. 4). At the same time a correlation was demonstrated between the presence of *H. pylori* DNA in water samples and phosphate, ammonia and iron concentrations.

In analyzing the results of water sampling conducted in the framework of the project "Detection of Helicobacter pylori in drinking water samples. In what way is the water contaminated and what is the source of contamination?" we have reached the conclusion that we cannot yet say with certainty whether water can be considered as a source of *H. pylori* infection. Questions, therefore, arise to which the answers would be helpful in solving the abovementioned problem.

As the results of our study confirmed the presence of the bacteria in tap water only (i.e., after the process of purification/water treatment), but was not found in rivers, reservoirs and in wells where the water is completely untreated, the first question concerns the existence of a link between the amount of bacteria and the degree and process of the water treatment. The link between the amount of bacteria present in tap water and the distance from the point of chlorination can also be taken into consideration (the farther from the treatment, the smaller the concentration of bactericidal chlorine).

On the basis of these results it can be concluded that the presence of *H. pylori* in water is affected by the season. Confirmation of the presence of *H. pylori* in the water samples taken in June, while there was no evidence of it in October, may also result from the fact that each of the water treatment plants in Krakow uses a number of technological processes for water treatment, depending on the quality of the water collected. Accordingly, further examinations should be conducted to ascertain whether the presence of *H. pylori* is actually related to the time of year, or to other factors.

This raises the question - if the bacteria can survive for so long in distilled water, does this mean that the physiologically important endogenous pool of metals is enough for them?

If so we can expect that the metals in the water around them will be important for their survival? On the other hand, there is no doubt about the effects of toxic metals, but these levels are continuously monitored in water - as is the bacterial cell toxicity of heavy metals. And do the levels of acceptable standards for drinking water have anything to do with this.

6. Further research

1. Determination of *H. pylori* interaction with co-occurring elements in water by enriching their culture media with in the laboratory experiment.

2. Understanding the effects of dissolved organic carbon in the survival of bacteria during water treatment.

3. Taking into account the differences in the composition and concentration studied seasonal elements for the possible coexistence of *H. pylori*.

These relationships can be used to develop a better method of treating water in order to minimize the exposure of humans to infection

Acknowledgements

The study was a part of the project of National Center of Science in Poland entitled "Detection of *Helicobacter pylori* in drinking water samples. In what way is the water contaminated and what is the source of contamination?" to Drs. Plonka, Targosz and Brzozowski as principal investigators. This work was supported by grant No 2011/01/B/NZ/01539.

Author details

Malgorzata Plonka[1,2], Aneta Targosz[2] and Tomasz Brzozowski[2*]

*Address all correspondence to: mpbrzozo@cyf-kr.edu.pl

1 University School of Physical Education, Cracow, Poland

2 Department of Physiology Jagiellonian University Medical College, Cracow, Poland

References

[1] Brown LM. Helicobacter pylori: epidemiology and routes of transmission. Epidemiol. Rev. 2000; 22: 283–297.

[2] Percival SL, Thomas JG. Transmission of Helicobacter pylori and the role of water and biofilms. J. Water Health 2009; 7(3): 469-477.

[3] Mazari-Hiriart M, Lopez-Vidal Y, Ponce de Leon S, Castillo-Rojas G, Hernandez-Eugenio C, Rojo F. Bacteria and disinfection byproducts in water from southern Mexico City. Arch. Environ. Health 2003; 58: 233–237.

[4] Baker KH, Hegarty JP, Redmond B, Reed NA, Herson DS. Effect of oxidizing disinfectants (chlorine monochloramine and ozone) on Helicobacter pylori. Appl. Environ. Microbiol. 2002; 68: 981–984.

[5] Moreno Y, Piqueres P, Alonso JL, Jimenez A, Gonzalez A, Ferrus MA. Survival and viability of Helicobacter pylori after inoculation into chlorinated drinking water. Water Res. 2007; 41: 3490–3496.

[6] Frenck RW, Clemens J. Heliocobacter in the developing world. Microbes Infect. 2003; 5: 705–713.

[7] Konturek PC, Konturek SJ, Brzozowski T. Helicobacter pylori infection in gastric cancerogensesis. J Physiol. Pharmacol. 2009; 60(3): 3-21.

[8] Lee A, Fox JG, Otto G, Dick EH, Krakowka S. Transmission of Helicobacter spp. A challenge to the dogma of fecal-oral spread. Epidemiol Infect. 1991; 107(1): 99–109.

[9] Cave DR. How is Helicobacter pylori transmitted? Gastroenterology 1997; 113(6): 9-14.

[10] Malaty HM, Graham DY, Klein PD, Evans DG, Adam E, Evans DJ. Transmission of Helicobacter pylori infection. Studies in families of healthy individuals. Scand. J Gastroenterology 1991; 26: 927–932.

[11] Drum B, Perez-Perez GI, Blaser MJ, Sherman PM. Intrafamilial clustering of Helicobacter pylori infection. N Engl J Med.1990; 322: 359–63.

[12] Brenner H, Rothenbacher D, Bode G, Dieudonne P, Adler G. Active infection with Helicobacter pylori in healthy couples. Epidemiol Infect.1999; 122: 91-95.

[13] Parente F, Maconi G, Sangaletti O, et al. Prevalence of Helicobacter pylori and related gastroduodenal lesions in spouses of Helicobacter pylori positive patients with duodenal ulcer. Gut 1996; 39: 629–33.

[14] Rothenbacher D, Bode G, Berg G, Knayer U, Gonser T, Adler G, Brenner H, Helicobacter pylori among preschool children and their parents: evidence of parent- child transmission. J Infect Dis.1999; 179 (2): 398-402.

[15] Brenner H, Rothenbacher D, Bode G, Adler G. Parental history of gastric or duodenal ulcer and Helicobacter pylori infection among pre-school children: evidence for mother-infant transmission. BMJ 1998; 316: 665.

[16] Lambert JR, Lin SK, Sievert W, Nicholson L, Schembri M, Guest C. High prevalence of Helicobacter pylori antibodies in an institutionalized population: evidence for person-to-person transmission. Am J Gastroenterol. 1995; 90 (12): 2167-71.

[17] Böhmer CJ, Klinkenberg-Knol EC, Kuipers EJ, Niezen-de Boer MC, Schreuder H, Schuckink-Kool F, Meuwissen SG. The prevalence of Helicobacter pylori infection among inhabitants and healthy employees of institutes for the intellectually disabled. Am J Gastroenterol 1997; 92 (6):1000-4.

[18] Kimura A, Matsubasa T, Kinoshita H, Kuriya N, Yamashita Y, Fujisawa T, Terakura H, Shinohara M. Helicobacter pylori seropositivity in patients with severe neurologic impairment. Brain Dev.1999; 21(2):113-7.

[19] Harris AW, Douds A, Meurisse EV, Dennis M, Chambers S, Gould SR. Seroprevalence of Helicobacter pylori in residents of a hospital for people with severe learning difficulties. Eur J Gastroenterol Hepatol. 1995; 7(1):.21-3.

[20] Lewindon PJ, Lau D, Chan A, Tse P, Sullivan PB. Helicobacter pylori in an institution for disabled children in Hong Kong. Dev Med Child Neurol. 1997; 39(10): 682-5.

[21] Malaty HM, Paykov V, Bykova O, Ross A, Graham DP, Anneger JF, Graham DY. Helicobacter pylori and socioeconomic factors in Russia. Helicobacter.1996; 1(2): 82-7.

[22] Vincent P, Gottrand F, Pernes P, Husson MO, Lecomte-Houcke M, Turck D, Leclerc H. High prevalence of Helicobacter pylori infection in cohabiting children. Epidemiology of a cluster, with special emphasis on molecular typing. Gut. 1994; 35(3): 313–316.

[23] Mégraud F. Transmission of Helicobacter pylori: faecal-oral versus oral-oral route. Aliment Pharmacol Ther. 1995; 9(2): 85-91.

[24] Pytko-Polończyk J, Konturek SJ, Karczewska E, Bielański W, Kaczmarczyk A. Oral cavity as permanent reservoir of Helicobacter pylori and potential source of reinfection. J Physiol Pharmacol.1996; 47(1):121–129.

[25] Parsonnet J, Shmuely H, Haggerty T. Fecal and Oral Shedding of Helicobacter pylori From Healthy Infected Adults JAMA. 1999; 282(23): 2240-2245.

[26] Thomas JE, Gibson GR, Darboe MK, Dale A, Weaver LT. Isolation of Helicobacter pylori from human faeces. Lancet 1992; 340(14):1194-5.

[27] Graham DY. Helicobacter pylori: Future Direction in Research Helicobacter pylori. Gastritis and Peptic Ulcer 1990:463-470.

[28] Klein PD, Graham DY, Gaillour A, Opekun AR, Smith EO. Water source as risk factor for Helicobacter pylori infection in Peruvian children. Gastrointestinal Physiology Working Group. Lancet. 1991; 337(22):1503-6.

[29] Tytgat GN. Endoscopic transmission of Helicobacter pylori. Aliment Pharmacol Ther. 1995; 9(2): 105-10.

[30] Lin SK, Lambert JR, Schembri MA, Nicholson L, Johnson IH. The prevalence of Helicobacter pylori in practicing dental staff and dental students. Aust Dent J. 1998; 43(1): 35-9.

[31] Lin SK, Lambert JR, Schembri MA, Nicholson L, Korman MG. Helicobacter pylori prevalence in endoscopy and medical staff. J Gastroenterol Hepatol. 1994; 9(4): 319-24.

[32] Handt LK, Fox JG, Dewhirst FE, Fraser GJ, Paster BJ, Yan LL, Rozmiarek H, Rufo R, Stalis IH. Helicobacter pylori isolated from the domestic cat: public health implications. Infect Immun. 1994; 62(6): 2367-74.

[33] Fox JG. Non-human reservoirs of Helicobacter pylori. Aliment Pharmacol Ther.1995; 9(2):93-103.

[34] Grubel P, Hoffman JS, Chong FK, Burstein NA, Mepani C, Cave DR. Vector potential of houseflies (Musca domestica) for Helicobacter pylori. J Clin Microbiol. 1997; 35(6): 1300-3.

[35] Grubel P, Huang L, Masubuchi N, Stutzenberger FJ, Cave DR. Detection of helicobacter-pylori DNA in houseflies (musca-domestica) on 3 continents. Lancet 1998: 352: 788-789.

[36] Vaira D, Holton J. Vector potential of houseflies (Musca domestica) for Helicobacter pylori. Helicobacter.1998; 3(1):65-6.

[37] Goodman KJ, Correa P, Tenganá Aux HJ, Ramírez H, DeLany JP, Guerrero Pepinosa O, López Quiñones M, Collazos Parra T. Helicobacter pylori infection in the Colombian Andes: a population-based study of transmission pathways. Am J Epidemiol. 1996, 144(3): 290-9.

[38] Dore MP, Bilotta M, Vaira D, Manca A, Massarelli G, Leandro G, Atzei A, Pisanu G, Graham DY, Realdi G. High prevalence of Helicobacter pylori infection in shepherds. Dig Dis Sci. 1999;.44(6):1161-4.

[39] Papiez D, Konturek PC, Bielanski W, Plonka M, Dobrzanska M, Kaminska A, Szczyrk U, Bochenek A, Wierzchos E. Prevalence of Helicobacter pylori infection in Polish shepherds and their families. Dig Liver Dis. 2003; 35(1):10-5.

[40] Plonka M, Bielanski W, Konturek SJ, Targosz A, Sliwowski Z, Dobrzanska M, Kaminska A, Sito E, Konturek PC, Brzozowski T. Helicobacter pylori infection and serum gastrin, ghrelin and leptin in children of Polish shepherds. Dig Liver Dis. 2006; 38(2): 91-7.

[41] Teh BH, Lin JT, Pan WH, Lin SH, Wang LY, Lee TK, Chen CJ. Seroprevalence and associated risk factors of Helicobacter pylori infection in Taiwan. Anticancer Res. 1994; 14, (3B): 1389-92.

[42] Hopkins RJ, Vial PA, Ferreccio C, Ovalle J, Prado P, Sotomayor V, Russell RG. Wasserman SS. Glenn J, Morris J. Seroprevalence of Helicobacter pylori in Chile: Vegetables May Serve as One Route of Transmission. J Infect Dis. 1993; 168(1): 222-226.

[43] She FF, Lin JY, Liu JY, Huang C, Su DH. Virulence of water-induced coccoid Helicobacter pylori and its experimental infection in mice. World Journal of Gastroenterology 2003; 9: 516–520.

[44] Nabwera HM, Logan RP. Epidemiology of Helicobacter pylori: transmission, translocation and extragastric reservoirs. Journal of Physiology and Pharmacology 1999; 50: 711–722.

[45] Velazquez M, Feirtag JM. Helicobacter pylori: characteristics, pathogenicity, detection methods and mode of transmission implicating foods and water. International Journal of Food Microbiology 1999; 53: 95–104.

[46] Vale FF, Vítor JMB.. Transmission pathway of Helicobacter pylori: Does food play a role in rural and urban areas? International Journal of Food Microbiology 2010; 138: 1–12.

[47] Lu Y, Redlinger TE, Avitia R, Galindo A, Goodman K. Isolation and genotyping of Helicobacter pylori from untreatedmunicipal wastewater. Applied and Environmental Microbiology 2002; 68: 1436–1439.

[48] Cellini L, Di CE, Grand R, Di BS, Prenna M., Pasquantonio M, Pane L. Detection of Helicobacter pylori associated with zooplankton. Aquatic Microbial Ecology: International Journal 2005; 40: 115–120.

[49] Cellini L, Del VA, Di CM, Di CE, Favaro M, Donelli G. Detection of free and plankton-associated Helicobacter pylori in seawater. Journal of Applied Microbiology 2004; 97: 285–292.

[50] Samra ZQ, Javaid U, Ghafoor S, Batool A, Dar N, Athar MA. PCR assay targeting virulence genes of Helicobacter pylori isolated from drinking water and clinical samples in Lahore metropolitan, Pakistan. J Water Health 2011; 9(1): 208-16.

[51] Mazari-Hiriart M, Lopez-Vidal Y, Calva JJ. Helieobaeter pylori in water systems for human use in Mexico City. Water Sei. Tech. 2001; 43: 93-98.

[52] Nurgalieva Z. Heiicobacter pylori infection in Kazakhstan: effect of water source and household hygiene. Am. J. Trop. Med. Hyg. 2002; 67: 201-206.

[53] Azevedo NF, Almeida C, Fernandes I, Cerqueira L, Dias S, Keevil CW, Vieira MJ. Survival of gastric and enterohepatic Helicobacter spp. in water: implications for transmission. Applied and Environmental Microbiology 2008; 74: 1805–1811.

[54] Queralt N, Araujo R. Analysis of the survival of H. pylori within a laboratory based aquatic model system using molecular and classical techniques. Microbial Ecology 2007; 54: 771–777.

[55] Shahamat M,Mai U, Paszko-Kolva C, Kessel M, Colwell RR. Use of autoradiography to assess viability of Helicobacter pylori in water. Applied and Environmental Microbiology 1993; 59: 1231–1235.

[56] Percival SL, Thomas JG. Transmission of Helicobacter pylori and the role of water and biofilms. Journal of Water and Health 2009; 7: 469–477.

[57] Giao MS, Azevedo NF, Wilks SA, Vieira MJ, Keevil CW. 2008. Persistence of Helicobacter pylori in heterotrophic drinking-water biofilms. Applied and Environmental Microbiology 74, 5898–5904.

[58] Gouider, M., Bouzid, J., Sayadi, S., Montiel, A. Impact of orthophosphate addition on biofilm development in drinking water distribution systems. Journal of Hazardous Materials 2009; 167: 1198–1202.

[59] Stoodley P, Wilson S, Hall-Stoodley L, Boyle JD, Lappin-Scott HM., Costerton JW. Growth and detachment of cell clusters from mature mixed-species biofilms. Applied and Environmental Microbiology 2001; 67: 5608–5613.

[60] Degnan AJ, Sonzogni WC, Standridge JH. Development of a plating medium for selection of Helieobaeter pylori from water samples. App. Environ. Mierobiol. 2003; 69(5): 2914-2918.

[61] Fernández M, Contreras M, Suárez P, Gueneau P, García-Amado MA. Use of HP selective medium to detect Helicobacter pylori associated with other enteric bacteria in seawater and marine mollusks. Lett Appl Microbiol 2007; 45(2): 213-8.

[62] Rowan NJ. Viable but non-culturable forms of food and waterborne bacteria: quo vadis? Trends Food Sci. Technol. 2004; 15: 462–467.

[63] Moreno Y, Ferrus MA, Alonso JL, Jimenez A, Herandez J. Use of fluorescent in situ hybridization to evidence the presence of Helicobacter pylori in water. Water Res. 2003; 37: 2251–2256.

[64] Hegarty JP, Dowd MT, Baker KH. Occurrence of Helicobacter pylori in surface water in the United States. J. Appl. Microbiol. 1999; 87: 697–701.

[65] Azevedo NF, Pacheco AP, Keevil CW, Vieira MJ. Adhesion of water stressed Helicobacter pylori to abiotic surfaces. J. Appl. Microbiol. 2006; 101: 718–724.

[66] Sen K, Schable NA, Lye DJ. Development of an internal control for evaluation and standardization of a quantitative PCR assay for detection of Helicobacter pylori in drinking water. Appl. Environ. Microbiol. 2007; 73: 7380–7387.

[67] Mizoguchi H, Fujioka T, Nasu M. Evidence for viability of coccoid forms of Helicobacter pylori. J. Gastroenterol. 1999; 34(Suppl.11): 32–36.

[68] Zheng PY, Hua J, Ng HC, Ho B. Unchanged characteristics of Helicobacter pylori during its morphological conversion. Microbios 1999; 98: 51–64.

[69] Moreno Y, Ferrus MA, Alonso JL, Jimenez A, Herandez J. Use of fluorescent in situ hybridization to evidence the presence of Helicobacter pylori in water. Water Res. 2003; 37: 2251–2256.

[70] Nayak AK, Rose JB. Detection of Helicobacter pylori in sewage and water using a new quantitative PCR method with SYBR green. J. Appl. Microbiol. 2007; 103: 1931–1941.

[71] Janzon A, Sjoling A, Lothigius A, Ahmed D, Qadri F, Svennerholm AM. Failure To Detect Helicobacter pylori DNA in Drinking and Environmental Water in Dhaka,

Bangladesh, Using Highly Sensitive Real-Time PCR Assays. Appl. Environ. Microbiol. 2009; 75(10): 3039–3044.

[72] Costerton JW, Stewart PS, Greenberg EP. Bacterial biofilms: a common cause of persistent infections. Science 1999; 284:1318–1322.

[73] Percival SL, Walker J, Hunter PR. Microbiological Aspects of Biofilms and Drinking Water. CRC Press, New York 2000.

[74] Sibille I, Sime-Ngando T, Mathieu L, Block JC. Protozoan bacterivory and Escherichia coli survival in drinking water distribution systems. Appl. Environ. Microbiol. 1998; 64: 197–202.

[75] Percival SL, Chalmers RM, Embrey M, Hunter PR, Sellwood J, Wyn-Jones P. Microbiology of Waterborne Diseases. Elsevier Academic Press 2004, London.

[76] MacKay WG, Gribbon LT, Barer MR, Reid DC. Biofilms in drinking water systems: a possible reservoir for Helicobacter pylori. J. Appl. Microbiol. 1999; 85: 52s–59s.

[77] Andersen LP, Rasmussen L. Helicobacter pylori-coccoid forms and biofilm formation. FEMS Immunol Med Microbiol. 2009; 56 (2): 112-5.

[78] Park SR., MacKay WG, Reid DC. Helicobacter sp. recovered from drinking water biofilm sampled from a water distribution system. Water Res. 2001; 35: 1624–1626.

[79] Bunn JE, MacKay WG, Thomas JE, Reid DC, Weaver LT. Detection of Helicobacter pylori DNA in drinking water biofilms: implications for transmission in early life. Lett. Appl. Microbiol. 2002; 34: 450–454.

[80] Watson CL, Owen RJ, Said B, Lai S, Lee JV, Surman-Lee S, Nichols G. Detection of Helicobacter pylori by PCR but not culture in water and biofilm samples from drinking water distribution systems in England. J. Appl. Microbiol. 2004; 97: 690–698.

[81] Adams BL, Bates TC, Oliver JD. Survival of Helicobacter pylori in a natural freshwater environment. Appl. Environ. Microbiol. 2003; 69: 7462–7466.

[82] Azevedo NF, Vieira MJ, Keevil CW. Establishment of a continuous model system to study Helicobacter pylori survival in potable water biofilms. Water Sci. Technol. 2003; 47:155–160.

[83] Azevedo NF, Pinto AR, Reis NM, Vieira MJ, Keevil CW. Shear stress, temperature, and inoculation concentration influence the adhesion of water-stressed Helicobacter pylori to stainless steel 304 and polypropylene. Appl. Environ. Microbiol. 2006; 72: 2936–2941.

[84] Azevedo NF, Almeida C, Cerqueira L, Dias S, Keevil CW, Vieira MJ. Coccoid form of Helicobacter pylori as a morphological manifestation of cell adaptation to the environment. Appl. Environ. Microbiol. 2007; 73:3423–3427.

[85] Shahamat M, Alavi M, Watts JEM, Gonzalez JM, Sowers KR, Maeder GW, Robb FT. Development of two PCR-based techniques for detecting helical and coccoid forms of Helicobacter pylori. J. Clin. Microbiol. 2004; 3613-3619.

[86] Lu JJ, Perng CI, Shyu RY, Chen CH, Lou Q, Chong SKF, Lee CH. Comparison of five methods for detection of Helicobacter pylori DNA in gastric tissues. J. Clin. Microbiol 1999; 37: 772-774.

[87] Twing KI, Kirchman DL, Campbell BJ. Temporal study of Helicobacter pylori presence in coastal freshwater, estuary and marine waters. Water Research 2011; 45: 1897-1995.

Section 3

H. pylori and Gastric Cancer: Molecular Epidemiology and Possibilities of Prevention

Chapter 4

Molecular Epidemiology of *Helicobacter pylori* in Brazilian Patients with Early Gastric Cancer and a Review to Understand the Prognosis of the Disease

Bruna Maria Roesler and
José Murilo Robilotta Zeitune

Additional information is available at the end of the chapter

http://dx.doi.org/10.5772/58328

1. Introduction

Helicobacter pylori (*H. pylori*) is an universally distributed bacterium that affects more than half of the world population and is considered an important public health problem. Although colonization with *H. pylori* is not actually a disease, it is a condition that affects the relative risk of developing various clinical disorders of the upper gastrointestinal tract, as chronic gastritis, peptic ulcer disease, mucosa-associated lymphoid tissue (MALT lymphoma) and gastric adenocarcinoma, and, possibly, extradigestive diseases.

Colonization with *H. pylori* virtually leads to infiltration of the gastric mucosa in both antrum and corpus with neutrophilic and mononuclear cells. Gastritis can be classified as an acute or chronic gastritis and it can involve all parts of the stomach or just the fundus, corpus or antrum. The chronic active gastritis is the primary condition related to *H. pylori* colonization, and other *H. pylori*-associated disorders, in particular, resulting from this chronic inflammatory process, as atrophic gastritis, causing an elevated risk of gastric cancer. Considering this association, in 1994 the bacterium was classified as a group I carcinogen by the International Agency for Research on Cancer, World Health Organization.

Molecular techniques have revealed that *H. pylori* possesses a remarkable degree of genetic diversity, which could be responsible for its adaptation in the host stomach and for its pathological characteristics, in addition to the clinical outcome of the infection, although this aspect remains unclear.

In Brazil, it is estimated that only about 10 to 15% of the gastric cancer cases are diagnosed at an early stage, aspect that directly impact the prognosis of the disease, which presents low survival rates. Unlike patients with advanced gastric cancer, that ones diagnosed at the early stage of the disease present an excellent prognostic, in which a five-year survival rate is more than 90%.

Many early gastric cancers are believed to go through a life cycle consisting of ulcerations, followed by healing, then reulceration, and some tumors remain at this early stage for years even without treatment. Nevertheless, some of these tumors rapidly advanced, perhaps one of the principal questions concerning the gastric carcinogenesis.

Consequently, some questions can be considered about it. Is the *H. pylori* presence important for the evolution of the early lesions in advanced ones? To what extent *H. pylori* eradication could prevent the progression of lesions from one to another stage? Are the genetic characteristics of *H. pylori* strain that is colonizing the patient with early gastric cancer important for the progression of the disease in a faster or in a slower way?

The principal aim of our book chapter is to identify the genetic characteristics of *H. pylori* strains in Brazilian patients diagnosed with early distal type intestinal gastric adenocarcinoma, trying to determine the genotypic pattern of bacterium in our population through molecular techniques. Besides, other aim of our study is to discuss the principal aspects of the *H. pylori* infection and then correlate them with the development of the precancerous lesions and the development of the early gastric cancer properly, trying to understand to what extent the microorganism eradication treatment could be important to preventing the disease progression.

2. *Helicobacter pylori*

2.1. General characteristics

Helicobacter pylori (H. pylori) is a spiral-shaped Gram-negative flagellate bacterium that colonizes the human stomach and can establish a long-term infection of the gastric mucosa [1]. In gastric biopsy specimens, *H. pylori* organisms are 2.5 to 5.0 μm long and 0.5 to 1.0 μm wide, with four to six unipolar sheated flagella, which are essential for bacterial motility. When cultured on solid medium, the bacteria assume a rod-like shape and spiral shapes are infrequent or absent [2]; after prolonged culture on solid or liquid medium, coccoid forms, that are metabolically active, tipically predominate [3].

Gastric colonization with *H. pylori* affects at least half the world´s population, and, while the infection is on a fast decline in most of the western countries, mainly due to the success of therapeutic regimens and improved personal and community hygiene that prevents re-infection, the situation is exactly opposite in many of the developing countries due to failure of treatment and emergence of drug resistance [4,5]. Most studies suggest that males and females are infected at approximately the same rates [6] and, probably, the infection occurs in the childhood. In developed countries, persons of higher socioeconomic status have lower infection rates, although among certain ethnic minorities, high rates persist despite economic advancement [7].

http://dx.doi.org/10.5772/58328

The routes of transmission of *H. pylori* still remain unclear. Person-to-person transmission and intrafamilial spread seem to be the main route, based on the intrafamilial clustering observed in some studies [8,9]. Children are often infected by a strain which a genetic fingerprint identical to that of their parents, and they maintain this genotype even after moving to a different environment [10]. Animals harbor organisms that resemble *H. pylori,* but with the exception of nonhuman primates [11] and, under particular circumstances, perhaps cats [12] and houseflies (*Musca domestica*) [13], none harbor *H. pylori.* In the same way, food-borne transmission has not been substantiated [14]. Nevertheless, the waterborne infection remains possible [15,16].

H. pylori remains one of the most common worldwide human infections and its isolation by Marshall and Warren (1984) [17] has markedly improved our understanding about the nature of chronic gastritis and other important upper gastrointestinal disorders, such as peptic ulcer disease, mucosa-associated lymphoid tissue (MALT) lymphoma and gastric adenocarcinoma [18]. In 1994, the bacterium was classified as a group I carcinogen by the International Agency for Research on Cancer and is regarded as a primary factor for gastric cancer development [19]. For their revolutionary discovery, Marshall and Warren received the Nobel Prize in Physiology or Medicine in 2005.

In addition, in the last years, *H. pylori* infection has also been associated with some extradigestive diseases, such as iron-deficiency anemia [20], idiopathic thrombocytopenic purpura [21,22], cardiovascular diseases [23,24], hepatobiliary diseases [25,26], and diabetes mellitus [27], among others.

2.2. Virulence factors of *H. Pylori*

H. pylori populations are highly diverse and constantly change their genome, which can be an important factor in its adaptation to the host stomach and also for the clinical outcome of the infection. The changes in its genome occur mainly due to point mutations, substitutions, insertions, and/or deletions of their genome. Moreover, mixed infections are frequent and lead to exchange of DNA fragments between different *H. pylori* strains in a single host [28,29]. Experience with other bacterial pathogens suggests that *H. pylori*-specific factors may exist that influence the microorganism pathogenicity, and, these factors, together with the host genetic characteristics and the external environment, can contribute to the clinical outcome of the infection. Among the most studied virulence factors of *H. pylori* are the urease gene, the vacuolating cytotoxin gene (vacA), the cytotoxin associated gene-Pathogenicity Island (cagPAI) and the duodenal ulcer promoting gene (dupA).

Urease is an important enzyme which is produced by *H. pylori* to counteract the acidic environment of the stomach. Urease causes damage to the epithelium through the production of ammonia, that, in conjunction with neutrophil metabolites, forms carcinogenic agents that might participate in the development of gastric malignances [30,31]. Ammonia is capable to cause different cell alterations, including swelling of intracellular acidic compartments, alterations of vesicular membrane transport, repression of protein synthesis and ATP production, and cell-cycle arrest [32]. Urease might also help to the recruitment of neutrophils and monocytes in the mucosa and to the production of proinflammatory cytokines

[33]. It has been demonstrated that this enzyme plays and important hole in the *H. pylori* colonization, being observed that urease-defective bacteria mutants are not able to colonize the gastric environment [32].

VacA is a cytotoxin secreted from *H. pylori* as a large 140kd polypeptide and latter trimmed at both ends to finally deliver it in an active form to host cells, where it exerts its activity [34]. The gene encoding VacA is present in all *H. pylori* strains and displays allelic diversity in three main regions: s (signal), i (intermediate) and m (middle); consequently, the activity of the toxin varies between strains [35]. Different combinations of two major alleles of each region (s1, s2, i1, i2, m1, m2) may exist, which results in VacA toxins with distinct capability of inducing vacuolating in epithelial cells [36]. VacA induces multiple cellular activities, including the alteration in the endosomal maturation which consequently leads to vacuolating of epithelial cells, the induction of membrane-channel formation, the cytochrome c releasing from mitochondria and the binding to cell-membrane receptors activating a proinflammatory response [35].

The cagPAI is a 40kb region of chromosomal DNA encoding approximately 31 genes that forms a type IV secretion system that forms a pilus that delivers CagA, an oncoprotein, into the cytosol of gastric epithelial cells through a rigid needle structure covered by CagY, a VirB10-homologous protein and CagT, a VirB7-homologous protein, at the base [37,38]. cagA is a polymorphic gene that presents different numbers of repeat sequences located in its 3′region and each repeat region of the CagA protein contains Glu-Pro-IIe-Tyr-Ala (EPIYA) motifs, including a tyrosine phosphorylation site [39]. Upon delivery into host cells, CagA undergoes Src-dependent tyrosine phosphorylation and activates an eukaryotic phosphatase (SHP-2), leading to dephosphorylation of host cell proteins and cellular morphologic changes [40]. CagA has also been shown to dysregulate β-catenin signaling [41] and apical-junctional complexes [42], events that have been linked to increased cell motility and oncogenic transformation in a variety of models [43]. In addition, some studies have been reported that the cagPAI appears to be involved in the induction of gastric interleukin-8 (IL-8) production, a potent neutrophil-activating chemokine [44]. Consequently, the presence of the cagA gene has been associated with higher grades of inflammation, which may lead to the development of the most severe gastrointestinal diseases, such as peptic ulcer disease and gastric cancer [45-48].

H. pylori duodenal ulcer promoting gene (dupA), located in the plasticity region of bacterium genome, has been initially described as a risk marker for duodenal ulcer development and a protective factor against gastric cancer [49]. It was the first putative specific marker whose association was described using strains obtained from in both Asian (Japan and Korea) and Western (Colombia) regions and it is though to be a *vir*B4 homologue [49, 50]. dupA gene encompasses two continuous sequences, jhp0917 and jhp0918, as described in strain J99. The jhp0917 gene encodes a protein of 475 amino acids, but lacks a region homologous to the C-terminus of *vir*B4, while jhp0918 gene encodes a product of 140 amino acids that is homologous to the missing *vir*B4 region [51]. Since its discovery, dupA gene has been studied by various authors, and the results of their researches suggest that, in some places, dupA gene is not associated with an specific disease [52], or it is suggested that it can be associated with gastric cancer development [53-55], or it is directly associated with the development of duodenal ulcer disease [50,56]. Considering all these results, it is suggested that there must be diversity in gene content that can contribute to bacterial adaptation to genetically different ethnic groups that make up de human population [57].

3. Gastric cancer

3.1. Epidemiology

Cancer is a worldwide full-scale problem as it will affect one in three men and one in four women during their lifetime [58]. Nowadays, this disease represents one in eight deaths around the world. The global cancer rate has doubled in the last 30 years of the 20th century, and will almost triple by 2030, a year in which it is foreseen that 20.3 million people will be diagnosed cancer and 13.2 million will die as a result of this disease [59].

World Health Organization estimates that 43% of cancer deaths are due tobacco, diet and infection. One-fifth of cancers worldwide are due to chronic infections, mainly from hepatitis viruses (liver), papillomaviruses (cervix), *H. pylori* (stomach), schistosomes (bladder), the liver fluke (bile duct), and human immunodeficiency virus (Kaposi sarcoma and lymphoma) [60].

Gastric cancer continues to be a major global health problem [61] and, despite the decreasing incidence and mortality rates observed worldwide over the last 50 years, it still ranks as a leading cause of cancer-related deaths in many parts of the world [62]. As symptoms are often absent or nonspecific in patients with the early stages of the disease, gastric cancer is usually diagnosed in an advanced stage, when curative options are limited. With exceptions in countries that have developed screening programs for early diagnoses, as example Japan, most patients reach treatment with cancers already in advanced stages [63]. Consequently, gastric cancer carries a poor prognosis, with an overall five-year survival rate of less than 20% [64].

Besides, one study assessed the survival of gastric cancer in population-based registries obtained in cities from four continents and concluded that the large differences observed among these areas were exclusively due to the different types of stomach cancer, highlighting the importance of the stage of the disease as an indicator of the effect of delayed diagnosis on the prognosis of these patients [65].

In Brazil, in 2005, the highest incidence rates, adjusted by age, were found in São Paulo (male, 38,8/100.000; female, 15,0/100.000) and the Federal District (male, 32,7/100.000; female 14,7/100.000) [66]. The National Institute of Cancer in Brazil estimates that, in 2014, there will occur 580.000 new cases of cancer. The most frequent cancers in Brazilian population will be non-melanoma skin (182.000), prostate (69.000), breast (57.000), colon and rectum (33.000), lung (27.000) and stomach (20.000). Considering Brazilian regions and gender, gastric cancer will be the fourth most common cancer in Brazil. In male gender, it is the second most common tumour in the North (11/100.000 cases) and Northeast (10/100.000 cases) regions; it is the fourth most common tumour in the Midwest (11/100.000 cases) and in the South (16/100.000) regions and the fifth most common in the Southeast region (15/100.000 cases). Concerning the female gender, gastric cancer is the fifth most common cancer in Brazil, the third most frequent in the

North region (6/100.000 cases), and the fifth most frequent in the Northeast (6/100.000 cases) and Southeast (8/100.000 cases) regions [67].

The chances of surviving the onset of some common cancers depend largely on how early they are detected and how well they are treated. Early detection is based on the observation that treatment is more effective when cancer is detected early. It includes awareness of early signs and symptoms of cancer and screening, which is the mass testing of people who appear to be healthy. In many developing countries, where these are not feasible, several other low technology approaches are being studied and look promising. The success of public health programmes in detecting cancer early depends on the allocation of resources, availability of qualified specialists and access to follow-up treatment [60].

3.2. Classification of gastric cancer

The vast majority of gastric cancers are adenocarcinomas. Two histologically distinct variants of gastric adenocarcinoma have been described, each with different pathophysiological features: the diffuse type and the intestinal type [68], which corresponds, respectively, to the undifferentiated or poorly-differentiated type and to the well-differentiated type, in the Japanese classification [69].

Diffuse type gastric adenocarcinoma is often associated with familial distribution and more commonly affects younger people. It consists of individually infiltrating neoplastic cells that do not form glandular structures and arises closer to the advancing border of inflammation but without any identifiable histological precursor lesion [62,70,71].

Gastric adenocarcinoma of the intestinal type is preceded by a prolonged precancerous process. In 1975, Correa and colleagues proposed a model of gastric carcinogenesis, postulating that the intestinal type of gastric cancer was the end result of progressive changes in the gastric mucosa, starting with chronic gastritis, followed by multifocal atrophic gastritis and intestinal metaplasia [72]. This model was updated in 1988 and 1992 [73,74] and the following steps were recognized: normal gastric mucosa → superficial gastritis (later renamed non-atrophic gastritis) → multifocal atrophic gastritis without intestinal metaplasia → intestinal metaplasia of the complete (small intestine) type → intestinal metaplasia of the incomplete (colonic) type → low-grade dysplasia (low-grade noninvasive dysplasia) → high-grade dysplasia (high-grade noninvasive dysplasia) → invasive adenocarcinoma [75]. These lesions are well-characterized histopathologically and represent a continuum of changes depicting multiple events that increase in intensity and extension with time [76].

Both diffuse and intestinal types are associated with *H. pylori* infection, which plays an initiating role in the pathogenesis of gastric cancer by changing many important factors, including antioxidant agents, reactive oxygen metabolites, and the balance between epithelial cell proliferation and apoptosis [77]. *H. pylori* infection induces cell apoptosis, stimulates cell proliferation in the gastric epithelium, and causes alterations or mutations of apoptosis/ proliferation-related genes [78].

3.3. *Helicobacter pylori* and gastric cancer — The precancerous cascade

Exposure of gastric epithelial cells to *H. pylori* results in an inflammatory reaction with the production of reactive oxygen species and nitric oxide that, in turn, deaminates DNA causing mutations [62]. The complex interplay among *H. pylori* strain, inflammation and host characteristics, besides the external environment, may directly promote diffuse type gastric cancer or induce the cascade of morphological events that leads to intestinal type gastric cancer.

Specifically regarding to intestinal type gastric adenocarcinoma, evidence that *H. pylori* increases the risk of gastric cancer development via the sequence of atrophy and metaplasia originates from various studies, in which it was shown that *H. pylori* positive subjects develop these conditions more often than do uninfected controls [79]. Consequently, since *H. pylori* isolation, many investigators have emphasized its role in gastric carcinogenesis [80,81]. Epidemiological studies have determined that the attributable risk for gastric cancer conferred by *H. pylori* is approximately 75% [82]. Besides, in respect to localization in the stomach, premalignant lesions are most frequently localized in the antrum in the transitional zone between the antrum and corpus [83].

As explained before, Correa and colleagues (1975) proposed a model of gastric carcinogenesis, considering that the intestinal type gastric cancer probably is the result of histological continuum changes that occur especially due to *H. pylori* infection: chronic active nonatrophic gastritis, multifocal atrophic gastritis, intestinal metaplasia, dysplasia, and, finally, invasive adenocarcinoma. Consequently, the principal characteristics of each one of these stages are report below.

3.3.1. *Chronic active non-atrophic gastritis*

Gastritis is characterized by increased infiltration of the lamina propria with mononuclear leukocytes (chronic inflammation) and polymorphonuclear neutrophils (acute inflammation). Additionally, scattered eosinophils and mast cells can be observed. The gastritis is called "active" when polymorphonuclear neutrophils are found, representing acute inflammation. This phase of the precancerous process does not show loss of glands (atrophy) and is called "nonatrophic gastritis" in the updated Sydney classification of gastritis, adopted by most pathologists (Figure 1) [84].

The most frequent cause of gastritis is *H. pylori* infection and the severity of inflammation may vary according to the infected *H. pylori* strain [75].

3.3.2. *Multifocal atrophic gastritis*

Loss of normal glandular tissue is the first specific recognizable step in the precancerous cascade. Usually it is the result of a prolonged inflammatory process and tends to be multifocal, giving rise to the so-called multifocal atrophic gastritis (Figure 2). The foci of atrophy are present in the mucosa of gastric antrum and body, and their extension progresses with time [75]. More virulent bacterial strains and a permissive host immune response are strongly associated with atrophy and progression to severe disease [84].

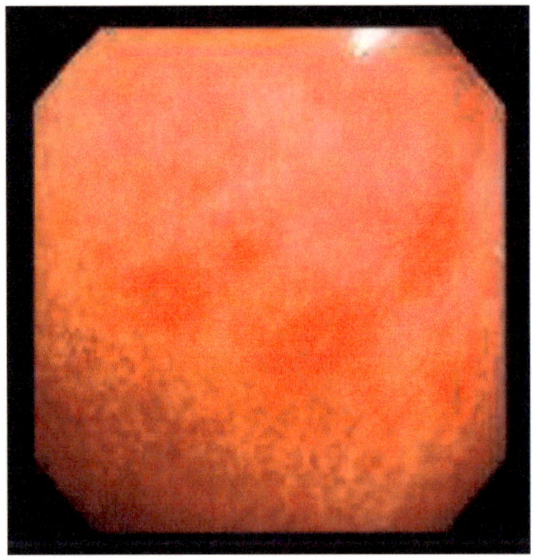

Figure 1. Chronic gastritis

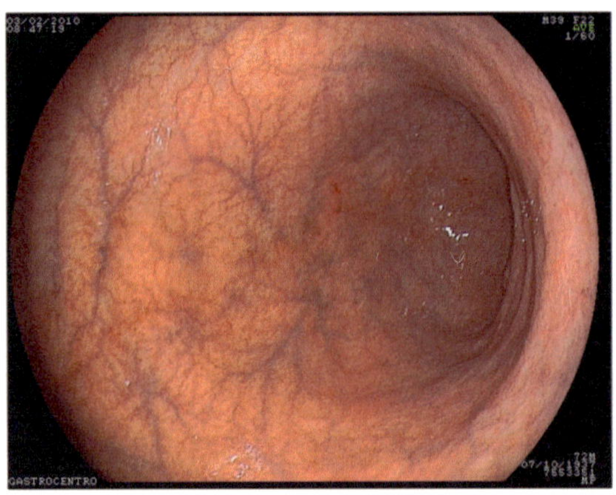

Figure 2. Atrophic gastritis

3.3.3. Intestinal metaplasia

At this stage of the gastric precancerous process, the original glands and the foveolar epithelium are replaced by cells with intestinal phenotype [84]. Intestinal metaplasia (Figure 3) is considered to be an advanced stage of atrophy because the metaplastic glands replace the original glands and chronologically the metaplastic glands appear after the gastric glands are lost. Intestinal metaplasia has been classified on the basis of morphology and enzyme histochemistry in two main types: the small intestine or complete type, and the colonic or incomplete type [75].

Up to this point in the cascade, the epithelium in the atrophic and metaplastic lesions remains well differentiated, with normal nuclear-cytoplasmic ratio, normal nuclear morphology, and normal tissue architecture. The dynamics of the precancerous process to this point shows a gradual phenotypic transformation from normal epithelium to metaplastic cells with small intestinal morphology and then to cells resembling colonic mucosa, additionally expressing gastric and colonic mucins. This process usually takes decades and is progressive, supporting the notion that although environmental alterations (bacterial factors and cytokine environment, loss of cell signaling) may have initially driven differentiation decisions, with time, permanent changes in the stem cell compartment have occurred. In some patients with incomplete metaplasia, a mild degree of nuclear atypia and architectural distortion is observed, leading some investigators to consider incomplete metaplasia as a mild form of dysplasia [84,85].

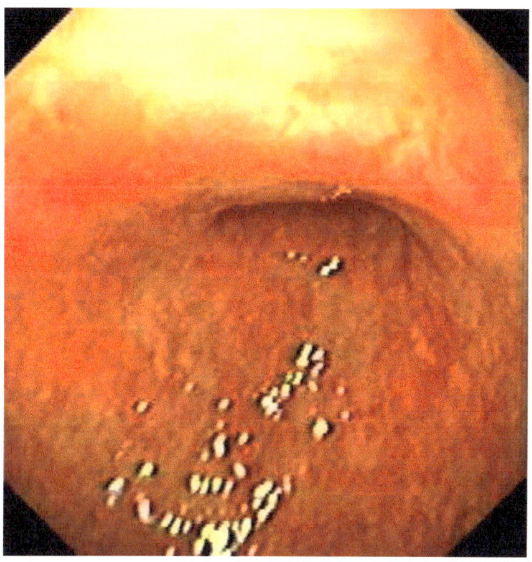

Figure 3. Intestinal metaplasia (antrum)

3.3.4. Dysplasia

Also called intraepithelial neoplasia or noninvasive neoplasia, dysplasia is characterized by a neoplastic phenotype, both in terms of cell morphology and architectural organization [75]. The nuclei of the dysplastic epithelium are enlarged, hyperchromatic, irregular in shape, and devoid of polarity [84]. The Padova classification is focused on gastric dysplasia and was developed by an international group of experienced gastrointestinal pathologists and recognizes five categories of lesions, utilizing mostly western nomenclature and grouping them numerically following the prevailing Japanese system: 1. negative for dysplasia; 2. indefinite for dysplasia; 3. noninvasive neoplasia (sub-classified in low grade or high grade); 4. suspicious for invasive carcinoma; and 5. invasive carcinoma [86].

The management of low-grade dysplasia is not well defined and there is a recommendation of annual endoscopic monitoring with rebiopsy [87]. Nevertheless, patients with high-grade dysplasia confirmed at least two gastrointestinal pathologists should undergo surgical or endoscopic resection because of the high probability of coexisting or metachronous invasive carcinoma [88].

3.3.5. Invasive adenocarcinoma

Invasive adenocarcinoma is the next stage in the cascade and requires the penetration of neoplastic cells into the surrounding stroma (Figure 4). Recent evidence suggests that this step demands that neoplastic cells acquire the capability of degrading the stromal matrix surrounding the neoplastic cells [75.

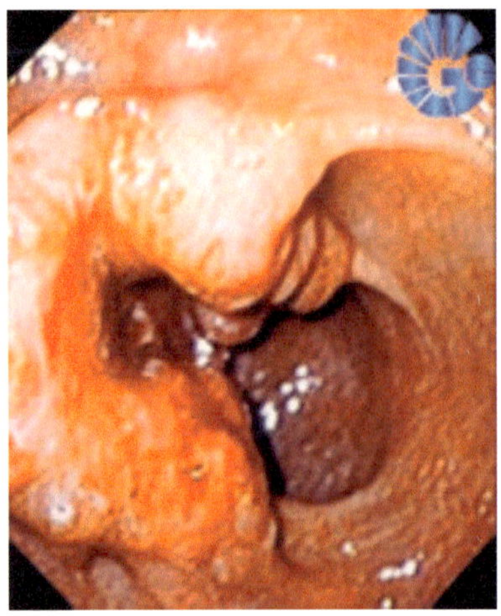

Figure 4. Gastric adenocarcinoma

3.4. Early and advanced lesions

Follow-up of patients with precursor lesions in populations at high gastric cancer risk has thrown light on the dynamics of the process. The progression of the precursor lesions described before follows a pattern of steady state, with episodes of progression to more advanced lesions and episodes of regression to less advanced lesions.

Unlike patients with advanced gastric cancer, patients diagnosed in an early stage of the disease present an excellent prognostic, in which a five-year survival rate is more than 90%. Early gastric cancer lesions are defined as the adenocarcinoma that is confined to the mucosa or submucosa, irrespective of lymphonode invasion (Figure 5). Many early gastric cancers are believed to go through a life cycle consisting of ulcerations, followed by healing, then reulceration, and some lesions remain at this early stage for years even without treatment [89]. Nevertheless, some early tumours rapidly became advanced and it is one of the principal questions concerning the gastric carcinogenesis. Are *H. pylori* virulence factors important to influence these alterations? To what extent *H. pylori* eradication treatment would be important to prevent the continued progression of the disease? To what extent *H. pylori* eradication in the early stage of cancer would be important to prevent the appearance of new lesions?

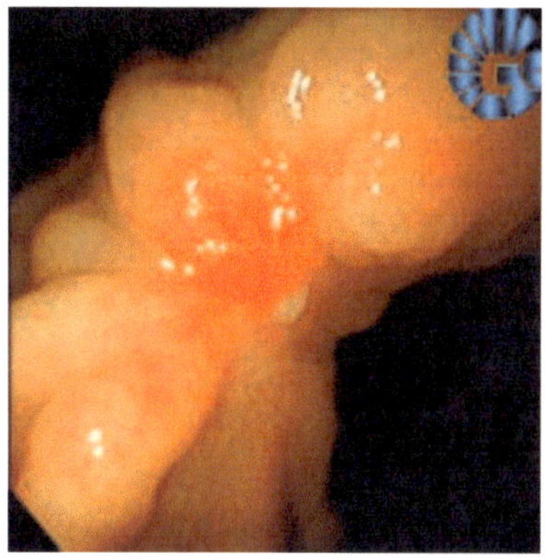

Figure 5. Early gastric adenocarcinoma

Considering these important questions, our chapter is divided into two sections: 1. the identification of the principal genetic characteristics of *H. pylori* strains in Brazilian patients with early distal type intestinal gastric adenocarcinoma, in order to determine the genotypic pattern of bacterium in our population through molecular techniques; 2. the discussion of the principal studies concerning *H. pylori* eradication and its importance to prevent the progression of precancerous lesions and the importance of *H. pylori* eradication in the early gastric cancer to prevent the development of new cancerous lesions.

4. Materials and methods

4.1. Determination of principal genotypes of *H. Pylori* in Brazilian patients with early gastric adenocarcinoma

4.1.1. Clinical samples

Clinical isolates of *H. pylori* analyzed in this study were obtained from the Laboratory of Pathology of the Center of Diagnosis of Digestive Diseases, Faculty of Medical Sciences, State University of Campinas (Campinas, São Paulo, Brazil). Third one paraffin wax-embedded specimens of gastric tissue were analyzed from a total of 31 patients with early distal type intestinal gastric adenocarcinoma. All the gastric tissue samples were obtained from endoscopic biopsy and were positive for *H. pylori* by histological analysis. Samples from gastric tissue obtained from endoscopic biopsy of patients with chronic gastritis and peptic ulcer disease and positive for *H. pylori* were used as positive controls for all the reactions carried out in this study. The study was approved by the Ethics Committee of the Faculty of Medical Sciences, State University of Campinas.

4.1.2. Methods

Paraffin wax-embedded tissue DNA extraction was carried out with xylene and ethanol washes for paraffin removal; successive steps using proteinase K, phenol, chloroform, and isoamyl alcohol were carried out in order to isolate and purify the DNA [90]. Quantification of the obtained product and polymerase chain reaction (PCR) for human betaglobin gene [91] were carried out to guarantee the quality of all the results.

After DNA extraction, PCR for ureaseC [92], vacA (s and m) [93,94,95], cagA [96], cagT [97] and dupA (jhp0917 and jhp0918) [49] genes were performed. Primers pairs for all the genes as well as the length of the fragments are described in Table 1. PCR for ureaseC gene was carried out to confirm the positivity for *H. pylori* in all the samples.

After amplification, each PCR product was analyzed by eletrophoresis on a 2% agarose gel stained with ethidium bromide with a 0.5 X tris-acetate-EDTA buffer. A 100-bp ladder was used as standard.

Gene	Strand	Primer sequence (5´ - 3´)	Length (bp)
betaglobin	+	ACAAACTGTGTTCACTAGC	110
	-	CAACTTCATCCACGTTTCACC	
ureaseC	+	AAGCTTTAGGGGTGTTAGGGGTTT	294
	-	AAGCTTACTTTCTAACACTAACGC	
vacA (s1/s2)	+	ATGGAAATACAACAAACACAC	s1: 259
	-	CTGCTTGAATGCGCCAAAC	s2: 286
vacA m1	+	GGTCAAAATGCGGTCATGG	290
	-	CCATTGGTACCTGTAGAAAC	
vacA m2	+	ATGCTTTAATATCGTTGAGA	198
	-	GAACATGTTTTAGTGAAAGC	
cagA	+	GATAACAGGCAAGCTTTTGAGG	349
	-	CTGCAAAAGATTGTTTGGCAGA	
cagT	+	CCATGTTTATACGCCTGTGT	301
	-	CATCACCACACCCTTTTGAT	
dupA (jhp0917)	+	TGGTTTCTACTGACAGAGCGC	307
	-	AACACGCTGACAGGACAATCTCCC	
dupA (jhp0918)	+	CCTATATCGCTAACGCGCGCTC	276
	-	AAGCTGAAGCGTTTGTAACG	

Table 1. Sequence of synthetic oligonucleotide primers used to characterization of *H. pylori* strains

Then, for each specific reaction, products obtained were classified in vacA s1m1, s2m1, s1m2 or s2m2; cagA positive or negative; cagT positive or negative; and dupA positive or negative. dupA gene was considered positive when its two regions (jhp0917 and jhp0918) were positive simultaneously.

After all amplifications, a table with absolute frequencies (n) and percentages (%) was made in order to determine genotypes combinations.

4.2. Analysis of the principal manuscript references concerning the study of eradication treatment of *H. pylori* in precancerous lesions and early gastric cancer

After determination of the principal genotype presented in Brazilian patients with early gastric cancer, a review concerning the importance of eradication of *H. pylori* in precancerous lesions and in early gastric adenocacinoma was done.

5. Results

5.1. Determination of principal genotypes of *H. Pylori* in Brazilian patients with early gastric adenocarcinoma

PCR for ureaseC gene of *H. pylori* was positive for all 31 samples obtained from patients with early distal type intestinal gastric adenocarcinoma. As regards to vacA gene region s, of 31 samples, 71.0% (22 cases) were s1 and 29.0% (9 cases) were s2. Related to the vacA region m, all the samples were m1. Following this analysis, samples were classified in s1m1 or s2m1. So, 71.0% (22 cases) were s1m1 and 29.0% (9 cases) were s2m1.

Classification	
UreaseC	31 (100.0%)
vacA s1	22 (71.0%)
vacA s2	9 (29.0%)
vacA m1	31 (100.0%)
vacA m2	0 (0.0%)
vacA s1m1	22 (71.0%)
vacA s2m1	9 (29.0%)
cagA positive	19 (61.3%)
cagA negative	12 (38.7%)
cagT positive	17 (54.8%)
cagT negative	14 (45.2%)
dupA (jhp0917/jhp0918) positive	11 (35.5%)
dupA (jhp0917/jhp0918) negative	20 (64.5%)
Total	31 (100.0%)

Table 2. Frequencies and percentages of the principal genes of *H. pylori* studied in samples of early gastric cancer

As regards to gene cagA, 61.3% (19 cases) were cagA positive and, for cagT gene, 54.8% (17 cases) were positive. For dupA (jhp0917/jhp0918) gene, there were 35.5% (11 cases) of positivity. All these results can be seen in Table 2.

Genotypes combinations where then analyzed and the most prevalent genotype for gastric samples obtained from Brazilian patients with early distal type intestinal gastric adenocarcinoma was vacA s1m1, cagA positive, cagT positive and dupA negative (Table 3).

Genotype combinations: **vacA s/m cagA cagT dupA (jhp0917/jhp0918)**	**Early gastric cancer**
s1m1 neg neg neg	4 (12.90)
s1m1 neg neg pos	1 (3.23)
s2m1 neg neg neg	1 (3.23)
s2m1 neg neg pos	0 (0.00)
s1m1 neg pos neg	2 (6.45)
s1m1 neg pos pos	1 (3.23)
s2m1 neg pos neg	2 (6.45)
s2m1 neg pos pos	1 (3.23)
s1m1 pos neg neg	3 (9.68)
s1m1 pos neg pos	2 (6.45)
s2m1 pos neg neg	2 (6.45)
s2m1 pos neg pos	1 (3.23)
s1m1 pos pos neg	5 (16.13)
s1m1 pos pos pos	4 (12.90)
s2m1 pos pos neg	2 (6.45)
s2m1 pos pos pos	0 (0.00)
Total	**31**

Table 3. Genotype combinations for early gastric adenocarcinoma samples

5.2. Analysis of the principal manuscript references concerning the study of eradication treatment of *H. pylori* in precancerous lesions and early gastric cancer

Epidemiological studies have established a strong causal relationship between *H. pylori* infection and gastric cancer. *H. pylori* eradication is therefore likely to be one of the most promising approaches to gastric cancer prevention. Animal studies have shown that eradication of *H. pylori* infection, especially at the early stage, is effective in preventing *H. pylori*-related gastric carcinogenesis. However, the available data from human studies show that *H. pylori* eradication does not completely prevent gastric cancer and that it might be useful in patients without atrophic gastritis or intestinal metaplasia at baseline [77].

Considering these important issues, the present chapter book analized and discussed some studies that assessed the possible relationship between the eradication of *H. pylori* infection and the prevention of gastric cancer even if the precancerous cascade has started. Obviously, there should be a point which there is no return in this process and the presence of *H. pylori* could not be more decisive to continue the progression of the precancerous lesions. With the aim to analyze these topics, we discussed some important questions concerning *H. pylori* infection, precancerous cascade and *H. pylori* eradication treatment, both in the precancerous lesions (atrophic gastritis, metaplasia intestinal and dysplasia) and in the early gastric cancer stage.

6. Discussion

Molecular techniques may be applied to the measurement of host or agent factors and of exposures. Molecular techniques help to stratify and to refine data by providing more sensitive and specific measurements, which facilitate epidemiologic activities, including disease surveillance, outbreak investigations, identifying transmission patterns and risk factors among apparently disparate cases, characterizing host-pathogen interactions, detecting uncultivatable organisms, providing clues for possible infectious causes of cancer and other chronic diseases, and providing better understanding of disease pathogenesis at the molecular level [98].

Our study determined the principal genotype of *H. pylori* strains in Brazilian patients with early distal type intestinal gastric adenocarcinoma, which is vacA s1m1, cagA positive, cagT positive and dupA negative. It provides to the scientific community important information concerning the epidemiology of gastric cancer in Brazil, as regards to the infecting strains. This principal *H. pylori* genotype was also the principal found in advanced gastric cancer samples, but, when considering the cagA gene in an isolate evaluation, it was more incident in patients with advanced gastric cancer [48].

Many factors, including a high-salt diet [99], genetic abnormality [100] and autoimmune gastritis [101], among others, have been reported concerning gastric carcinogenesis; however, it is clear that *H. pylori* infection is the most important gastric carcinogen [60, 102].

Currently recommended anti-*H. pylori* infection therapies achieve eradication rates of up to 90% [103]. Several studies have indicated that *H. pylori* screening and eradication is a cost-effective strategy for the prevention of gastric cancer in middle-aged adults, even if the treatment prevents only 20%-30% of *H. pylori*-associated cancers, and that the strategy is particularly beneficial in high-risk populations and in the long term [77,104,105,106], although the feasibility, safety and appropriated timing of this strategy for cancer prevention in the general population remains to be determined [77].

Some studies focused on patients with gastric precancerous lesions such as gastric atrophy, intestinal metaplasia and dysplasia and evaluated the effect of eradicating *H. pylori* on the intermediate lesions in the carcinogenic cascade rather than using gastric cancer as the primary end points [107].

Conflicting results have been reported on whether or not these precancerous lesions were reversible following successful eradication of *H. pylori* infection.

The investigation of Uemura et al. (2001) [108] is considered the first study providing some evidence that *H. pylori* eradication has an impact in gastric cancer. In this study, none of the 253 treated patients developed cancer, whilst there were 36 gastric cancer cases among 993 untreated patients. However, it is of note that the mean duration of follow-up after eradication was significantly shorter than the mean duration for patients who were not treated (4,8 vs. 8,5 years; $p < 0.001$). Therefore, the risk of gastric cancer development could have been understated in the treated group [107].

In a randomized placebo controlled study in China, gastritis (acute and chronic) decreased in both the antrum and the corpus at one year after *H. pylori* eradication and a slight regression of intestinal metaplasia was observed [109]. With similar results, a follow-up study developed by Zhou et al. (2003) [110] demonstrated that *H. pylori* eradication significantly reduced the severity and activity of chronic gastritis. Besides, while the proportion of intestinal metaplasia in the *H. pylori* positive group increased significantly, intestinal metaplasia in the antrum either regressed or had no progression in the *H. pylori* negative group.

In Colombia, a randomized, controlled chemoprevention trial with patients with confirmed multifocal nonmetaplastic atrophy and/or intestinal metaplasia demonstrated that, after *H. pylori* eradication therapy and/or dietary supplementation with ascorbic acid or beta-carotene, or their placebos, it was observed a significant increase in the rate of regression of the precursos lesions [111].

Other follow-up studies also identified that *H. pylori* eradication in patients with intestinal metaplasia could be important in the regression of the lesions [112-118]. In the same way, other randomized studies identified that *H. pylori* eradication in intestinal metaplasia could be important in the regression of this precancerous lesion [76,109-111,119,120]. Oppositely, other trials, both follow-up and randomized control, had not identified regression of intestinal metaplasia when *H. pylori* eradication was administrated [121-129].

Concerning to patients with gastric atrophy, the most part of the studies have identified that this lesion presents a regression when *H. pylori* eradication occurs [76, 109, 111, 119, 120, 128-130]. In Japan, where there is a significant ability in diagnostic, with a detection of 94% of early gastric cancers, one important multicenter randomized controlled trial by the Japan Gast Study Group enrolled patients undergoing previous endoscopic therapy for gastric cancer and demonstrated that eradication therapy significantly reduced the prevalence of secondary gastric cancer in a 3-year follow-up period [131]. However, this study does not demonstrate that eradication therapy can prevent newly developed gastric cancer even in secondary cancer, because the follow-up period was too short.

As well as other authors mentioned before, Ito (2009) [132] considered that theoretically *H. pylori* eradication therapy should be beneficial for cancer prevention. However, attention should be drawn to the fact that the gastric cancer risk is not similar between noninfected and eradicated people. Until now, many human studies have demonstrated that some patients develop gastric cancer even if they have undergone successful eradication therapy [133]. Considering it, we can conclude that eradication therapy may have an effect on cancer prevention if the therapy is administrated before a single cancer cell has transformed or before cancer tissue shows invasive growth. It is likely that eradication therapy has no effect if the cancer has progressed to an advanced stage.

Wong et al. (2004) [134], with the aim to determine whether eradication of *H. pylori* infection reduces the incidence of gastric cancer, carried out a randomized, placebo controlled trial with 1630 *H. pylori* infected patients in a high-risk region of China. Their results indicated that *H. pylori* eradication can reduce the incidence of gastric cancer in patients without precancerous lesions at entry. Besides, the eradication therapy had no statistically significant effect on the incidence of gastric cancer in patients with precancerous lesions on presentation. It appears that there is a point of no return for patients with precancerous lesions and a chemoprevention strategy may work only in a subset of *H. pylori* infected subjects [135].

As regards to animal models, they are useful because they represent tractable systems that permit insights into the effects of host, pathogen and environmental factors on gastric carcinogenesis [136]. Nevertheless, the use of animals does not completely reflect *H. pylori*-induced cancer in humans. Romero-Gallo et al. (2008) [137], using a population of gerbils that received antibiotics for *H. pylori* treatment, demonstrated that the timing of intervention influences the magnitude of suppression of pro-inflammatory cytokine expression, inflammation, pre-malignant, and neoplastic lesions. These findings have demonstrated that treatment of *H. pylori* decreases the incidence and the severity of pro-inflammatory cytokine expression, as well as premalignant and malignant lesions. However, the effectiveness of eradication is dependent upon the timing of intervention [137].

A 5-year study in Japanese monkeys (*Macaca fustata*) demonstrated that *H. pylori* infection can cause gastric atrophy, increased cell proliferation, and mutation of *p53* in gastric epithelial cells [138]. In other study, with Mongolian gerbils, it was demonstrated that the resulting pathological changes in gastric mucosa are similar to those in humans [139]. Some studies demonstrated that when the animals were infected with *H. pylori* together with a carcinogen (N-methyl-N-nitrosourea or N-methyl-N-nitro-N-nitrosoguanidine), they developed gastric cancer (both diffuse and intestinal types) that were at significantly higher frequencies than animals receiving either *H. pylori* or the carcinogen alone [140-142]. Gastric cancer incidence was reduced at 75 weeks to 6.7%, 27.3%, and 38.2% in Mongolian gerbils receiving eradication treatment at early (15 weeks), middle (35 weeks) and late (55 weeks) stages, respectively. These results suggest that eradication at an early stage might be effective in preventing carcinogenesis. Other study demonstrated that application of antimicrobial therapy at 8 weeks postinoculation of bacterium attenuated inflammation, but did not completely prevent the development of premalignant and malignant lesions, indicating that the *H. pylori* eradication therapy is effective when administered at an early stage after infection [143]. Nevertheless, it is important to remember that the carcinogenic potential of *H. pylori* is strain dependent and some results of these studies could be caused by the use of an *H. pylori* strain that lacked carcinogenic potential.

In the mouse model, both *H. pylori* infection and gastric atrophy increase the serum concentration of polypeptide hormone gastrin, a hormone that controls secretion of gastric acid by the stomach´s parietal cells and hypergastrinemia is regarded to play a role in the development.

The results obtained indicated that the timing of antimicrobial eradication therapy is very important as early application can prevent the progression of gastric cancer [144].

Finally, for cancers detected early, endoscopic mucosal resection can conserve the noncancerous gastric mucosa, but it can not eliminate the recurrence of metachronous gastric cancer [145]. Fukase et al. (2008) [131], in a randomized control trial, studied a group of patients submitted to *H. pylori* eradication therapy following endoscopic resection of early gastric cancer. These patients were monitored at different time intervals: at 3 years, metachronous gastric cancer had developed in 9 of 225 patients in the eradication group compared with 24 of 250 patients in the control group, suggesting that prophylactic eradication of *H. pylori* in a high-risk population can substantially reduce gastric cancer rates.

Briefly, the most part of the studies suggests that *H. pylori* eradication is able to induce regression of precancerous lesions in most of the treated subjects, and particularly in those with baseline, early and non-severe lesions. However, it also seems that a proportion of treated subjects will still show progression of preneoplastic lesions. So, we can consider that they really are other factors that contribute to the progression of these lesions. So, *H. pylori* eradication is an effective strategy in reducing the risk of gastric cancer; however, it is not efficient enough to eradicate gastric cancer. Prevention of the infection, *H. pylori* immunization, *H. pylori* eradication in the youth, selection of the high-risk population, and alternative chemopreventive measures may be essential for optimal management of malignancy of the stomach.

7. Conclusions

All the available evidence suggests that *H. pylori* eradication might represent a primary chemopreventive strategy in a subset of subjects. However, *H. pylori* eradication in those patients who have already developed advanced preneoplastic lesions does not prevent gastric cancer development, and endoscopic follow-up should always be performed.

More research is needed to elucidate mechanisms underlying the *H. pylori*-induced gastric carcinogenesis. As the infection usually depends on the characteristics of the infecting strain, studies that determine the genotypes in gastric cancer, as we presented in our study, are necessary. Besides, more trials concerning the interaction among the infecting strain, the host characteristics and the external environment are also needed to explaining the complex gastric carcinogenesis. An understanding of biochemical, genetic and epigenetic changes following eradication therapy would be helpful to develop strategies to identify high-risk individuals, thereby contributing to effective management in gastric cancer prevention.

Finally, it is important to gain more insight into the pathogenesis of H. pylori-induced gastric adenocarcinoma, not only to develop more effective treatments for this cancer, but also because it might serve as a paradigm for the role of chronic inflammation in the genesis of other malignancies.

http://dx.doi.org/10.5772/58328

Author details

Bruna Maria Roesler and José Murilo Robilotta Zeitune

*Address all correspondence to: roeslerbruna@gmail.com

Department of Internal Medicine, Center of Diagnosis of Digestive Diseases, Faculty of Medical Sciences – State University of Campinas – UNICAMP, Campinas, São Paulo, Brazil

References

[1] Kusters JG, van Vliet AHM, Kuipers EJ. Pathogenesis of *Helicobacter pylori* infection. Clinical Microbiology Reviews 2006; 19(3): 449-490.

[2] Goodwin CS, Armstrong JA. Microbiological aspects of *Helicobacter pylori* (*Campylobacter pylori*). European Journal of Clinical Microbiology 1990; 9(1): 1-13.

[3] Bode G, Mauch F, Malfertheiner P. The coccoid forms of *Helicobacter pylori.* Criteria for their viability. Epidemiology and Infection 1993; 111(3): 483-490.

[4] Blaser MJ. An endangered species in the stomach. Scientific American 2005; 292(2): 38-45.

[5] Ahmed N. 23 years of the discovery of *Helicobacter pylori:* Is the debate over? Annals of Clinical Microbiology and Antimicrobials 2005; 4: 17-19.

[6] Replogle ML, Glaser SL, Hiatt RA, Parsonnet J. Biologic sex as a risk factor for *Helicobacter pylori* infection in healthy young adults. American Journal of Epidemiology 1995; 142(8): 856-863.

[7] Graham DY, Malaty HM, Evans DG, Evans DJ, Klein PD, Adam E. Epidemiology of *Helicobacter pylori* in an asymptomatic population in the United States. Gastroenterology 1991; 100(6): 1495-1501.

[8] Urita Y, Watanabe T, Kawagoe N, Takemoto I, Tanaka H, Kijima S, Kido H, Maeda T, Sugasawa Y, Miyazaki T, Honda Y, Nakanishi K, Shimada N, Nakajima H, Sugimoto M, Urita C. Role of infected grandmothers in transmission of *Helicobacter pylori* to children in a Japanese rural town. Journal of Paediatrics and Child Health 2013; 49(5): 394-398.

[9] Bastos J, Carreira H, La Vecchia C, Lunet N. Childcare attendance and *Helicobacter pylori* infection: systematic review and meta-analysis. European Journal of Cancer Prevention 2013; 22(4): 311-319.

[10] Covacci A, Telford JL, Del Giudice G, Parsonnet J, Rapuolli R. *Helicobacter pylori* virulence and genetic geography. Science 1998; 284(5418): 1328-1333.

[11] Dubois A, Fiala N, Heman-Ackah LM, Drazek ES, Tarnawski A, Fishbein WN, Perez-Perez GI, Blaser MJ. Natural gastric infection with *Helicobacter pylori* in monkeys: a model for spiral bacteria infection in humans. Gastroenterology 1994; 106(6): 1405-1417.

[12] Fox JG, Batchelder M, Marini R, Yan L, Handt L, Li X, Shames B, Hayward A, Campbell J, Murphy JC. *Helicobacter pylori*-induced gastritis in the domestic cat. Infection and Immunity 1995; 63(7): 2674-2681.

[13] Grubel P, Hoffman JS, Chong FK, Burstein NA, Mepani C, Cave DR. Vector potential of houseflies (*Musca domestica*) for *Helicobacter pylori*. Journal of Clinical Microbiology 1997; 35(6): 1300-1303.

[14] Dunn BE, Cohen H, Blaser MJ. *Helicobacter pylori*. Clinical Microbiology Reviews 1997; 10(4): 720-741.

[15] Lu Y, Redlinger TE, Avitia R, Galindo A, Goodman K. Isolation and genotyping of *Helicobacter pylori* from untreated municipal wastewater. Applied and Environmental Microbiology 2002; 68(3): 1436-1439.

[16] Bahrami AR, Rahimi E, Ghasemian Safaei H. Detection of *Helicobacter pylori* in City Water, Dental Unit´s Water and Bottled Mineral Water in Isfahan, Iran. Scientific World Journal 2013.

[17] Marshall BJ, Warren JR. Unidentified curved bacilli in the stomach of patients with gastritis and peptic ulceration. Lancet 1984; 1(8390): 1311-1315.

[18] Ahmed N, Sechi LA. *Helicobacter pylori* and gastroduodenal pathology. New threats of the old friend. Annals of Clinical Microbiology and Antimicrobials 2005; 4:1-10.

[19] International Agency for Research on Cancer. Schistosomes, liver flukes and *Helicobacter pylori*. IARC Working Group on the Evaluation of Carcinogenic Risks to Humans. IARC monographs on the evaluation of carcinogenic risks to humans. World Health Organization, International Agency for Research on Cancer 1994; 61: 1-241.

[20] Capurso G, Lahner E, Marcheggiano A, Caruana P, Carnuccio A, Bordi C, Delle Fave G, Annibale B. Involvement of the corporal mucosa and related changes in gastric acid secretion characterize patients with iron deficiency anemy associated with *Helicobacter pylori* infection. Alimentary Pharmacology & Therapeutics 2001; 15(11): 1753-1761.

[21] Pelicano R, Franceschi F, Saracco G, Fagoonee S, Roccarina D, Gasbarrini A. *Helicobacters* and extragastric diseases. Helicobacter 2009; 14(Suppl 1): 58-68.

[22] Arnold DM, Bernotas A, Nazi I, Stasi R, Kuwana M, Liu Y, Kelton JG, Crowther MA. Platelet count response to *H. pylori* treatment in patients with immune thrombocytopenic purpura with and without *H. pylori* infection: a systematic review. Haematologica 2009; 94(6): 850-856.

[23] Franceschi F, Navarese EP, Mollo R, Giupponi B, De Marco G, Merra G, Gasbarrini G, Silveri NG. *Helicobacter pylori* and atherosclerosis. A review of the literature. Recenti Progressi in Medicina 2009; 100(2): 91-96.

[24] Rogha M, Nikvarz M, Poumoghaddas Z, Shirneshan K, Dadkhah D, Poumoghaddas M. Is *Helicobacter pylori* infection a risk factor for coronary heart disease? ARYA Atherosclerosis 2012; 8(1): 5-8.

[25] Isaeva GSh, Abuzarova ER, Valeeva IuV, Pozdeev OK, Murav'eva EV. *Helicobacter pylori* in patients with disorders of hepatobiliary system. Zh Mikrobiol Epidemiol Immunobiol 2009; 2: 96-101.

[26] Pirouz T, Zounubi L, Keivani H, Rakhshani N, Hormazdi M. Detection of *Helicobacter pylori* in paraffin-embedded specimens from patients with chronic liver diseases, using the amplification method. Digestive Diseases and Sciences 2009; 54(7): 1456-1459.

[27] Zhou X, Zhang C, Wu J, Zhang G. Association between *Helicobacter pylori* infection and diabetes mellitus: a meta-analysis of observational studies. Diabetes Research and Clinical Practice 2013; 99(2): 200-208.

[28] Blaser MJ, Berg DE. *Helicobacter pylori* genetic diversity and risk of human disease. The Journal of Clinical Investigation 2001; 107(7): 767-773.

[29] Suerbaum S, Michetti P. *Helicobacter pylori* infection. New England Journal of Medicine 2002; 347(15): 1175-1186.

[30] Megraud F, Neman-Simha, Brugmann D. Further evidence of the toxic effect of ammonia produced by Helicobacter pylori urease on human epithelial cells. Infection and Immunity 1992; 60(5): 1858-1863.

[31] Suzuki M, Miura S, Suematsu M, Fukumura D, Kurose I, Suzuki H, Kai A, Kudoh Y, Ohashi M, Tsuchiya M *Helicobacter pylori*-associated ammonia production enhances neutrophil-dependent gastric mucosal cell injury. American Journal of Physiology 1992; 263 (5 Pt 1): G719-725.

[32] Montecucco C, Rapuolli R. Living dangerously: how *Helicobacter pylori* survives in the human stomach. Nature Reviews. Molecular Cell Biology 2001; 2(6): 457-466.

[33] Harris PR, Mobley HL, Perez-Perez GI, Blaser MJ, Smith PD. *Helicobacter pylori* urease is a potent stimulus of mononuclear phagocyte activation and inflammatory cytokine production. Gastroenterology 1996; 111(2): 419-425.

[34] Leunk RD, Johnson PT, David BC, Kraft WG, Morgan DR. Cytotoxic activity in broth-culture filtrates of *Campylobacter pylori*. Journal of Medical Microbiology 1988; 26(2): 93-99.

[35] Amieva MR, El-Omar EM. Host-bacterial interactions in *Helicobacter pylori* infection. Gastroenterology 2008; 134(1): 306-323.

[36] Atherton JC, Cao P, Peek RMJr, Tummuru MK, Blaser MJ, Cover TL. Mosaicism in vacuolating cytotoxin alleles of *Helicobacter pylori*. Association of specific vacA types

with cytotoxin production and peptic ulceration. *Journal of Biological Chemistry 1995;* 270(30): 17771-17777.

[37] Covacci A, Rappuoli R. Tyrosine-phosphorylated bacterial proteins: Trojan horses for the host cell. Journal of Experimental Medicine 2000; 191(4): 587-592.

[38] Backert S, Selbach M. Role of type IV secretion in *Helicobacter pylori* pathogenesis. Cellular Microbiology 2008; 10(8): 1573-1581.

[39] Hatakeyama M. Oncogenic mechanisms of the *Helicobacter pylori* CagA protein. Nature Reviews. Cancer 2004; 4(9): 688-694.

[40] Higashi H, Tsutsumi R, Muto S, Sugiyama T, Azuma T, Asaka M, Hatakeyama M. SHP-2 tyrosine phosphatase as an intrancellular target of *Helicobacter pylori* CagA protein. Science 2002; 295(5555): 683-686.

[41] Murata-Kamiya N, Kurashima Y, Teishikata Y, Yamahashi Y, Saito Y, Higashi H, Aburatani H, Akiyama T, Peek RMJr, Azuma T, Hatakeyama M. *Helicobacter pylori* CagA interacts with E-cadherin and deregulates the β-catenin signal that promotes intestinal transdifferentiation in gastric epithelial cells. Oncogene 2007; 26(32): 4671-4626.

[42] Amieva MR, Vogelmann R, Covacci A, Tompkins LS, Nelson WJ, Falkow S. Disruption of the epithelial apical-junctional complex by *Helicobacter pylori* CagA. Science 2003; 300(5624): 1430-1434.

[43] Suzuki M, Mimuro H, Suzuki T, Park M, Yamamoto T, Sasakawa C. Interaction of CagA with Crk plays an important role in *Helicobacter pylori*-induced loss of gastric epithelial cell adhesion. Journal of Experimental Medicine 2005; 202(9): 1235-1247.

[44] Brandt S, Kwok T, Hartig R, Konig W, Backert S. NF-kappaB activation and potentiation of proinflammatory responses by the *Helicobacter pylori* CagA protein. Proceedings of the National Academy of Sciences of the United States of America 2005; 102(26): 9300-9305.

[45] Blaser MJ, Perez-Perez GI, Kleanthous H, Cover TL, Peek RM, Chyou PH, Stemmermann GN, Nomura A. Infection with *Helicobacter pylori* strains possessing cagA is associated with an increased risk of developing adenocarcinoma of the stomach. Cancer Research 1995; 55(10): 2111-2115.

[46] Parsonnet J, Friedman GD, Orentreich N, Vogelman H. Risk for gastric cancer in people with CagA positive or CagA negative *Helicobacter pylori* infection. Gut 1997; 40(3): 297-301.

[47] Figueiredo C, van Doorn LJ, Nogueira C, Soares JM, Pinho C, Figueira P, Quint WG, Carneiro F. *Helicobacter pylori* genotypes are associated with clinical outcome in Portuguese patients and show a high prevalence of infections with multiple strains. Scandinavian Journal of Gastroenterology 2001; 36(2): 128-135.

[48] Roesler BM, Costa SCB, Zeitune JMR. Virulence factors of *Helicobacter pylori* and their relationship with the development of early and advanced distal intestinal type gastric adennocarcinoma. In: Paola Tonino (ed.). Gastritis and gastric cancer. New insights in gastroprotection, diagnosis and treatments. Rijeka: InTech; 2011.

[49] Lu H, Hsu P, Graham DY, Yamaoka Y. Duodenal ulcer promoting gene of *Helicobacter pylori*. Gastroenterology 2005; 128(4): 833-848.

[50] Zhang Z, Zheng Q, Chen X, Xiao S, Liu W, Lu H. The *Helicobacter pylori* duodenal ulcer promoting gene, dupA in China. BMC Gastroenterology 2008; 8: 49-54.

[51] Yamaoka Y. Roles of the plasticity regions of *Helicobacter pylori* in gastroduodenal pathogenesis. Journal of Medical Microbiology 2008; 57(5): 545-553.

[52] Douraghi M, Mohammadi M, Oghalaie A, Abdirad A, Mohagheghi MA, Hosseini ME, Zeraati H, Ghasemi A, Esmaieli M, Mohajerani N. dupA as a risk determinant in *Helicobacter pylori* infection. Journal of Medical Microbiology 2008; 57 (Pt.5): 554-562.

[53] Argent RH, Burette A, Miendje Deyi VY, Atherton JC. The presence of dupA in *Helicobacter pylori* is not significantly associated with duodenal ulceration in Belgium, South Africa, China or North America. Clinical Infectious Diseases 2007; 45(9): 1204-1206.

[54] Schimidt HMA, Andres S, Kaakoush NO, Engstrand L, Eriksson L, Goh KL, Fock KM, Hilmi I, Dhamodaran S, Forman D, Mitchell H. The prevalence of the duodenal ulcer promoting gene (dupA) in *Helicobacter pylori* isolates varies by ethnic group and is not universally associated with disease development: a case-control study. Gut Pathogens 2009; 1(1): 5-13.

[55] Roesler BM, Oliveira TB, Costa SCB, Zeitune JMR. Is there any relationship between *Helicobacter pylori* dupA gene and the development of early and advanced gastric cancer in Brazilian patients? Journal of Medical Research and Science 2011; 2(1): 15-24.

[56] Arachchi HSJ, Kalra V, Lal B, Bhatia V, Baba CS, Chakravarthy S, Rohatgi S, Sarma PM, Mishra V, Das B, Ahuja V. Prevalence of duodenal ulcer promoting gene (dupA) of *Helicobacter pylori* in patients with duodenal ulcer in North Indian population. Helicobacter. 2007; 12(6): 591-597

[57] Gressmann H, Linz B, Ghai R, Pleissner KP, Schlapbach R, Yamaoka Y, Kraft C, Suerbaum S, Meyer TF, Achtman M. Gain and loss of multiple genes during the evolution of *Helicobacter pylori*. PLoS Genetics 2005; 1(4): e43.

[58] Siegel R, Ward E, Brawley O, Jemal A. Cancer statistics, 2011. The impact of eliminating socioeconomic and racial disparities on premature cancer deaths. CA. a cancer journal for clinicians 2011; 61(4): 212-236.

[59] Bray F, Jemal A, Grey N, Ferlay J, Forman D. Global cancer transition according to the Human Development Index (2008-2030): a population-based study. Lancet Oncology 2012, 13(8): 790-801.

[60] World Health Organization. Global action against cancer. Global cancer control. WHO Library Cataloguing-in-Publication Data. Switzerland 2005. http://www.who.int/cancer/media/en/GlobalActionCancerEnglfull.pdf (accessed 01 december 2013).

[61] Malfertheiner P, Bornschein J, Selgrad M. Role of *Helicobacter pylori* infection in gastric cancer pathogenesis: a chance for prevention. Journal of Digestive Diseases 2010; 11(1): 2-11.

[62] Nardone G, Rocco A, Malfertheiner P. Review article: *Helicobacter pylori* and molecular events in precancerous gastric lesions. Alimentary pharmacology & therapeutics 2004; 20(3): 261-270.

[63] Hoehnberger P, Gretschel S. Gastric cancer. Lancet 2003; 362(9380): 305-315.

[64] Bowles MJ, Benjamin IC. ABC of the upper gastrointestinal tract. Cancer of the stomach and pancreas. BMJ 2001; 323(7326): 1413-1416.

[65] Verdecchia A, Mariotto A, Gatta G, Bustamante-Teixeira MT, Ajiki W. Comparison of stomach cancer incidence and survival in four continents. European Journal of Cancer 2003; 39(11): 1603-1609.

[66] Guerra MR, Gallo CVM, Mendonça GAS. The risk of cancer in Brazil: tendencies and recent epidemiologic studies. Revista Brasileira de Cancerologia 2005; 51(3): 227-234.

[67] Ministério da Saúde. Instituto Nacional do Câncer José Alencar Gomes da Silva. Estimativa 2014 – Incidência de Câncer no Brasil. MS: http://www2.inca.gov.br (accessed 29 November 2013).

[68] Lauren P. The two histological main types of gastric carcinoma: Diffuse and so-called intestinal type carcinoma. Acta Pathologica et Microbiologica Scandinavica 1975; 64: 31-49.

[69] Sugiyama T, Asaka M. *Helicobacter pylori* infection and gastric cancer. Medical Electron Microscopy 2004; 37(3): 149-157.

[70] Yoshimura T, Shimoyama T, Fukuda S, Tanaka M, Axon AT, Munakata A. Most gastric cancer occurs on the distal side of the endoscopic atrophic border. Scandinavian Journal of Gastroenterology 1999; 34(11): 1077-1081.

[71] Polk DB; Peek Jr RM. *Helicobacter pylori*: gastric cancer and beyond. Nature Reviews. Cancer 2010; 10(6): 403-414.

[72] Correa P, Haenszel W, Cuello C, Tannenbaum S, Archer M. A model for gastric cancer epidemiology. Lancet 1975; 2(7924): 58-60.

[73] Correa P. A human model of gastric carcinogenesis. Cancer Research 1988; 48(13): 3554-3560.

[74] Correa P. Human gastric carcinogenesis: a multistep and multifactorial process – First American Cancer Society Award lecture on cancer epidemiology and prevention. Cancer Research 1992; 52(24): 6735-6740.

[75] Correa P, Piazuelo MB. The gastric precancerous cascade. Journal of Digestive Diseases 2012; 13(1): 2-9.

[76] Mera R, Fontham ET, Bravo LE, Bravo JC, Piazuelo MB, Camargo MC, Correa P. Long term follow up of patients treated for *Helicobacter pylori* infection. Gut 2005; 54(11): 1536-1540.

[77] Cheung TK, Xia HH, Wong BCY. *Helicobacter pylori* eradication for gastric cancer prevention. Journal of Gastroenterology 2007; 42(Suppl. 17): 10-15.

[78] Yang Y, Deng CS, Peng JZ, Wong BC, Lam SK, Xia HH. Effect of *Helicobacter pylori* on apoptosis and apoptosis related genes in gastric cancer cells. Molecular Pathology 2003; 56(1): 19-24.

[79] Kuipers EJ. Review article: relationship between *Helicobacter pylori*, atrophic gastritis and gastric cancer. Alimentary pharmacology & therapeutics 1998; 12(Suppl 1): 25-36.

[80] Forman D, Newell DG, Fullerton F, Yarnell JW, Stacey AR, Wald N, Sitas F. Association between infection with *Helicobacter pylori* and risk of gastric cancer: evidence from a prospective investigation. BMJ 1991; 302(6788): 1302-1305.

[81] Danesh J. *Helicobacter pylori* infection and gastric cancer: systemic review of the epidemiological studies. Alimentary pharmacology & therapeutics 1999; 13(7): 851-856.

[82] Herrera V, Parsonnet J. *Helicobacter pylori* and gastric adenocarcinoma. Clinical Microbiology and Infection 2009; 15(11): 971-976.

[83] de Vries AC, Haringsma J, Kuipers EJ. The detection, surveillance and treatment of premalignant gastric lesions related to *Helicobacter pylori* infection. Helicobacter 2007; 12(1): 1-15.

[84] Correa P, Houghton J. Carcinogenesis of *Helicobacter pylori*. Gastroenterology 2007; 133(2): 659-672.

[85] Filipe MI, Potet F, Bogomoletz WV, Dawson PA, Fabiani B, Chauveinc P, Fenzy A, Gazzard B, Goldfain D, Zeegen R. Incomplete sulphomucin-secreting intestinal metaplasia for gastric cancer. Preliminary data from a prospective study from three centres. Gut 1985; 26(12): 1319-1326.

[86] Rugge M, Correa P, Dixon MF, Haltori T, Leandro G, Lewin K, Riddeli RH, Sipponen P, Watanabe H. Gastric dysplasia: the Padova international classification. The American journal of surgical pathology 2000; 24(2): 167-176.

[87] Lauwers GY, Srivastava A. Gastric preneoplastic lesions and epithelial dysplasia. Gastroenterology clinics of North America 2007; 36(4): 813-829.

[88] Hirota WK, Zuckerman MJ, Adler DG, Davila RE, Egan J, Leighton JA, Qureshi WA, Rajan E, Fanelli R, Wheeler-Harbaugh J, Baron TH, Faigel DO. ASGE guideline: the role of endoscopy in the surveillance of premalignant conditions of the upper GI tract. Gastrointestinal Endoscopy 2006; 63(4): 570-580.

[89] Everett SM, Axon ATR. Early gastric cancer: disease or pseudo-disease? Lancet 1998; 351(9112): 1350-1352.

[90] Goelz SE, Hamilton SR, Vogelstein B. Purification of DNA from formaldehyde fixed and paraffin embedded human tissue. Biochemical and Biophysical Research Communications 1985; 130(1): 118-126.

[91] Saiki RK, Gelfand DH, Stoffel S, Scharf SJ, Higuchi R, Horn GT, Mullis KB, Erlich HA. Primer-directed enzymatic amplification of DNA with a termostable DNA polymerase. Science 1988; 239(4839): 487-491.

[92] Lage AP, Godfroid P, Fauconnier A, Burette A, Butzler JP, Bollen A, Glupczynski Y. Diagnosis of *Helicobacter pylori* infection by PCR: comparison with other invasive techniques and detection of cagA gene in gastric biopsy specimens. Journal of Clinical Microbiology 1995; 33(10): 2752-2756.

[93] Atherton JC, Peek RM, Tham KT, Cover TL, Blaser MJ. Clinical and pathological importance of heterogenicity in vacA, the vacuolating cytotoxin gene of *Helicobacter pylori*. Gastroenterology 1997; 112(1): 92-97.

[94] Atherton JC, Cover TL, Twells RJ, Morales MR, Hawkey CJ, Blaser MJ. Simple and accurate PCR-based system for typing vacuolating cytotoxin alleles of *Helicobacter pylori*. Journal of Clinical Microbiology 1999; 37(9): 2979-2982.

[95] Thomazini CM, Pinheiro NA, Pardini MI, Naresse LE, Rodrigues MAM. Infecção por *Helicobacter pylori* e câncer gástrico: freqüência de cepas patogênicas cagA e vacA em pacientes com câncer gástrico. Jornal Brasileiro de Patologia e Medicina Laboratorial 2006; 42(1): 25-30.

[96] Faundez G, Troncoso M, Figueroa G. cagA and vacA in strains of *Helicobacter pylori* from ulcer and non-ulcerative dyspepsia patients. BMC Gastroenterology 2002; 2:20-24.

[97] Mattar R, Marques SB, Monteiro MS, Santos AF, Iriya K, Carrilho FJ. *Helicobacter pylori* cag pathogenicity island genes: clinical relevance for peptic ulcer disease development in Brazil. Journal of Medical Microbiology 2007; 56(1): 9-14.

[98] Foxman B, Riley L. Molecular Epidemiology: Focus on Infection. American Journal of Epidemiology 2001; 153(12): 1135-1141.

[99] Nozaki K, Shimizu N, Inada K, Tsukamoto T, Inoue M, Kumagai T, Sugiyama A, Mizoshita T, Kaminishi M, Tatematsu M. Synergistic promoting effects of *Helicobacter*

pylori infection and high-salt diet on gastric carcinogenesis in Mongolian gerbils. Japanese Journal of Cancer Research 2002; 93(10): 1083-1089.

[100] Humar B, Blair V, Charlton A, More H, Martin I, Guilford P, E-cadherin deficiency initiates gastric signet-ring cell carcinoma in mice and man. Cancer Research 2009; 69(5): 2050-2056.

[101] Fukayama M, Hino R, Uozaki H. Epstein-Barr vírus and gastric carcinoma: vírus-host interactions leading to carcinoma. Cancer Science 2008; 99(9): 1726-1733.

[102] Suzuki H, Hibi T, Marshall BJ. *Helicobacter pylori:* present status and future prospects in Japan. Journal of Gastroenterology 2007; 42(1): 1-15.

[103] Xia HH, Yu Wong BC, Talley NJ, Lam SK. Alternative and rescue treatment regimens for *Helicobacter pylori* eradication. Expert Opinion of Pharmacotherapy 2002; 3(9): 1301-1311.

[104] Parsonnet J, Harris RA, Hack HM, Owens DK. Modelling cost-effectiveness of *Helicobacter pylori* screening to prevent gastric cancer: a mandate for clinical trials. Lancet 1996; 348(9021): 150-154.

[105] Fendrick AM, Chernew ME, Hirth RA, Bloom BS, Bandekar RR, Scheiman JM. Clinical and economic effects of population-based *Helicobacter pylori* screening to prevent gastric cancer. Archives of Internal Medicine 1999; 159(2): 142-148.

[106] Roderick P, Davies R, Raftery J, Crabbe D, Pearce R, Patel P et al. Cost-effectiveness of population screening for *Helicobacter pylori* in preventing gastric cancer and peptic ulcer disease, using simulation. Journal of Medical Screening 2003; 10(3): 148-156.

[107] Fuccio L, Zagari RM, Minardi ME, Bazzoli F. Systematic review. *Helicobacter pylori* eradication for the prevention of gastric cancer. Alimentary Pharmacology & Therapeutics 2007; 25(2): 133-141.

[108] Uemura N, Okamoto S, Yamamoto S, Matsumura M, Yamaguchi S, Yamakido M, Taniyama K, Sasaki N, Schlemper RJ. *Helicobacter pylori* infection and the development of gastric cancer. New England Journal of Medicine 2001; 345(11): 784-789.

[109] Leung WK, Lin SR, Ching JY, To KF, Ng EK, Chan FK, Lau JY, Sung JJ. Factors predicting progression of gastric intestinal metaplasia. Results of a randomized trial on *Helicobacter pylori* eradication. Gut 2004; 53(9): 1244-1249.

[110] Zhou L, Sung JJ, Lin S, Jin Z, Ding S, Huang X, Xia Z, Guo H, Liu J, Chao W. A five-year follow-up study on the pathological changes of gastric mucosa after *H. pylori* eradication. Chinese Medical Journal 2003; 116(1): 11-14.

[111] Correa P, Fontham ET, Bravo JC, Bravo LE, Ruiz B, Zarama G, Realpe JL, Malcom GT, Li D, Johnson WD, Mera R. Chemoprevention of gastric dysplasia: randomized trial of antioxidant supplements and anti-*Helicobacter pylori* therapy. Journal of the National Cancer Institute 2000; 92(23): 1881-1888.

[112] Genta RM, Lew GM, Graham DY. Changes in the gastric mucosa following eradication of *Helicobacter pylori*. Modern Pathology 1993; 6(3): 281-289.

[113] Ciok J, Dzieniszewski J, Lucer C. *Helicobacter pylori* eradication and antral intestinal metaplasia – two years follow-up study. Journal of Physiology and Pharmacology 1997; 48(Suppl. 4): 115-122.

[114] Uemura N, Mukai T, Okamoto S, Yamaguchi S, Mashiba H, Taniyama K, Sasaki N, Haruma K, Sumii K, Kajiyama G. Effect of *Helicobacter pylori* eradication on subsequent development of cancer after endoscopic resection of early gastric cancer. Cancer Epidemiology, Biomarkers & Prevention 1997; 6(8): 639-642.

[115] Kim N, Lim SH, Lee KH, Choi SE, Jung HC, Song IS, Kim CY. Long-term effects of *Helicobacter pylori* eradication on intestinal metaplasia in patients with duodenal and benign gastric ulcers. Digestive Diseases and Sciences 2000; 45(9): 1754-1762.

[116] Ohkusa T, Fujiki K, Takashimizu I, Kumagai J, Tanizawa T, Eishi Y, Yokoyama T, Watanabe M. Improvement in atrophic gastritis and intestinal metaplasia in patients in whom *Helicobacter pylori* was eradicated. Annals of Internal Medicine 2001; 134(5): 380-386.

[117] Kokkola A, Sipponen P, Rautelin H, Härkönen M, Kosunen TU, Haaapiainen R, Puolakkainen P. The effect of *Helicobacter pylori* eradication on the natural course of atrophic gastritis with dysplasia. Alimentary Pharmacology & Therapeutics 2002; 16(3): 515-520.

[118] Ito M, Haruma K, Kamada T, Mihara M, Kim S, Kitadai Y, Sumii M, Tanaka S, Yoshihara M, Chayama K. *Helicobacter pylori* eradication therapy improves atrophic gastritis and intestinal metaplasia: a 5-year prospective study of patients with atrophic gastritis. Alimentary Pharmacology & Therapeutics 2002; 16(8): 1449-1456.

[119] You WC, Brown LM, Zhang L, Li JY, Jin ML, Chang YS, Ma JL, Pan KF, Liu WD, Hu Y, Crystal-Mansour S, Pee D, Blot WJ, Fraumeni JF Jr, Xu GW, Gail MH. Randomized double-blind factorial trial of three treatments to reduce the prevalence of precancerous gastric lesions. Journal of the National Cancer Institute 2006; 98(14): 974-983.

[120] Ley C, Mohar A, Guarner J, Herrera-Goepfert R, Figueroa LS, Halperin D, Johnstone I, Parsonnet J. *Helicobacter pylori* eradication and gastric preneoplastic conditions: a randomized, double-blind, placebo-controlled trial. Cancer Epidemiology, Biomarkers & Prevention 2004; 13(1): 4-10.

[121] Witteman EM, Mravunac M, Becx MJ, Hopman WP, Verschoor JS, Tytgat GN, de Koning RW. Improvement of gastric inflammation and resolution of epithelial damage one year after eradication of *Helicobacter pylori*. Journal of Clinical Pathology 1995; 48(3): 250-256.

[122] Forbes GM, Warren JR, Glaser ME, Cullen DJ, Marshall BJ, Collins BJ. Long-term follow-up of gastric histology after *Helicobacter pylori* eradication. Journal of Gastroenterology and Hepatology 1996; 11(7): 670-673.

[123] van der Hulst RW, van der Ende A, Dekker FW, Ten Kate FJ, Weel JF, Keller JJ, Kruizinga SP, Dankert J, Tytgat JN. Effect of *Helicobacter pylori* eradication on gastritis in relation to cagA: a prospective 1-year follow-up study. Gastroenterology 1997; 113(1): 25-30.

[124] Satoh K, Kimura K, Takimoto T, Kihira K. A follow-up study of atrophic gastritis and intestinal metaplasia after eradication of *Helicobacter pylori*. Helicobacter 1998; 3(4): 236-240.

[125] Kyzekova J, Mour J. The effect of eradication therapy on histological changes in the gastric mucosa in patients with non-ulcer dyspepsia and *Helicobacter pylori* infection. Prospective randomized intervention study. Hepatogastroenterology 1999; 46(27): 2048-2056.

[126] Annibale B, Aprile MR, D´Ambra G, Caruana P, Bordi C, Delle Fave G. Cure of *Helicobacter pylori* infection in atrophic body gastritis patients does not improve mucosal atrophy but reduces hypergastrinemia and its related effects on body ECL-cell hyperplasia. Alimentary Pharmacology & Therapeutics 2000; 14(5): 625-634.

[127] Sung JJ, Lin SR, Ching IY, Zhou LY, To KF, Wang RT, Leung WK, Ng EK, Lau JY, Lee YT, Yeung CK, Chao W, Chung SC. Atrophy and intestinal metaplasia one year after cure of *H. pylori* infection: a prospective, randomized study. Gastroenterology 2000; 119(1): 7-14.

[128] Kamada T, Haruma K, Hata J, Kusunoki H, Sasaki A, Ito M, Tanaka S, Yoshihara M. The long-term effect of *Helicobacter pylori* eradication therapy on symptoms in dyspeptic patients with fundic atrophic gastritis. Alimentary Pharmacology & Therapeutics 2003; 18(2): 245-252.

[129] Kuipers EJ, Nelis GF, Klinkenberg-Knol EC, Snel P, Goldfain D, Kolkman JJ, Festen HP, Dent J, Zeitoun P, Havu N, Lamm M, Walan A. Cure of *Helicobacter pylori* infection in patients with reflux oesophagitis treated with long term omeprazole reverses gastritis without exacerbation of reflux disease: results of a randomised controlled trial. Gut 2004; 53(1): 12-20.

[130] Ruiz B, Garay J, Correa P, Fontham ET, Bravo JC, Bravo LE, Realpe JL, Mera R. Morphometric evaluation of gastric antral atrophy: improvement after cure of *Helicobacter pylori* infection. American Journal of Gastroenterology 2001; 96(12): 3281-3287.

[131] Fukase K, Kato M, Kikuchi S, Inoue K, Uemura N, Okamoto S, Terao S, Amagai K, Hayashi S, Asaka M, Japan Gast Study Group. Effect of eradication of *Helicobacter pylori* on incidence of metachronous gastric carcinoma after endoscopic resection of early gastric cancer: an open-label, randomized controlled trial. Lancet 2008; 372(9636): 350-352.

[132] Ito M, Takata S, Tatsugami M, Wada Y, Imagawa S, Matsumoto Y, Takamura A, Kitamura S, Matsuo T, Tanaka S, Haruma K, Chayama K. Clinical prevention of gastric cancer by *Helicobacter pylori* eradication therapy: a systematic review. Journal of Gastroenterology 2009; 44(5): 365-371.

[133] Takata S, Ito M, Yoshihara M, Tanaka S, Imagawa S, Haruma K, Chayama K. Host factors contributing to the discovery of gastric cancer after successful eradication therapy of *Helicobacter pylori:* preliminary report. Journal of Gastroenterology and Hepatology 2007; 22(4): 571-576.

[134] Wong BC, Lam SK, Wong WM, Chen JS, Zheng TT, Feng RE, Lai KC, Hu WH, Yuen ST, Leung SY, Fong DY, Ho J, Ching CK, Chen JS, China Gastric Cancer Study Group. *Helicobacter pylori* eradication to prevent gastric cancer in a high-risk region of China: a randomized controlled trial. JAMA 2004; 291(2): 187-194.

[135] Kabir S. Effect of *Helicobacter pylori* eradication on incidence of gastric cancer in human and animal models: underlying biochemical and molecular events. Helicobacter 2004; 14(3): 159-171.

[136] Rogers AB, Fox JG. Inflammation and Cancer. Rodent models of infectious gastrointestinal and liver cancer. American Journal of Physiology. Gastrointestinal and Liver Physiology 2004; 286(3): G361-G366.

[137] Romero-Gallo J, Harris EJ, Krishna U, Washington MK, Perez-Perez GI, Peek Jr RM. Effect of *Helicobacter pylori* eradication on gastric carcinogenesis. Laboratory Investigation 2008; 88(3): 328-336.

[138] Oda T, Murakami K, Nishizono A, Kodama M, Nasu M, Fujioka T. Long-term *Helicobacter pylori* infection in Japanese monkeys induces atrophic gastritis and accumulation of mutations in the *p53* tumor suppressor gene. Helicobacter 2002; 7(3): 143-151.

[139] Hirayama F, Takagi S, Kusuhara H, Iwao E, Yokoyama Y, Ykeda Y. Induction of gastric ulcer and intestinal metaplasia in mongolian gerbils infected with *Helicobacter pylori*. Journal of Gastroenterology 1996; 31(5): 755-757.

[140] Shimizu N, Inada K, Nakanishi H, Tsukamoto T, Ikehara Y, Kaminishi M, Kuramoto S, Sugiyama A, Katsuyama T, Tatematsu M. *Helicobacter pylori* infection enhances glandular stomach carcinogenesis in Mongolian gerbils treated with chemical carcinogens. Carcinogenesis 1999; 20(4): 669-676.

[141] Sugiyama A, Maruta F, Ikeno T, Ishida K, Kawasaki S, Katsuyama T, Shimizu N, Tatematsu M. *Helicobacter pylori* infection enhances N-methyl-N-nitrosourea-induced stomach carcinogenesis in the Mongolian gerbil. Cancer Research 1998; 58(10): 2067-2069.

[142] Tokieda M, Honda S, Fujioka T, Nasu M. Effect of *Helicobacter pylori* infection on the N-methyl-N-nitro-N-nitrosoguanidine-induced gastric carcinogenesis in Mongolian gerbils. Carcinogenesis 1999; 20(7): 1261-1266.

[143] Franco AT, Israel DA, Washington MK, Krishna U, Fox JG, Rogers AB, Neish AS, Collier-Hyams L, Perez-Perez GI, Hatakeyama M, Whitehead R, Gaus K, O'Brien DP, Romero-Gallo J, Peek RM Jr. Activation of beta-cateninby carcinogenic *Helicobacter pylori*. Proceedings of the National Academy of Sciences of the United States of America 2005; 102(30): 10646-10651.

[144] Cai X, Carlson J, Stoicov C, Li H, Wang TC, Houghton J. *Helicobacter felis* eradication restores normal architecture and inhibits gastric cancer progression in C57BL/6 mice. Gastroenterology 2005; 128(7): 1937-1952.

[145] Ono H, Kondo H, Gotoda T, Shirao K, Yamaguchi H, Saito D, Hosokawa K, Shimoda T, Yoshida S. Endoscopic mucosal resection for treatment of early gastric cancer. Gut 2001; 48(2): 225-229.

Chapter 5

Helicobacter pylori Infection and Gastric Cancer — Is Eradication Enough to Prevent Gastric Cancer

Aleksandra Sokic-Milutinovic, Dragan Popovic,
Tamara Alempijevic, Sanja Dragasevic,
Snezana Lukic and Aleksandra Pavlovic-Markovic

Additional information is available at the end of the chapter

http://dx.doi.org/10.5772/57412

1. Introduction

Helicobacter pylori (H. pylori) is a gram negative, microaerophilic spiral bacterium with a clear role in the pathogenesis of gastric and duodenal ulcer, low grade B cell gastric lymphoma (MALT lymphoma) and gastric cancer. The bacterium was successfully cultivated by Warren and Marshall in 1982. Their discovery led to completely different therapeutic approach to patients with peptic ulcer disease and gastric MALT lymphoma. Despite initial skepticism concerning *H. pylori* role in gastric carcinogenesis, in 1991 two epidemiological studies [1,2] confirmed previously published reports suggesting higher incidence of gastric cancer in *H. pylori* infected individuals [3-5]. Furthermore, cohort studies in California, Hawaii and Great Britain confirmed increased risk for gastric cancer in *H. pylori* infected individuals. As a result of accumulated scientific evidence *Helicobacter pylori* was marked as human carcinogen by International Agency for Research on Cancer in 1994. Gastric cancer is the third most common cancer among males and fifth most common among females. The incidence of gastric cancer is declining in developed countries, but the global burden is rising due to cases occurring in developing countries. The five-year survival for advanced stage gastric cancer is below 20% even in developed countries [6].

Different outcomes of *Helicobacter pylori* infection are to be expected depending on distinct patterns of gastritis that were identified and described in detail. Namely, antrum-predominant gastritis leads to duodenal ulcer formation while chronic corpus predominant and multifocal atrophic gastritis lead to increased risk for gastric cancer formation [7-9].

The outcome of *Helicobacter pylori* infection depends on characteristics of the microorganism, characteristics of the host and environmental factors.

2. *Helicobacter pylori* virulence factors

Helicobacter pylori virulence depends on different factors enabling it to colonize gastric mucosa and induce tissue damage. Epidemiological studies revealed so far six distinct *H. pylori* strains (hpEurope, hpEastAsia, hpAsia2, hpAfrica 1, hpAfrica2 and hpNEAfrica) that are related to geographic regions and correlate well with the incidence of gastric cancer [10].

H. pylori is a highly heterogeneous bacterium [11,12]. Several *H. pylori* virulence factors are thought to contribute to gastric cancer development and this review will focus on cytotoxin-associated gene A and CagA protein (CagA), vacuolating cytotoxin (VacA) and outer inflammatory protein (OipA) (Figure 1) with a brief comment on possible role of duodenal ulcer–promoting gene (dupA).

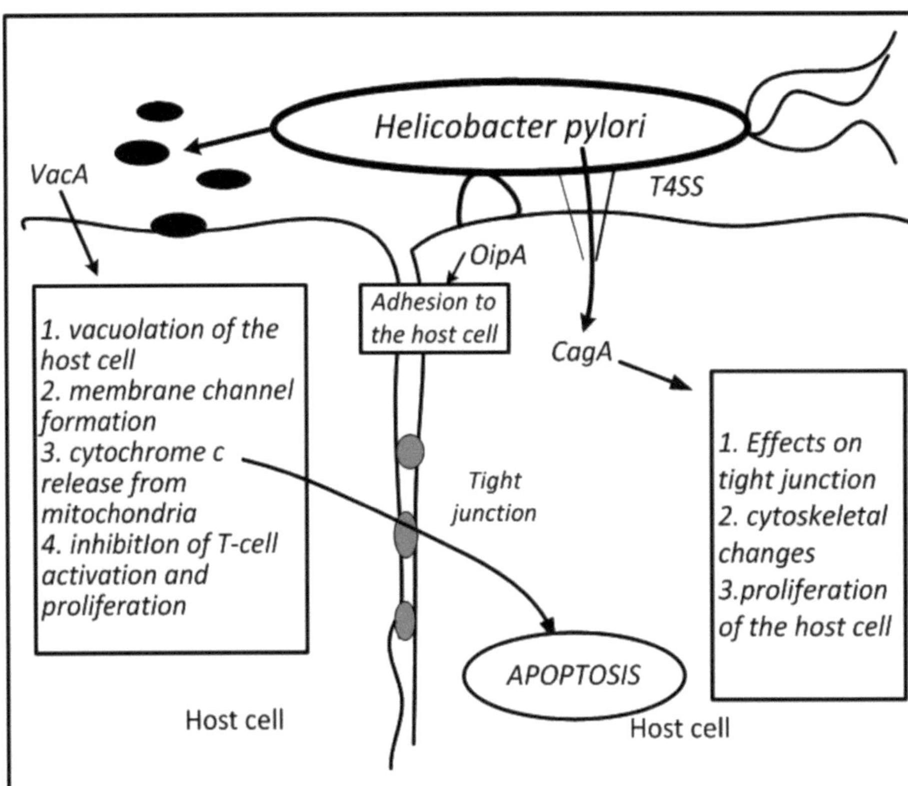

Figure 1. Mechanism of *Helicobacter pylori* induced host cell injury

2.1. *cagA*

There are two types of clinical *H. pylori* isolate: CagA-producing (*cagA* positive) strains and CagA-nonproducing (*cagA* negative) strains. Results of studies obtained on animal model revealed that gastric cancer developed only in animals infected with *cagA* positive *H. pylori* strains or when CagA protein was artificially introduced into the host [13,14] and authors concluded that CagA protein was important factor in gastric carcinogenesis. Further investigations revealed that *cagA* gene polymorphisms could at least partly explain why only some *cagA* positive individuals develop gastric cancer. Namely, there are different number of repeat sequences located on 3` region of the cagA gene in different *H. pylori* strains. It is now well known that sequences of these repeat regions differ significantly between strains isolated in East Asia and Western strains [15]. Each repeat region of the CagA protein contains Glu-Pro-Ile-Tyr-Ala (EPIYA) motifs. The first repeat region is termed EPIYA-A and EPIYA-B and second repeat region EPIYA-C or EPIYA-D segments [11]. Western type CagA has EPIYA ABC, ABCC or ABCCC, while East Asian CagA has EPIYA ABD segments [11].

CagA protein is composed of a disordered C-terminal region that contains the EPIYA motifs and a structured N-terminal region with several conserved regions. When the bacterium contacts the host cell CagA is injected into the host cell via the *cag* pathogenicity island (*cag*PAI)-encoded type IV secretion system (T4SS). Upon injection, CagA is linked to the inner leaflet of the cell membrane probably via an electrostatic interaction with phosphatidylserine [16]. When injected into the cytoplasm via the T4SS, CagA can be phosphorylated by the host and alter host cell signaling in both phosphorylation-dependent and phosphorylation-independent manner. CagA is phosphorylated on EPIYA motifs [17]. Induction of heme oxygenase 1, which exhibits anti-inflammatory and antioxidant effects, reduced CagA phosphorylation during *H. pylori* infection of gastric epithelial cells *in vitro*. However, there is data suggesting that the bacterium developed a strategy to diminish heme oxygenase 1 gene expression in gastric epithelial cells [18].

Recently it was demonstrated that another protein component of T4SS termed CagL induces hypergastrinemia, which is a major risk factor for the development of gastric adenocarcinoma [17].

2.2. *vacA*

VacA induces vacuolation of the host cell, membrane-channel formation, cytochrome *c* release from mitochondria leading to apoptosis, induces autophagy and alters host immune response [17,20,21]. VacA also inhibits T-cell activation and proliferation [22]. All *H. pylori* strains have a functional *vacA* gene. There is a variation in the vacuolating activity among different *H. pylori* strains [23] related to differences in the *vacA* gene structure at the signal (s1 and s2) region, middle region (m1 and m2) and intermediate (i1 and i2) region. Combination of subtype of these three regions influences the levels of VacA activity and is related to risks for different gastrointestinal diseases.

The most cytotoxic are s1/m1 strains, followed by s1/m2 strains, whereas s2/m2 strains have no cytotoxic activity and s2/m1 strains are rare [24]. Individuals infected with s1 or m1 *H. pylori* strains have an increased risk of peptic ulcer or gastric cancer compared with individuals infected with s2 or m2 strains [11]. In East Asia most *H. pylori* strains are s1 type that led to conclusion (based on epidemiological data) that in East Asia presence of m1 region leads to increased risk for gastric cancer [11] and its typing is the best marker for gastric cancer risk out of all *vacA* regions.

Intermediate region of *vacA* is identified between s and m regions few years ago. All s1/m1 strains belong to the type i1, and all s2/m2 strains are type i2. Strains tha contain s1/m2 can be type i1 or i2. Strains with i1 region are more pathogenic. In some populations typing of i-region is superior in predicting gastric cancer risk than typing of s region, while in other populations it has no predictive value [25].

The deletion (d) region—was identified between the i-region and the m region [26]. The d region is divided into d1 and d2. The study of Western strains demonstrated that d1 was a risk factor for gastric mucosal atrophy; however, almost all East Asian strains are classified as s1/i1/d1 [11].

2.3. oipA

Outer membrane proteins (OMPs) are coded by different genes in *Helicobacter pylori* genome. One of the OMPs that can function as adhesin is OipA, which was identified in 2000 [11].

OipA is a protein that induces proinflammatory response and its activity leads to increase in mucosal interleukin-8 (IL8) levels. OipA is involved in the attachment of *H. pylori* to gastric epithelial cells *in vitro* [27]. Results from animal studies demonstrated that OipA alone plays a role in the development of gastric cancer [13].

The production of CagA, VacA and OipA is linked and the majority of *H. pylori* strains produce either all of these proteins or none of them. Almost all East Asian strains of *H. pylori* are classified as CagA-producing, VacA-producing (*vacA* s1), and OipA-producing strains and are highly pathogenic. In addition, CagA, VacA and OipA are all thought to be involved in the development of both gastric cancer and duodenal ulcer [11].

2.4. *dupA*

Duodenal ulcer–promoting gene *dupA* was described in 2005. It is localized in the plasticity zone and it is involved in T4SS formation. Initial report suggested it to be the first disease-specific *H. pylori* virulence factor that induced duodenal ulcer formation and had a suppressive action on gastric cancer (DupA) [28]. After this report multiple studies failed to demonstrate correlation between *dupA* gene and specific gastroduodenal disease [10,29,30]. This gene is,however, highly polymorphic, and that could explain the conflicting data obtained in different studies [17].

2.5. Geographic differences in gastric cancer incidence related to *Helicobacter pylori* strains

Multilocus sequence typing (MLST) of the housekeeping genes revealed six *H. pylori* strains (hpEurope, hpEastAsia, hpAsia2, hpAfrica 1, hpAfrica2 and hpNEAfrica) that are related to geographic regions and correlate well with the incidence of gastric cancer.

Sequence differences among the examined housekeeping genes of the six major genotypes probably have no influence on the disease outcome but serve as a marker for other virulence factors related to the disease outcome (i.e *cagA* and *vacA*) [10]. In 2003, Falush et al analyzed 370 *H. pylori* isolates and assigned the strains to four main clusters: hpEurope, hpEastAsia, hpAfrica1 and hpAfrica2 due to their obvious geographical associations [31]. HpEurope is common in Europe and countries colonized by Europeans and most isolates from East Asia belong to hpEastAsia. HpAfrica2 is very distinct and has only been isolated in South Africa. Four years later Linz et al expanded the analysis using 769 *H. pylori* isolates and assigned the isolates to six distinct groups, adding to previously descried clusters (hpEurope, hpEastAsia, hpAfrica1 and hpAfrica2) two new clusters termed hpAsia 2 and hpNEAfrica. Cluster hpAsia2 was isolated in South and Southeast Asia. Cluster hpNEAfrica is predominant among isolates from Northeast Africa [12].

Populations with high rates of gastric cancer correspond with regions presenting hpEastAsia strains. In contrast, incidence of gastric cancer is very low in Africa, where most strains are hpNEAfrica, hpAfrica1 or hpAfrica2, and in South Asia, where most strains are hpAsia2. The differences in *H. pylori* isolates in different populations are considered to be an explanation of the both African and Asian enigma. Namely, populations with high incidences of *Helicobacter pylori* infection in East Asian countries have high incidences of gastric cancer, as opposed to low incidence of gastric cancer in other highly infected populations in Africa (African enigma) and South Asia (Asian enigma) [10].

3. Host factors

Host characteristics and immune response to *Helicobacter pylori* infection also play a role in gastric carcinogenesis. Different gene polymorphisms that affect host immune response and extent of cell proliferation are described and linked to gastric carcinogenesis together with gene polymorphisms for growth factors and growth factor receptors. Majority of these polymorphisms are single nucleotide polymorphisms (SNP). In recent years, host genetic polymorphisms involved in inflammatory response, carcinogen metabolism, antioxidant protection, mucosal protection and cell proliferation regulation have been widely studied as potential biomarkers to predict gastric cancer risk.

4. Cytokine gene polymorphisms

Cytokines modulate inflammatory response to *Helicobacter pylori* infection and indirectly the risk for gastric cancer. Gene polymorphisms for interleukin-1 beta and its receptor antagonist, tumor necrosis factor alpha, interleukin-8 and interleukin-10 were extensively studied and reported as relevant in determining gastric cancer risk.

4.1. Interleukin-1

Interleukin-1 beta (IL-1β) is a potent inhibitor of gastric acid secretion. Reduced gastric acid secretion on the other hand promotes development of *H. pylori* induced pangastritis, gastric mucosa atrophy and subsequently, in a subset of individuals, gastric cancer development. El-Omar et al described in 2000 polymorphisms in the pro-inflammatory *IL-1B* gene (encoding IL-1β) and *IL-IRN* (encoding IL-1β receptor antagonist) associated with elevated risk for hypochlorhydria and gastric cancer in the persons with *H. pylori* infection [32] (El-Omar). Presence of *IL-1B*-31C or -511T and *IL-IRN**2/*2 polymorphisms is associated with a 2-3-fold increase in risk for intestinal and diffuse non-cardia gastric cancer among *H. pylori*-infected persons [33]. These genetic polymorphisms modulate gastric cancer risk by increasing expression of pro-inflammatory cytokine IL-1β. It was later established that these polymorphisms interact synergistically with bacterial virulence factors (*cagA* positive, *vacA* s1 and *vacA* m1). Gastric cancer risk is highest among those with both host and bacterial high-risk genotypes [34].

Results of meta-analysis provided by Persson et al. based on available data from epidemiological studies showed strongest association of IL1RN2 polymorphism with increased risk for gastric cancer [35] in non-Asian populations for both intestinal and diffuse cancers. The *IL1RN22* genotype has been reported to cause high circulating IL-1receptor antagonist and IL-1β levels resulting in a severe and prolonged inflammatory response. IL1B-511T carriers were found to have an increased risk of gastric cancer in non-Asian populations. Possible explanation is that stronger inflammatory reaction may increase the risk of cancer through damage to gastric cells and bacterial overgrowth and accumulation of toxic byproducts [32]. These findings are supported by results of some [36,37], but not all previously published meta-analysis [38]. Surprisingly, according to Persson et al *IL-1B*-31C polymorphism was associated with a reduced overall risk for gastric cancer in Asian populations [35].

4.2. Tumor necrosis factor alpha

Tumor necrosis factor alpha (TNF-α) is another proinflammatory cytokine produced in gastric mucosa in response to *H. pylori* infection. Polymorphisms in *TNF-A* gene, especially presence of the high producing A allele of *TNF-A* at position 308 (G→A) is considered to be associated with increased risk for non-cardia gastric cancer [6]. This finding is supported by majority [39-41], but not all of available meta-analysis [35].

4.3. Interleukin 10

Interleukin 10 is an anti-inflammatory cytokine that down-regulates *IL-1B, TNF-A,* and interferon-γ gene expression. Previously published studies suggested that individuals carrying the *IL-10* ATA haplotype associated with low IL-10 production (-592, -819, -1082) have an increased risk for non-cardia gastric cancer [33]. Nevertheless meta-analysis failed to confirm these observations except for *IL10*-1082G where the effect of polymorphism depends on ethnicity of the host. It seems that this polymorphism increases gastric cancer risk in Asians, but has no significant effect in non-Asian populations [39].

4.4. Interleukin 8

IL-8 is a CXC family cytokine that is a potent chemoattractant for neutrophils and lymphocytes affecting proliferation, migration, and tumor angiogenesis. However, not all studies have replicated the positive associations between pro-inflammatory cytokines polymorphisms and gastric cancer risk [42]. A polymorphisms in *IL-8* (-251 T→A) is associated with increased production of IL-8 in *H. pylori* infected gastric mucosa and with precancerous gastric abnormalities in Caucasians and gastric cancer in Asian populations [43]. Nevertheless, studies in Asian populations [44,45] have failed to confirm relevance of this polymorphism and meta-analysis supported this finding [35], but this can be attributable to small sample size in these studies and limited number of the high quality studies available for the meta-analysis.

4.5. Presence of multiple high-risk cytokine gene polymorphisms

Possession of multiple high-risk host polymorphisms is associated with increased risk for gastric cancer. Presence of 3-4 of the polymorphisms (*IL-B1*-511*T, *IL-IRN**2/*2, *TNF-A*-308*A and *IL-10* ATA/ATA) confers a 27-fold increase in risk of non-cardia gastric cancer [33].

5. Polymorphisms in innate immune response genes

H. pylori attaches to gastric epithelium via receptors. Thus, polymorphisms in the innate immune response genes, which interact with these receptors, could influence outcome of infection and potentially the risk of gastric cancer.

5.1. Toll like receptor 4 (TLR4)

TLR4 is a cell-surface signaling receptor involved in the recognition and host response to *Helicobacter pylori*. Toll-like receptor 4 gene codes for a lipopolysaccharide (LPS) receptor molecule involved in innate immune recognition of microbe pathogen-associated molecular patterns. The *TLR4*+896A>G polymorphism linked with impaired reactivity to bacterial lipopolysaccharide may play a role in gastric carcinogenesis [44] and is associtaed with hypochlorhydria and upper gastrointestinal cancer. *TLR4* 896 polymorphisms results in changed conformation of the extra cellular domain of the TLR4 receptor and carriers are unable to adequately respond to LPS challenge. The defective signaling through TLR4 leads to an exaggerated inflammatory response with severe tissue destruction that causes gastric atrophy and severe hypochlorhydria. Two independent case-control studies have demonstrated that *TLR4*+896G carriers have eightfold increase in odds ratio for hypochlorhydria and gastric atrophy, and over two-fold increase for gastric cancer [44,45]

6. Cell proliferation-related gene polymorphisms

Meta-analysis by Gao et al identified 23 polymorphisms significantly related to gastric cancer in at least one published study suggesting the importance of polymorphisms in genes implicated in cell proliferation in development of gastric cancer. The overall effect of these polymorphisms is probably modest but should not be neglected [46].

6.1. Cell cycle and apoptosis regulators

Cell cycle and apoptosis regulators are directly involved in the initiation of malignant proliferation of the cell. Polymorphisms of functional regulators of *TP53, TP53BP2* (tumor protein P53 binding protein 2) and *MDM2* (gene encoding Mouse double minute 2 homolog, an important negative regulator of the p53 tumor suppressor) were found to be related to the development of gastric cancer. *TP3* gene encodes a multi-purpose protein (P53) that takes part in regulating the cell cycle, carrying out programmed cell death, initiating DNA repair, and regulating the transcription of a large number of genes that cells use for various biological purposes. Given its many essential functions, P53 is frequently found inactivated in tumor cells. Results of meta-analysis confirm that association of *TP3* gene polymorphisms vary by population and type of gastric cancer. The *TP3* Arg allele carriers of Asian origin have an increased risk for gastric cancer, while same polymorphism seems to have protective effects in Caucasians [43]. Possible explanation is difference in environmental factors that act together with either apoptotic or DNA repairing mechanisms. Data obtained for other two polymorphisms in cell-cycle related genes that were extensively studied are inconsistent, both for *Lmyc* (nuclear oncogen) EcoRI polymorphism and *p21* (gene encoding P21/ cyclin-dependent kinase inhibitor 1) polymorphism (Arg31Ser), probably due to relatively small sample sizes and underestimated importance of environmental factors and their interplay with host genetics.

PPAR-γ (peroxisome proliferator-activated receptors γ) is a member of the nuclear hormone receptor family that plays an important role in cell differentiation and regulation of metabolism. A potential interplay between *PPAR-γ* Pro12Ala polymorphism and *H. pylori* infection was observed in the development of gastric cancer [47,48].

6.2. Growth factors and growth factor receptors

Polymorphisms determining higher level of growth factors and related receptors, which are important for tissue repair, were associated with reduced risk of gastric cancer. Such associations were observed for gene encoding epidermal growth factor (EGF) *EGF* 5′ UTR 61G>A, [49], polymorphisms for transforming growth factor beta (TGFB) i.e. *TGFB1* -509C>T, *TGFBR2*-875G>A [50] and gene encoding insulin-like growth factor-binding protein 3 *IGFBP3* -202A>C and Gly32Ala [51,52].

7. Environmental factors

Environmental regulation of virulence factors could be an interesting concept explaining why not all infected individuals develop severe complications of disease despite infection with pathogenic *Helicobacter pylori* strains.

Recent study demonstrated that high salt diet could influence *H. pylori* protein expression [53].

7.1. Diet

In 2007 World Cancer Research Fund declared that high intake of vegetables and fruit probably decrease risk of gastric cancer, and that high intakes of salt and salty food probably increase risk of gastric cancer [54]. The proposed underlying mechanism for the inverse association of gastric cancer risk with vegetable and fruit/rich diet is related to the presence of antioxidants. Salt on the other hand acts directly on the stomach lining, destroying the mucosal barrier, causes gastritis and increased epithelial cell proliferation [55]. A synergistic interaction between diet and *Helicobacter pylori* infection with risk of gastric cancer has been proposed [56]. Recent study demonstrated that high salt diet could influence *Helicobacter pylori* protein expression leading to increased risk of gastric cancer [53]. Salt responsive increase in *cagA* expression attributable to increased CagA transcription was described that could lead to increased risk of gastric cancer.

7.2. Smoking

Tobacco smoking is the risk factor associated with the largest number of cancer cases worldwide and the causal link with stomach cancer is recognized [54]. A recent meta-analysis found significant positive associations of smoking with risk of both cardia and non-cardia gastric cancer among the majority of studies, overall increasing risk by 62% for male and 20% for female current smokers [57]. It is possible that tobacco smoke carcinogens affect gastric cancer risk directly through contact with the stomach mucosa or indirectly through the blood flow [54]. In a large population-based study in Europe (EPIC), 17.6% of gastric cancer cases were attributed to smoking [56]. The cancer risk in past smokers can remain up to 14 years after cessation of smoking [57,58]. The effect of smoking on gastric cancer is dose-dependent and additive in the presence of other risk factors [59,60]. However, passive smoking does not seem to increase the risk [61].

7.3. Non-steroidal anti-inflammatory drugs

Protective effect of regular use of non-steroidal anti-inflammatory drugs (NSAIDs) and particularly aspirin on risk of gastric cancer was repeatedly reported in observational studies and then results of meta-analysis [62] confirmed these finding. According to Algra et al regular NSAID users have up to 20% reduced risk of gastric cardia adenocarcinoma and up to 36% reduced risk of distal gastric adenocarcinoma [62]. NSAIDs suppress the production of cyclooxygenase enzymes. Data on clinical efficacy of NSAIDs in prevention of gastric cancer first suggested that aspirin reduces risk for both proximal and distal gastric cancer [63]. Recent results from population-based intervention trial by Wong et al revealed that celecoxib treatment or *Helicobacter pylori* eradication alone had beneficial effects on the regression of advanced gastric lesions. Nevertheless no favourable effects were seen for *H. pylori* eradication followed by celecoxib treatment [64]. Meta-analysis by Tian et al suggests significant protective effects of NSAIDs against gastric cancer [65].

7.4. Socioeconomic status

Lower socioeconomic status is associated with at least two-fold greater risk of gastric cancer irrespective of the country incidence of gastric cancer [54]. Possible explanation is related to increased likelihood of transmission and re-infection with *H. pylori* (large family, poor sanitation, less frequent use of antibiotics). Also, low socioeconomic status is related to a diet lower in fresh fruits and vegetables.

8. Importance of *Helicobacter pylori* eradication in prevention of gastric cancer development-current knowledge and evidence

Helicobacter pylori infection is mainly associated with distal forms and intestinal-type gastric carcinoma [7-9]. Namely, there are two distinct sites of gastric adenocarcinoma: proximal (cardia) and distal (non-cardia), with different epidemiological and clinical characteristics. Main risk factors for cardia gastric cancer are obesity, gastro-oesophageal reflux disease and Barrett's oesophagus [66] and its incidence is increasing over last decades. On the contrary, main risk factors for development of distal gastric cancer are *H.pylori*, low socioeconomic status, smoking, salty and smoked food intake, low consumption of fruits and vegetables and a family history of gastric cancer. Clear decline in incidence of distal gastric cancer is observed in the last decades [67].

Histologically gastric cancer is, according to Lauren classification, divided into two subtypes: intestinal and diffuse type. The intestinal type is related to corpus-predominant gastritis with intestinal metaplasia and is closely related to long-lasting *H.pylori* infection, whereas the diffuse originates from superficial pangastritis without atrophy [7-9].

Intestinal type gastric adenocarcinoma results from a prolonged precancerous process. The link between gastric intestinal metaplasia and cancer was proposed by pathologists in Java and Sumatra in 1938. This idea was over time only occasionally revisited by scientists until in 1975 Correa et al proposed a model of gastric carcinogenesis. This model postulated that intestinal type of gastric cancer was a result of progressive changes in the gastric mucosa [68]. Authors updated their model in 1988 and 1992. In Correa cascade the following consecutive steps are now recognized: normal gastric mucosa, superficial (non-atrophic) gastritis, multi-focal atrophic gastritis (MAG), complete (small intestine type) intestinal metaplasia followed by intestinal metaplasia of the incomplete (colonic) type, low-grade dysplasia, high-grade dysplasia and invasive adenocarcinoma. [7-9, 68]. Loss of normal glandular tissue is the first specific recognizable step in the precancerous cascade. However, the changes of the precancerous lesions over time remain an issue difficult to assess leading to the fact that the point of no return, although of critical importance for timely eradication, still remains unidentified.

Five randomized controlled trials (RCT) reported effects of *H.pylori* infection eradication on invasive gastric cancer or premalignant histological lesions of gastric mucosa. [69-75]

Study by Wong et al. was designed as RCT conducted in a high-risk gastric cancer region in China that evaluated gastric cancer incidence as a primary outcome [69]. Authors identified healthy individuals with *H. pylori* infection and treated them either with eradication therapy or placebo. During a follow-up period of 7.5 years authors failed to demonstrate overall decrease in gastric cancer incidence. The study concluded that incidence of gastric cancer development in the general population was similar between subjects receiving *H. pylori* treatment and placebo. The study, however, suggested the possible protective role of *H. pylori* eradication in participants without precancerous lesions, including gastric atrophy, intestinal metaplasia, or dysplasia.

Other above cited trials were not designed to assess gastric cancer as a primary outcome [70, 71] or had low numbers of gastric cancer cases [69, 72] to provide an informative assessment of the effects of eradication on cancer occurrence. Nevertheless, recently an important study was published by Ma et al [74] with the long-term follow-up results of a randomized trial in which 2258 *H. pylori* seropositive adults from a general population in China were randomly assigned to three interventions (*H. pylori* eradication, garlic supplements, supplemental vitamins) or control groups. After 15 years there were 34 new gastric cancers in *H. pylori* eradication group and 52 in the corresponding control group (relative risk of 0.61, 95 % confidence interval 0.38-0.96) that clearly demonstrated benefit of eradication therapy in gastric cancer prevention.

This year Lee et al [76] evaluated the benefit of mass eradication of *H. pylori* infection started in Taiwanese population with high incidence of *H. pylori* infection. Individuals who were aged 30 years and older were tested for the presence of *H. pylori* infection and those positive underwent endoscopic screening and subsequent eradication therapy. Authors demonstrated the success of eradication in 78.7%. Gastric atrophy incidence decreased in over 77% after successful eradication of *H. pylori* with no significant change in intestinal metaplasia. Gastric cancer incidence during the chemoprevention period was reduced by 25%. Based on these findings authors suggest that ultimate benefit in reducing gastric cancer incidence and its mortality should be validated by a further long-term follow-up.

Over a decade ago Uemura et al. [77] first reported that *H. pylori* eradication could reduce the subsequent development of metachronous gastric cancer after endoscopic resection of early gastric carcinoma. Namely, 132 *H. pylori* serology-positive patients who underwent endoscopic resection were assigned to the *H. pylori*-treatment group or the no treatment group according to the patients' preference. Regular endoscopic follow-up for up to 4 years found no metachronous cancer in *H. pylori*-treated patients compared to 9% in the no treatment group.

Some years later, Fukase et al. [75] reported the results of a trial in which more than five hundred patients in Japan who had previously undergone endoscopic resection for treatment of early gastric cancer were randomized to either *H. pylori* eradication or usual care. They demonstrated statistically significant 65 % reduction in the risk of metachronous gastric carcinoma compared with the control group.

The evidence from more recent trial reports [74-76], taken together with the epidemiological and experimental evidence for the carcinogenic activity of chronic *H. pylori* infection, provides support for a protective effect of *H. pylori* eradication in gastric cancer.

9. Conclusion

H. pylori infection contributes 5.5% to global cancer burden and is the single most important cause of infection-associated cancer globally [6]. It is therefore reasonable to consider eradication therapy as optimal preventive approach in infected individuals. Interrupting transmission of infection is primary prevention, secondary should be eradication therapy and tertiary prevention includes identification of the individuals with early gastric cancer. However data from large study in China that included 1630 healthy carriers of *H. pylori* infection that were given eradication therapy or placebo detected no difference of gastric cancer incidence between these two groups [69]. Benefit would probably be seen in patients where gastric cancer cascade did not cross the point of no return, which would explain results of recently published studies [74,76]. Namely, intestinal-type gastric cancer results from a multistep process of mucosal alterations leading from chronic inflammation (gastritis) to glandular atrophy followed by development of intestinal metaplasia and dysplasia resulting in invasive carcinoma. Clinical studies should aim to identify a 'point of no return', a situation when mucosal alterations are no longer reversible after *H. pylori* eradication and progression to gastric cancer became independent of presence of the bacterium.

Higher risk for gastric cancer might be modulated by an overall pro-inflammatory host genetic profile in the adaptive and innate immune systems genes (e.g. *IL-1B, TNFA, IL-10, IL-8,* and *TLR4*) [77]. This pro-inflammatory profile might drive the immune response to *H. pylori* infection to a severe chronic inflammatory phenotype, reduced gastric acid secretion, bacterial overgrowth, and oxidative stress to the gastric mucosa.

Therefore timely eradication of *H pylori* infection especially in individuals with proinflammatory genetic profile could prevent development and in long term possibly decrease incidence of gastric cancer.

Author details

Aleksandra Sokic-Milutinovic[1,2], Dragan Popovic[1,2], Tamara Alempijevic[1,2], Sanja Dragasevic[2], Snezana Lukic[1,2] and Aleksandra Pavlovic-Markovic[1,2]

1 School of Medicine, University of Belgrade, Belgrade, Serbia

2 Clinic for Gastroenterology and Hepatology, Clinical center of Serbia, Belgrade, Serbia

References

[1] Talley NJ, Zinsmeister AR, Weaver A, DiMagno EP, Carpenter HA, Perez-Perez GI, Blaser MJ. Gastric adenocarcinoma and *Helicobacter pylori* infection. J Natl Cancer Inst 1991;83(23):1734-1739

[2] Parsonnet J, Friedman GD, Vandersteen DP, Chang Y, Vogelman JH, Orentreich N, Sibley RK. *Helicobacter pylori* infection and the risk of gastric carcinoma.N Engl J Med 1991;325(16):1127-1131.

[3] Scott N, Lansdown M, Diament R, Rathbone B, Murday V, Wyatt JI, McMahon M, Dixon MF, Quirke P. Helicobacter gastritis and intestinal metaplasia in a gastric cancer family. Lancet 1990;335(8691):728.

[4] Marwick C. Helicobacter: new name, new hypothesis involving type of gastric cancer. JAMA 1990;264(21):2724-2727.

[5] Caruso ML, Fucci L. Histological identification of *Helicobacter pylori* in early and advanced gastric cancer.J Clin Gastroenterol 1990;12(5):601-602.

[6] Mbulaiteye SM, Hisada M, El-Omar EM *Helicobacter pylori* associated global gastric cancer burden. Front Biosci (Landmark Ed). 2009;14:1490-1504.

[7] Correa P. A human model of gastric carcinogenesis. Cancer Res 1988; 48: 3554–3360.

[8] Correa P. Human gastric carcinogenesis: a multistep and multifactorial process – First American Cancer Society Award lecture on cancer epidemiology and prevention. Cancer Res 1992; 52: 6735–6740.

[9] Correa P, Piazzuelo MB. The gastric precancerous cascade. J Dig Dis 2012;13:2-9.

[10] Yamaoka Y, Kato M, Asaka M. Geographic differences in gastric cancer incidence can be explained by differences between *Helicobacter pylori* strains. Intern Med. 2008;47(12):1077-1083

[11] Yamaoka Y. Mechanisms of disease: *Helicobacter pylori* virulence factors. Nat Rev Gastroenterol Hepatol. 2010;7(11):629-641.

[12] Linz B, Balloux F, Moodley Y, Manica A, Liu H, Roumagnac P, Falush D, Stamer C, Prugnolle F, van der Merwe SW, Yamaoka Y, Graham DY, Perez-Trallero E, Wadstrom T, Suerbaum S, Achtman M.An African origin for the intimate association between humans and *Helicobacter pylori*. Nature 2007;445:915–918

[13] Franco AT, Johnston E, Krishna U, Yamaoka Y, Israel DA, Nagy TA, Wroblewski LE, Piazuelo MB, Correa P, Peek RM Jr. Regulation of gastric carcinogenesis by *Helicobacter pylori* virulence factors. Cancer Res 2008;68:379–387

[14] Ohnishi N, Yuasa H, Tanaka S, Sawa H, Miura M, Matsui A, Higashi H, Musashi M, Iwabuchi K, Suzuki M, Yamada G, Azuma T, Hatakeyama M.Transgenic expression of *Helicobacter pylori* CagA induces gastrointestinal and hematopoietic neoplasms in mouse. Proc Natl Acad Sci USA 2008;105:1003–1008.

[15] Yamaoka Y, Osato MS, Sepulveda AR, Gutierrez O, Figura N, Kim JG, Kodama T, Kashima K, Graham DY. Molecular epidemiology of *Helicobacter pylori*: separation of *H. pylori* from East Asian and non-Asian countries. Epidemiol Infect 2000;124:91–96.

[16] Hayashi T, Senda M, Morohashi H, Higashi H, Horio M, Kashiba Y, *et al.* Tertiary structure-function analysis reveals the pathogenic signaling potentiation mechanism of *Helicobacter pylori* oncogenic effector CagA. Cell Host Microbe 2012;12:20–33.

[17] Cid TP, Fernández MC, Benito Martínez S, Jones NL. Pathogenesis of *Helicobacter pylori* Infection. Helicobacter 2013;18 Suppl 1:12-17

[18] Gobert AP, Verriere T, de Sablet T, Peek RM Jr, Chaturvedi R, Wilson KT. Haem oxygenase-1 inhibits phosphorylation of the *Helicobacter pylori* oncoprotein CagA in gastric epithelial cells. Cell Microbiol 2013;15:145–156.

[19] Wiedemann T, Hofbaur S, Tegtmeyer N, Huber S, Sewald N, Wessler S, Backert S, Rieder G. *Helicobacter pylori* CagL dependent induction of gastrin expression via a novel alphavbeta5-integrin-integrin linked kinase signalling complex. Gut 2012;61:986–996.

[20] Atherton JC. The pathogenesis of *Helicobacter pylori*-induced gastro-duodenal diseases. Annu Rev Pathol Mech Dis 2006;1:63–96.

[21] Cover TL, Blanke SR. *Helicobacter pylori* VacA, a paradigm for toxin multifunctionality. Nat Rev Microbiol 2005;3:320–332

[22] Gebert B, Fischer W, Weiss E, Hoffmann R, Haas R. *Helicobacter pylori* vacuolating cytotoxin inhibits T lymphocyte activation. Science. 2003;301:1099–1102.

[23] Cover TL, Blaser MJ. Purification and characterization of the vacuolating toxin from *Helicobacter pylori*. J Biol Chem. 1992;267:10570–10575.

[24] Atherton JC, Cao P, Peek RM Jr, Tummuru MK, Blaser MJ, Cover TL. Mosaicism in vacuolating cytotoxin alleles of *Helicobacter pylori*Association of specific *vacA* types with cytotoxin production and peptic ulceration.

[25] Ogiwara H, Graham DY, Yamaoka Y. *vacA* i-region subtyping. Gastroenterology. 2008;134:1267.

[26] Ogiwara H, Sugimoto M, Ohno T, Vilaichone RK, Mahachai V, Graham DY, Yamaoka Y.Role of deletion located between the intermediate and middle regions of the *Helicobacter pylori vacA* gene in cases of gastroduodenal diseases. J Clin Microbiol. 2009;47:3493–3500.

[27] Yamaoka Y, Kita M, Kodama T, Imamura S, Ohno T, Sawai N, Ishimaru A, Imanishi J, Graham DY. *Helicobacter pylori* infection in mice: Role of outer membrane proteins in colonization and inflammation. Gastroenterology. 2002;123:1992–2004.

[28] Lu H, Hsu PI, Graham DY, Yamaoka Y. Duodenal ulcer promoting gene of *Helicobacter pylori*. Gastroenterology. 2005;128:833–848.

[29] Douraghi M, Mohammadi M, Oghalaie A, Abdirad A, Mohagheghi MA, Hosseini ME, Zeraati H, Ghasemi A, Esmaieli M, Mohajerani N. *dupA* as a risk determinant in *Helicobacter pylori* infection. J Med Microbiol. 2008;57:554–562.

[30] Nguyen LT, Uchida T, Tsukamoto Y, Kuroda A, Okimoto T, Kodama M, Murakami K, Fujioka T, Moriyama M.*Helicobacter pylori dupA* gene is not associated with clinical outcomes in the Japanese population. Clin Microbiol Infect. 2010;16:1264–1269.

[31] Falush D, Wirth T, Linz B, Pritchard JK, Stephens M, Kidd M, Blaser MJ, Graham DY, Vacher S, Perez-Perez GI, Yamaoka Y, Mégraud F, Otto K, Reichard U, Katzowitsch E, Wang X, Achtman M, Suerbaum S.Traces of human migrations in *Helicobacter pylori* populations. Science 2003;299: 1582-1585.

[32] El-Omar EM, Carrington M, Chow WH, McColl KE, Bream JH, Young HA, Herrera J, Lissowska J, Yuan CC, Rothman N, Lanyon G, Martin M, Fraumeni JF, Jr, Rabkin CS. Interleukin-1 polymorphisms associated with increased risk of gastric cancer. Nature. 2000;404:398–402.

[33] El-Omar EM, Rabkin CS, Gammon MD, Vaughan TL, Risch HA, Schoenberg JB, Stanford JL, Mayne ST, Goedert J, Blot WJ, Fraumeni JF, Jr, Chow WH. Increased risk of noncardia gastric cancer associated with proinflammatory cytokine gene polymorphisms. Gastroenterology 2003;124:1193–201.

[34] Figueiredo C, Machado JC, Pharoah P, Seruca R, Sousa S, Carvalho R, Capelinha AF, Quint W, Caldas C, van Doorn LJ, Carneiro F, Sobrinho-Simoes M. *Helicobacter pylori* and interleukin 1 genotyping: an opportunity to identify high-risk individuals for gastric carcinoma. J Natl Cancer Inst 2002;94:1680–7

[35] Persson C, Canedo P, Machado JC, El-Omar EM, Forman D. Polymorphisms in Inflammatory Response Genes and Their Association With Gastric Cancer: A HuGE Systematic Review and Meta-Analyses. Am J Epidemiol. 2011 February 1; 173(3): 259–270.

[36] Wang P, Xia HH, Zhang JY, Dai LP, Xu XQ, Wang KJ.Association of interleukin-1 gene polymorphisms with gastric cancer: a meta-analysis. Int J Cancer 2007;120(3): 552–562.

[37] Camargo MC, Mera R, Correa P, Peek RM Jr, Fontham ET, Goodman KJ, Piazuelo MB, Sicinschi L, Zabaleta J, Schneider BG.Interleukin-1β and interleukin-1 receptor antagonist gene polymorphisms and gastric cancer: a meta-analysis. Cancer Epidemiol Biomarkers Prev 2006;15(9):1674–1687

[38] Kamangar F, Cheng C, Abnet CC, Rabkin CS.Interleukin-1B polymorphisms and gastric cancer risk—a meta-analysis. Cancer Epidemiol Biomarkers Prev 2006;15(10): 1920–1928.

[39] Loh M, Koh KX, Yeo BH, Song CM, Chia KS, Zhu F, Yeoh KG, Hill J, Iacopetta B, Soong R.Meta-analysis of genetic polymorphisms and gastric cancer risk: variability in associations according to race. Eur J Cancer 2009;45(14):2562–2568.

[40] Gorouhi F, Islami F, Bahrami H, Kamangar F.Tumour-necrosis factor-A polymorphisms and gastric cancer risk: a meta-analysis. Br J Cancer 2008;98(8):1443–1451.

[41] Zhang J, Dou C, Song Y, et al. Polymorphisms of tumor necrosis factor-alpha are associated with increased susceptibility to gastric cancer: a meta-analysis. J Hum Genet 2008;53(6):479–489.

[42] Kamangar F, Abnet CC, Hutchinson AA, Newschaffer CJ, Helzlsouer K, Shugart YY, Pietinen P, Dawsey SM, Albanes D, Virtamo J, Taylor PR. Polymorphisms in inflammation-related genes and risk of gastric cancer (Finland) Cancer Causes Control 2006;17:117–25.

[43] Canedo P, Castanheira-Vale AJ, Lunet N, Pereira F, Figueiredo C, Gioia-Patricola L, Canzian F, Moreira H, Suriano G, Barros H, Carneiro F, Seruca R, Machado JC. The interleukin-8-251*T/*A polymorphism is not associated with risk for gastric carcinoma development in a Portuguese population. Eur J Cancer Prev 2008;17:28–32.

[44] Hold GL, Rabkin CS, Chow WH, Smith MG, Gammon MD, Risch HA, Vaughan TL, McColl KE, Lissowska J, Zatonski W, Schoenberg JB, Blot WJ, Mowat NA, Fraumeni JF, Jr, El-Omar EM. A functional polymorphism of toll-like receptor 4 gene increases risk of gastric carcinoma and its precursors. Gastroenterology 2007;132:905–12.

[45] Arbour NC, Lorenz E, Schutte BC, Zabner J, Kline JN, Jones M, Frees K, Watt JL, Schwartz DA. TLR4 mutations are associated with endotoxin hyporesponsiveness in humans. Nat Genet2000; 25: 187-191

[46] Gao L, Nieters A, Brenner H. Cell proliferation-related genetic polymorphisms and gastric cancer risk: systematic review and meta-analysis. Eur J Hum Genet. 2009;17:1658-67.

[47] Liao SY, Zeng ZR, Leung WK, Zhou SZ, Chen B, Sung JJ, Hu PJ.Peroxisome proliferator-activated receptor-gamma Pro12Ala polymorphism, *Helicobacter pylori* infection and non-cardia gastric carcinoma in Chinese. Aliment Pharmacol Ther. 2006;23:289–294.

[48] Prasad KN, Saxena A, Ghoshal UC, Bhagat MR, Krishnani N. Analysis of Pro12Ala PPAR gamma polymorphism and *Helicobacter pylori* infection in gastric adenocarcinoma and peptic ulcer disease. Ann Oncol 2008;19:1299–1303

[49] Hamai Y, Matsumura S, Matsusaki K, K, Kitadai Y, Yoshida K, Yamaguchi Y, Imai K, Nakachi K, Toge T, Yasui W. A single nucleotide polymorphism in the 50 untranslated region of the EGF gene is associated with occurrence and malignant progression of gastric cancer. Pathobiology 2005;72: 133 – 138.

[50] Jin G, Wang L, Chen W, Hu Z, Zhou Y, Tan Y, Wang J, Hua Z, Ding W, Shen J, Zhang Z, Wang X, Xu Y, Shen H. Variant alleles of TGFB1 and TGFBR2 are associated with a decreased risk of gastric cancer in a Chinese population.Int J Cancer 2007;120: 1330 – 1335.

[51] Zhang ZW, Newcomb PV, Moorghen M Zhang ZW, Newcomb PV, Moorghen M, Gupta J, Feakins R, Savage P, Hollowood A, Alderson D, Holly JM.Insulin-like growth factor binding protein-3: relationship to the development of gastric pre-ma-

lignancy and gastric adenocarcinoma (United Kingdom). Cancer Causes Control 2004;15:211 – 218.

[52] Chen W, Wang L, Ke Jin G, Tan Y, Zhou Y, Hu Z, Ma H, Wang J, Hua Z, Ding W, Shen J, Xu Y, Shen H. The role of IGFBP3 functional polymorphisms in the risk of gastric cancer in a high-risk Chinese population.Eur J Cancer Prev 2008;17: 82 – 87.

[53] Loh JT, Friedman DB, Piazuelo MB, Bravo LE, Wilson KT, Peek RM Jr,Correa P, Cover TL. Analysis of *Helicobacter pylori cag*A promoter elements required for salt-induced upregulation of CagA expression. Infect Immun 2012;80:3094–106.

[54] Blanca Piazuelo M, Epplein M, Correa P. Gastric cancer: An infectious disease. Infect Dis Clin North Am 2010; 24(4): 853–869

[55] Fox JG, Dangler CA, Taylor NS, King A, Koh TJ, Wang TC. High-salt diet induces gastric epithelial hyperplasia and parietal cell loss, and enhances *Helicobacter pylori* colonization in C57BL/6 mice. Cancer Res 1999;59(19):4823–8.

[56] Yamaguchi N, Kakizoe T. Synergistic interaction between *Helicobacter pylori* gastritis and diet in gastric cancer. Lancet Oncol 2001;2(2):88–94.

[57] Ladeiras-Lopes R, Pereira AK, Nogueira A, Pinheiro-Torres T, Pinto I, Santos-Pereira R, Lunet N. Smoking and gastric cancer: systematic review and meta-analysis of cohort studies. Cancer Causes Control 2008; 19:689 – 701.

[58] Koizumi Y, Tsubono Y, Nakaya N, Kuriyama S, Shibuya D, Matsuoka H, Tsuji I. Cigarette smoking and the risk of gastric cancer: a pooled analysis of two prospective studies in Japan. Int J Cancer 2004; 112: 1049 – 1055.

[59] Sjodahl K, Lu Y, Nilsen TI, Ye W, Hveem K, Vatten L, Lagergren J. Smoking and alcohol dinking in relation to risk of gastric cancer: a population-based,prospective cohort study. Int J Cancer 2007; 120: 128 – 132.

[60] Moy KA, Fan Y, Wang R, Gao YT, Yu MC, Yuan JM. Alcohol and tobacco use in relation to gastric cancer: a prospective study of men in Shanghai,China. Cancer Epidemiol Biomarkers Prev 2010; 19: 2287 – 2297.

[61] Duan L, Wu AH, Sullivan-Halley J, Berstein L. Passive smoking and risk of oesophageal and gastric adenocarcinomas. Br J Cancer 2009;100: 1483 – 1485

[62] Algra AM, Rothwell PM. Effects of regular aspirin on long-term cancer incidence and metastasis: a systematic comparison of evidence from observational studies versus randomised trials. Lancet Oncol 2012;13(5):518-27.

[63] Bosetti C, Rosato V, Gallus S, Cuzick J, La Vecchia C. Aspirin and cancer risk: a quantitative review to 2011. Ann Oncol 2012;23(6):1403-15.

[64] Wong BC, Zhang L, Ma JL, Pan KF, Li JY, Shen L, Liu WD, Feng GS, Zhang XD, Li J, Lu AP, Xia HH, Lam S, You WC. Effects of selective COX-2 inhibitor and *Helicobacterpylori* eradication on precancerous gastric lesions. Gut 2012;61(6):812-8.

[65] Tian W, Zhao Y, Liu S, Li X. Meta-analysis on the relationship between nonsteroidal anti-inflammatory drug use and gastric cancer. Eur J Cancer Prev. 2010 ;19(4):288-98

[66] Conteduca V, Sansonno D, Ingravallo G, Marangi S, Russi S, Lauletta G, Dammacco F. Barrett's esophagus and esophageal cancer: an overview. Int J Oncol 2012; 41:414–424.

[67] Fuccio L, Eusebi LH, Bazzoli F. Gastric cancer, *Helicobacterpylori* infection and other risk factors. World J Gastrointest Oncol 2010; 2:342–347.

[68] Correa P, Haenszel W, Cuello C, Tannenbaum S, Archer M. A model for gastric cancer epidemiology. Lancet 1975; 2: 58–60.

[69] Wong BC, Lam SK, Wong WM, Chen JS, Zheng TT, Feng RE, Lai KC, Hu WH, Yuen ST, Leung SY, Fong DY, Ho J, Ching CK. *Helicobacterpylori* eradication to prevent gastric cancer in a high-risk region of China: a randomized controlled trial. JAMA 2004;291:187–194.

[70] Leung WK, Lin SR, Ching JY, To KF, Ng EK, Chan FK, Lau JY, Sung JJ. Factors predicting progression of gastric intestinal metaplasia: results of a randomised trial on *Helicobacterpylori* eradication.Gut 2004;53(9):1244–1249

[71] Correa P, Fontham ET, Bravo JC, Bravo LE, Ruiz B, Zarama G, Realpe JL, Malcom GT, Li D, Johnson WD, Mera R. Chemoprevention of gastric dysplasia: randomized trial of antioxidant supplements and anti-*Helicobacterpylori* therapy. J Natl Cancer Inst 2000;6;92:1881–1888.

[72] Mera R, Fontham ET, Bravo LE, Bravo JC, Piazuelo MB, Camargo MC, Correa P. Long term follow up of patients treated for *Helicobacterpylori* infection. Gut 2005;54(11):1536–1540.

[73] You WC, Brown LM, Zhang L, Li JY, Jin ML, Chang YS, Ma JL, Pan KF, Liu WD, Hu Y, Crystal-Mansour S, Pee D, Blot WJ, Fraumeni JF Jr, Xu GW, Gail MH. Randomized double-blind factorial trial of three treatments to reduce the prevalence of precancerous gastric lesions. J Natl Cancer Inst 2006; 98:974-983.

[74] Ma JL, Zhang L, Brown LM, Li JY, Shen L, Pan KF, Liu WD, Hu Y, Han ZX, Crystal-Mansour S, Pee D, Blot WJ, Fraumeni JF Jr, You WC, Gail MH. Fifteen-year effects of *Helicobacterpylori*, garlic, and vitamin treatments on gastric cancer incidence and mortality. J Natl Cancer Inst 2012;104:488-492.

[75] Fukase K, Kato M, Kikuchi S, Inoue K, Uemura N, Okamoto S, Terao S, Amagai K, Hayashi S, Asaka M; Japan Gast Study Group.Effect of eradication of *Helicobacterpylori* on incidence of metachronous gastric carcinoma after endoscopic resection of early gastric cancer: an open-label, randomised controlled trial. Lancet 2008;372:392-397.

[76] Lee YC, Chen TH, Chiu HM, Shun CT, Chiang H, Liu TY, Wu MS, Lin JT. The benefit of mass eradication of *Helicobacterpylori* infection: a community-based study of gastric cancer prevention. Gut 2013;62:676-82

[77] El-Omar EM. Role of host genes in sporadic gastric cancer. Best Pract Res Clin Gastroenterol. 2006;20:675–86.

Section 4

H. pylori Infection in Children and Possible Causes of Iron Deficiency Anemia

Chapter 6

Particulars of the *Helicobacter pylori* Infection in Children

Florica Nicolescu

Additional information is available at the end of the chapter

http://dx.doi.org/10.5772/58326

1. Introduction

Helicobacter pylori (*H. pylori*) is an important pathogen in human gastroenterology. *H. pylori* is commonly acquired during early childhood and it is more common among people in developing countries. Globally, over 50% of the population is infected with this bacteria, being practically evenly distributed between the two genders, in spite of a few studies showing a slight predisposition in males.

The clinical consequences of *H. pylori* infection in children are yet to be fully understood. *H. pylori* infection in children differs from the same infection in adults, both in terms of the percentage of infected individuals, symptoms, degree of complication towards peptic ulcer disease or malignancy, the gastric areas affected, the degree of compliance to therapeutic management or bacterial resistance to treatment.

2. Context

Helicobacter pylori (*H. pylori)* is a Gram - negative bacillus responsible for one of the most commonly diagnosed infections, namely gastritis, in humans worldwide. [1]

In 1983 Robin Warren, an Australian pathologist, described an S-shaped bacteria for the first time, that was found in the gastric mucosa. Together with Barry Marshall, they managed to isolate thid micro-organism from biopsy samples taken during endoscopy, and called it *Campylobacter pyloridis*, to be called *H. pylori* later on. [2]

Although the presence of bacteria in the stomach had been known as early as the 19th century, these microbes were considered simply a consequence of gastric mucosa contamination from food intake and not colonizing species in the true sense of the word. The current in thinking had been so controversial from the very beginning, that, about 30 years later, when *H. pylori* was discovered and proposed as the causative agent for gastritis and peptic ulcer disease, the scientific community rejected and even ridiculed the new theory. Survival of microbes in the acidic pH conditions of the stomach was considered impossible.

In one of the boldest scientific approaches of the last century, Barry Marshall self-administered an *H. pylori* dose in 1984. Although the researcher physician expected to develop peptic ulcer disease in the coming months, the symptoms emerged much sooner: only 3 days later, Marshall displayed dizziness, halitosis and vomiting, and in another 8 days, pangastritis was diagnosed endoscopically, meaning inflammation of a large areas of the stomach.

Shortly after the publication of results in Warren and Marshall's research, *H. pylori* was also detected in biopsy specimens taken during digestive endoscopy performed in children with chronic gastritis and / or duodenal ulcers; at the same time, resolution of gastric pathology in children was also demonstrated with bacterial eradication. [3] Overall, these discoveries have demonstrated the important role of *H. pylori* in gastric pathology both in adults and children.

The discovery of *H. pylori,* the demonstration of causality between the infection and gastric pathology and improvement of the bacteria eradication methodology increased the living quality for a large number of patients. If, in the past, peptic ulcer disease surgery used to be one of the most common forms of surgery performed, management of ulcers by eradication of *H. pylori* is so effective nowadays that very few patients require surgery. The merit of Warren and Marshall's pioneering research was awarded the Nobel Prize for medicine in 2005.

Goals of current and future research of *H. pylori* equally require better understanding of immune-pathogenics of gastric disease associated with *H. pylori* infection, clarification of modes of transmission, as well as improving the safety and effectiveness of vaccines for prevention of *H. pylori* infection.

Children are different from adults regarding *H. pylori* infection, in terms of the prevalence of the infection, the complication rate, the almost complete absence of gastric malignancy, age-specific issues, with diagnostic tests and medication as well as a higher rate of resistance to antibiotics. The former and other differences as well can explain why some of the recommendations for adults cannot be applied to children. [4]

3. Description of *H. pylori*

Phylogenetic classification of *H. pylori* is: *Helicobacter* genus, *Helicobacteraceae* family, *Campylobacterales* order, *Proteobacteria* subdivision.

H. pylori is a Gram - negative type bacterium, able to colonize the gastric mucosa in the majority of the population in the context of very low pH and low partial pressure of oxygen (pO_2). *H. pylori* has a curved shape and is 2-4 microns long and 1 micron wide. It displays 2-6 flagella of about 3 microns in length, ensuring it high mobility. [5] Optimal development of this organism requires reduced O_2 pressure, high humidity, 37° C temperature and neutral pH. The metabolism of the microbe can process glucose but not any other sugars.

The bacterium displays a range of extraordinary adaptations needed for survival in the extreme conditions of the gastric environment. *H. pylori* is one of the most efficient animal species, capable of degrading urea. The abundance of the *urease* enzyme allows rapid urea hydrolysis in the gastric environment, with release of bicarbonate and ammonia, which neutralize the gastric pH and provide for the optimum conditions for bacterial life. At the same time, the ammonia generated is used in the metabolism of the bacterium for the synthesis of amino acids. [6] Initially, the *urease* enzyme is solely localized in the cytoplasm, however, in the case of exposure to acid *in vivo,* autolysis of the cell wall takes place and release of the enzyme, which is subsequently fixed on the *H. pylori* surface. At the same time, increased motility allows the bacterium to penetrate and become fixed in the layers of the gastric mucosa. [7]

Outside the host organism, however, *H. pylori* is fragile and unable to survive when stored at low and ultra-low temperatures as compared with other intestinal bacteria. Although healthy individuals' manner of infection of is not yet fully understood, it is assumed that transmission is largely by direct contact of individuals and less by contaminated objects.

4. The rate of *H. pylori* infection

H. pylori infection global rate differs by region, ethnicity, age, and socio-economic level of the population. The percentage of infected individuals is higher in disadvantaged socio-economic categories and increases with age. Large infection percentages (about 80%) may be found in Asian countries, in Eastern and South-Eastern Europe, in Latin America, whereas much smaller percentages (about 40%) are characteristic to Western countries. [8-10]

Regardless of the geographic area analysed, one finds that *H. pylori* infection is usually acquired in early childhood both in developed and developing countries.

5. Prevalence

Overall, about one third of the population is infected with *H. pylori*, and the frequency increases with age.

In general, the prevalence is higher in developing countries, and the infection is contacted at an early age. The incidence is 3-10% of the population every year in developing countries, as compared to 0.5% in developed countries. [11]

The prevalence of *H. pylori* infection is not only lower in industrialized countries than in developing countries, but the incidence of *H. pylori* infection, gastric cancer, peptic ulcer disease and related diseases are also declining. Worldwide, more than 1 billion people are estimated to be infected with *H. pylori*. [4]

6. Possibility of transmission

H. pylori does not tolerate increased O_2 partial pressure, high temperatures or nutrients poor environments outside the host organism. In other words, *H. pylori* is excellently adapted to gastric existing parameters, but it is a fragile organism, non-viable outside the host. One study highlights the possibility for *Helicobacter pylori* infection from a water supply. For these reasons, although the exact *H. pylori* mode of transmission is not completely understood, the type of transmission is accepted by primarily direct contact of healthy individuals with an infected person. Transmission of infection may also be the result of transport vectors.

H. pylori isolated strains are found more often in staff performing endoscopies than the general population.

H. pylori has been isolated and cultivated from faeces, indicating the possibility of faecal-oral transmission. Also, *H. pylori* was found in the oral cavity in both saliva and the plaque, suggesting oral-oral transmission variant. Therefore, transmission of *H. pylori* can occur by oral-oral, faecal-oral transmission or a combination thereof. [12]

Horizontal transmission is favoured by overcrowding found in densely populated human communities. This version is the most likely in the case of infection transmission among family members. Thus, children of *H. pylori* infected mothers run an 8 times higher risk of acquiring the bacterium. [13]

7. Diagnosis of *H. pylori*

Correct diagnosis of *H. pylori* is possible through a wide range of working methods. However, the opportunity to diagnose *H. pylori* and the working method chosen should be evaluated according to the specificity of each case.

H. pylori infection generated symptoms is nonspecific, including abdominal pain, gastro-oesophageal reflux with or without heartburn, halitosis, vomiting or hematemesis.

Because symptoms caused by *H. pylori* are general (nonspecific), the *H. pylori* infection may overlap with another digestive or abdominally located disorder. Therefore, the primary purpose of investigating gastrointestinal symptoms should be elucidating their real ethyology and not just determining the presence of *H. pylori* infection. This consideration is especially important in the case of *H. pylori* infection in children under the age of 12, because the latter are unable to accurately describe the location, nature or intensity of their discomfort. [14]

Assessment of patients infected with *H. pylori* should pay particular attention to anorexia and weight loss, pallor or laboratory tests to identify anaemia, vomiting, abdominal pain or pain associated with meals and night-time, as well as to any descriptions of gastrointestinal haemorrhage.

In children suspected of *H. pylori* infection, history should include the following:

- Abominable pain nature, location, frequency, duration, severity, exacerbation and alleviating factors;
- The intestinal transit and description of the stool;
- Appetite, diet, changes in weight;
- Halitosis, vomiting and description of the gastric material;
- Ulcer disease or gastrointestinal disorders (e.g. Crohn's disease) running in the family;
- Medications (on-prescription and OTC);
- Previous diagnostic tests and gastrointestinal tract specific therapy.

Physical examination of an asymptomatic *H. pylori* infected child usually ends in confusing results. In children with chronic gastritis, duodenal and peptic ulcer, important findings include epigastric tenderness or gastrointestinal bleeding (e.g., positive guaiac stools, tachycardia, pallor).

Children with peptic ulcer can develop complications (e.g., severe blood loss in the gastrointestinal tract, perforation, obstruction) and may show signs of hemodynamic instability or signs of acute abdomen. Children with long-term peptic ulcer caused by *H. pylori* may become anaemic from undetected and asymptomatic chronic bleeding. In such children, the following should be considered:

- The child's overall appearance;
- Assessment of perfusion, paying special attention to the child's mental status, heart rate, pulse as well as *refill of capillaries*.
- Evaluation of *the child's skin as well as* conjunctivae in order to check pallor.
- Careful cardiac and pulmonary scrutiny.
- Abdomen inspection, auscultation and palpating.
- Making a rectal exam and the guaiac test of the stool. [4]

For accurate diagnosis of *H. pylori* infection, several methods are available with varying degrees of accuracy:

7.1. Histopathological methods

Isolation and cultivation of *H. pylori* in biopsy specimens taken during endoscopy is the golden standard in diagnosing the infection. In addition, this method also has the advantage of providing information about tissue pathology as caused by *H. pylori* infection. Since distribution of *H. pylori* concentration on the gastric mucosa is not uniform but has rather the appearance of distinct lower or higher concentration islands, taking at least 2 biopsies is recommended, one of the gastric body and the other from the antrum. [15]

7.2. Breath analysis

Diagnosis of *H. pylori* infection may also be performed by breath analysis after oral administration of a urea solution. If the urea used is provided with a ^{13}C- labelled carbon atom, this isotope dosage can be performed, but the method is both very precise and demanding in terms of the equipment involved. Alternatively, unmarked urea can be administered to qualitatively detect the presence of *H. pylori* by identification of NH_3 (ammonia) in the air expired. [4]

7.3. Immunological methods

H. pylori infection causes emergence of specific antibodies: anti - *H. pylori* antibodies (IgA and IgG) in serum, blood, urine and / or saliva. Although cheap and fast, detection of these antibodies is not relevant to assess the current status of infection or success of the eradication therapy. Because of immunological memory, antibodies may persist for months and years even in the host organism after eradication of the infection. [16-18]

7.4. Detection of antigens

Identification of *H. pylori* antigen in faeces is an accurate way of establishing the diagnosis, as a non-invasive method and easier to apply in children than administration of urea solution or endoscopy.

In addition, the method has the advantage that even after the passage of five days from sample harvest, diagnosing *H. pylori* is as accurate. Thus, sampling of biological material can be performed without the active participation of children and their visit to the medical centre, as the sample may be dispatched by courier. [4]

Colonization of gastric mucosa by *H. pylori* does not automatically mean onset of the disease, but the infection correlates with increased risk of infection during the onset of peptic ulcers and gastric cancer. The materialization of this risk depends on a summation of factors related to the genome of the bacterium, the host and environmental factors.[19]

A wide range of extra-gastrointestinal disorders are thought to be associated with *H. pylori* infection, e.g. otitis media, upper respiratory tract infections, periodontitis, food allergies, Sudden Infant Death Syndrome (SIDS). However, there is currently no convincing scientific evidence regarding the causal relationship between *H. pylori* infection and such disorders.

Symptoms associated with *H. pylori* infection may be absent even in some cases where the presence of *H. pylori* was proved by histological analysis. In other cases however, infection is followed by the occurrence of peptic ulcer and its complications. The general pathology of *H. pylori* includes phenomena such as dyspepsia and refractory anaemia. [15]

http://dx.doi.org/10.5772/58326

8. Incriminatory factors

To determine their causal relationship with *H. pylori* infection, epidemiological studies have addressed various factors such as a bacterial cause, the host, genetic and environmental factors. Data are related to the spread of infection from person to person (e. g. dental plaque), but the origin and the mode of transmission is incomplete known. [4]

H. pylori infection causes include the following:

- We can observe that the transmission of *H. pylori* is possible person to person.

Groups of infection are under observation, particularly within families of infected children. Possible routes are faecal-oral, oral-oral and gastro-oral. Mother to child transmission has been suggested in a study analysing DNA of *H. pylori* strains. [20] Studies have shown identical *H. pylori* strains in mothers and their younger children. Maternal symptoms of nausea and vomiting and pacifier use were associated with the risk of *H. pylori* infection in children.

Cervantes et al. participated a study performed at the US-Mexico border and they have shown that a younger brother is 4 times more prone to *H. pylori* infection if the mother was *H. pylori* infected, compared to an uninfected mother. Younger brothers are 8 times more likely to acquire the infection if an older brother had persistent *H. pylori* infection. [13]

Absence or poor personal hygiene may also play a role. Increase in *H. pylori* infection may be observed in developing countries, which may reflect the combined effects of poor living conditions, poor hygiene and overcrowded cities.

The status of *H. pylori* infection in the United States, a comparatively higher socio-economic setting, shows that the higher the social and economic level, the lower the incidence of *H. pylori* infection, a finding that may reflect also the same factors as those mentioned in the case of developing countries.

- In the clinical manifestations of *H. pylori* infection the bacterial factors may play an important role. Patients infected with *H. pylori* may have two basic phenotypes reported the presence or absence of cytotoxin vacuole.

Inflammation is more pronounced in people with cytotoxin - positive infection, confirmed at endoscopy, than in those infected with *H. pylori* cytotoxin - negative.

As far as bacterial factors are involved, presence of two fundamental phenotypes has been shown in *H. pylori* infected patients, i.e. vacuolating cytotoxin positive and negative, respectively. Endoscopy performed on cytotoxin-positive infected patients has proved inflammation more marked than in patients where the cytotoxin was absent.[13]

The significance of host dependent factors has been demonstrated by such observations as the fact that adults are less capable of solving acute infections than children.

A different such factor may be the presence of hypochlorhydria in the host, which allows specific *H. pylori* colonization of the stomach.

In addition, *H. pylori may only persist if the* metaplastic epithelium of the stomach is atrophied.[4]

- One study highlights the possibility for *H. pylori* infection from a water supply. [21]
- Transmission of infection may also be the result of transport vectors. [22]
- *H. pylori* isolated strains are found more often in staff performing endoscopies than the general population.

9. Pathophysiology

H. pylori organisms are spiral Gram - negative bacteria, highly mobile due to their multiple unipolar flagella. They are microaerophilic powerful urease producers. These organisms inhabit the mucus adjacent to the gastric mucosa.

Important adaptive features improve survival of the organism in an acidic environment include its shape and motility, its low oxygen needs, its adhesion molecules serving a feeding role in certain gastric cells and *urease* production. Bacterial *urease* converts urea to ammonia and bicarbonate, therefore neutralizing gastric acid and providing protection from a hostile environment. Some of the lipopolysaccharides of the organism mimic the Lewis blood group antigens structure. This molecular mimicry also helps the survival of *H. pylori* in the unfavourable gastric environment. [23]

H. pylori generates disease triggers, including *urease*, vacuolating cytotoxin, catalase and lipopolysaccharide (LPS). *Urease* is a potent antigen inducing increased production of immunoglobulin G and immunoglobulin A. Expression of vacuolating cytotoxin generating inflammatory cytokines may be associated with more pronounced inflammation and marked tendency of disease triggering.

The most important virulence factor in *H. pylori* infection is cytotoxin - associated antigen (CagA). A person infected with CagA -negative strains is likely to develop chronic gastritis and have little chance to develop peptic ulcer disease or gastric cancer.

On the other hand, infection with CagA -positive strains greatly increases the risk of peptic ulcer and gastric cancer. Movement of CagA protein into gastric epithelial cells leads to rearrangement of the host cytoskeleton, alters signalling cell and disturbs the cell cycle control. [24]

In children with *H. pylori* infection, who have peptic ulcer disease, *in situ* expression of CagA is increased and may play an important role in the pathogenesis of peptic ulcer disease. [25]

The bacteria *H. pylori* localises in the stomach, induces inflammatory cytokines formation and causes gastric inflammation. People with *H. pylori* gastritis associated with increased gastric acid gastritis are prone to peptic ulcer disease. [26] In contrast, people infected with *H. pylori* associated with corpus gastritis, with decreased gastric acid production are more prone to developing gastric atrophy (intestinal metaplasia and gastric adenocarcinoma).

The infection with *H. pylori* has been associated with iron deficiency anaemia. The two main assumptions underlying this theory are iron sequestration because of antral *H. pylori* infection and decrease of non- hemin iron absorption caused by hypochlorhydria.

H. pylori infection and its association with gastric malignancies have been well described in several epidemiological studies. [27] However, the evolution from inflammation to cancer remains unclear.

There exists a model describing the progressive evolution of *H. pylori* infection to hypochlorhydria, chronic gastritis, atrophic gastritis, dysplasia, intestinal metaplasia and gastric cancer. [28, 29, 30, 31]

A newer hypothesis suggests that *H. pylori* infection may protect against self - inflammatory diseases such as asthma or inflammatory bowel disease. For instance, epidemiological data suggest that infection with *Helicobacter pylori* is less common in patients with inflammatory bowel disease, which leads to research for defining potential mechanisms underlying these clinical findings. [27]

10. Morbidity

Most *H. pylori* infected children are asymptomatic. Antral gastritis is the most common manifestation in children. Duodenal and gastric ulcers may be associated with *H. pylori* gastritis in adults, but is less common in children. The risk of gastric cancer, including non - Hodgkin lymphoma (i.e. associated to the lymphoid tissue mucosa MALT]) and adenocarcinoma is increased in adults.[4]

The relationship between *H. pylori* gastritis and recurrent abdominal pain (RAP) is controversial. The incidence of *H. pylori* gastritis in patients with RAP is not significantly higher than the incidence of *H. pylori* infection in the general population. Although certain studies have shown an improvement in symptoms in children with RAP and *Helicobacter pylori* gastritis after eradication therapy for *H. pylori,* data from a recent double-blind controlled trial have not confirmed this finding. [32]

According to the North American Society for Paediatric Gastroenterology, Hepatology and Nutrition no results were sufficiently reliable to support routine testing for *H. pylori in* children with RAP. [33]

Data published so far highlight an association between *H. pylori* infection and gastrointestinal symptoms in children, but no association has been found between RAP and *H. pylori* infection. Conflicting evidence has been found however concerning the association of *H. pylori* infection with epigastric pain. [34]

There are studies suggesting that *H. pylori* protects the human body from developing gastroesophageal reflux disease, while others affirm a causal association between them. Analysis of studies in conducted in adults has found no association between *H. pylori* eradication and development of new cases of gastroesophageal reflux disease in dyspeptic patients. [35]

According to a pediatric retrospective study, there was a significantly higher prevalence of reflux esophagitis in *H. pylori* infected children. [36]

H. pylori infection was also associated with extraintestinal manifestations such as short stature, immune thrombocytopenic purpura and migraine, with different levels of causation. [37, 38]. This infection is also associated with coronary diseases, iron-deficiency anemia and hepato-biliary diseases among others. [39, 40, 41, 42, 43, 44]

11. Dissemination (population category)

The predominance *H. pylori* infection is increased in black, Hispanic, Asian, and Native American populations.

The infection with *H. pylori* affect more than a half of the world's population, which is acquired almost always within the first 5 years of life [45]. In the developed world, the prevalence rates vary from 1.2% to 12.2% [46-49]. In developing countries, the prevalence rates are much higher. The serological prevalence rates of *H. pylori* were 45% among Indian children [40,51]. In Bolivia and Alaska, at the age of 9 years, the seroprevalence was 70% and 69%, respectively [52]. The seroprevalence in preschoolers in Brazil was found to be 69.7% [53]. An age-related increase of the prevalence of *H. pylori*, irrespective of the economic state of the country, was observed by several independent studies across the world [47-51, 54, 55].

In a study of Prof Dr Sibille Koletzko et al [15] was presented that during the first years of life in both developing and industrialized countries the *H. pylori* infection is usually acquired.The epidemiology of *H. pylori* infection in children, in Europe and North America has changed in recent decades. In the northern and western European countries are founding low incidence rates, resulting in prevalence far below 10% in children and adolescents. In contrast, the infection is still common in certain geographic areas such as southern or eastern Europe, Mexico, and certain immigrant populations from South America, Africa, and most Asian countries, and aboriginal people in North America. The different prevalence of infection and the corresponding effect on health care resources in industrialized compared with developing countries require different recommendations with respect to testing and treating children. These guidelines apply only to children living in Europe and North America, but not to those living in other continents, particularly in developing countries with a high *H. pylori* infection rate in children and adolescents and with limited resources for health care [15].

Infection rates are similar in men and women alike.

Many study present that less than 10% of children under 12 years of age are infected in developed countries, but seropositivity increases with age, to a rate of 0.3-1% per year. Seropositivity studies in developed countries in adults showed a prevalence of 30-50%.

In the US, estimated prevalence is 20% for people under 30 and 50% for persons over 60. In developing countries, prevalence rates are much higher. *H. pylori* serological prevalence rates have been 15% and 46% for Gambian children under 20 months and 40-60 months, respectively. [56]

http://dx.doi.org/10.5772/58326

12. Laboratory methodology

An important study of Prof Dr Sibille Koletzko et al was presented by using the testing guidelines recently provided by the European Society for Paediatric Gastroenterology Hepatology and Nutrition (ESPGHAN) and the North American Society for Paediatric Gastroenterology, Hepatology and Nutrition (NASPGHAN) for *H. pylori* infection in children [15]. These recommendations are:

- The primary purpose of clinical investigation of gastrointestinal symptoms is to determine the primary cause of the symptoms, and not the presence of *H. pylori* infection only.
- Diagnostic tests for *H. pylori* infection are not recommended in children with functional abdominal pain. Currently, in the absence of ulcer disease, there is insufficient evidence to justify a causal relationship between *H. pylori* gastritis and abdominal symptoms. Therefore, cases of abdominal pain consistent with diagnostic criteria for functional pain should not be investigated for *H. pylori,* unless upper endoscopy is conducted during diagnostic, in search of some organic disease.
- In children with first-degree relatives with gastric cancer, *H. pylori* testing may be considered.
- In children with refractory iron deficiency anaemia in whom other causes have been excluded, *H. pylori* testing can be considered.
- There is insufficient evidence that *H. pylori* infection is causally linked with otitis media, respiratory tract infections, periodontal diseases, food allergies, sudden infant death syndrome, idiopathic thrombocytopenic purpura and short stature.
- To confirm eradication in children selected with disease complicated by peptic ulcer or lymphoma and in children who remain symptomatic.

For diagnostic tests to be applied, the recommendations are as follows:

- For the diagnosis of *H. pylori* infection during esophagogastroduodenoscopy (EGD), it is recommended to obtain gastric biopsy samples (antrum and corpus gastritis).
- It is recommended that the initial diagnosis of *H. pylori* infection rely on positive histopathology examination and a rapid *urease* positive test or a positive culture.
- The ^{13}C - urea breath test (UBT) is a non-invasive test to determine successful eradication of *H. pylori*.
- A positive enzyme immunoassay (ELISA) for the detection of *H. pylori* antigen in the stool is a noninvasive test to determine whether *H.pylori* has been eradicated. Several methods are available for detection of the *H. pylori* antigen in stool, such as the enzyme immunoassay test (EIA) based on polyclonal or monoclonal antibodies and immunochromatographic tests (the so-called rapid tests).

Stool tests are generally much more convenient in children than UBT. Neither storage of evidence at room temperature for up to 5 days nor freezing them for months or even years appears to influence the accuracy of the stool tests. So far, only EIA based on monoclonal antibodies has equalled UBT accuracy.

- Tests relying on antibody detection (IgG, IgA) against *H. pylori* in the blood serum, urine and saliva are not viable for use in the clinic setting.
- Physicians are recommended to wait for at least 2 weeks after end of the proton pump inhibitors (IPP) therapy and for 4 weeks after end of antibiotics before conducting biopsy and non-invasive tests (UBT, stool test) for *H. pylori.*

It should be noted that these guidelines only apply to children in Europe and North America, not in other continents, particularly developing countries, with a high rate of paediatric *H. pylori* infection and limited health resources.

Another studies / tests

- Imaging studies are not useful in the diagnosis of *H. pylori* infection. They can be useful in patients with complicated diseases (e.g., ulcer, gastric cancer, MALToma).
- Urea breath test: The patient ingests a test meal containing carbon-13 (^{13}C) labelled urea, which is a nonradioactive isotope. *H. pylori urease* activity produces ^{13}C-labelled carbon dioxide, detectable in the breath. A positive result confirms *urease* activity and *H. pylori* infection. This is a highly specific test, sensitive in patients over 6 years of age. It is useful to check eradication of *H. pylori* after treatment. Experience in children 5 years or younger, in infants particularly, is relatively limited and needs further validation.

Detection of *Helicobacter pylori*

The procedure of choice for detecting gastritis, duodenitis and PUD in the paediatric population is upper endoscopy (EGD)

- EGD allows direct visualization of the mucosa, for locating the source of bleeding, to detect *H. pylori* by biopsy, culture and cytology analysis and DNA testing using PCR.
- In addition, a rapid test based on detection of *urease* activity (a *H. pylori* highly specific marker) may be performed. The test, called the *Campylobacter test* (CLO) allows diagnosis of *H. pylori* infection within 24 hours.
- Two modified urea rapid test kits are currently available on the market and reported as more accurate, with shorter reaction time and of better value for money than the CLO test.
- Endoscopy in children may reveal a nodular appearance in the gastric antrum resulting from lymphoid hyperplasia [34]. Approximately 50% of affected children have displayed endoscopic evidence of changes of *H. pylori* gastritis.

The appearance of an active ulcer is round or oval lesion in shape, the perforated base being smooth and white, with a red and oedematous surrounding mucosa. In *H. pylori* infection, the most common site for ulcer is the duodenal bulb.

http://dx.doi.org/10.5772/58326

Biopsy obtained from the prepiloric antrum has the highest yield in *H. pylori* infection. Often, tissue samples are also obtained from the body and the transition areas of the stomach, especially when the patient has recently taken acid suppressing medications.

- Endoscopic biopsy is indicated for the following reasons:
- Histological examination of gastric tissue;
- Rapid *urease* test (e.g. CLO test)
- Culture of organisms;
- PCR test for identification of *H. pylori* DNA
- Histological findings include infiltration of a substantial number of plasma cells and lymphocytes into the gastric mucosa and Giemsa, Diff-Quick visible bodies or haematoxylin and eosin. Sensitive colouring of a small number of bacteria is possible with a silver staining method such as Genta or Warthin-Starry.

Stages

- Multiple stages in the progression of the disease are well described in the literature, although no stages system for *H. pylori* infection has been established.
- The first step is chronic gastritis, followed by a second step, atrophic gastritis. The third step is intestinal metaplasia, which can evolve to dysplasia. The last step in this process is gastric adenocarcinoma.
- This is a very slow process (which may take decades, for example), and can stop at any step because gastric cancer probably requires several other factors to grow, not just *H. pylori* infection.

Treatment measures of *Helicobacter pylori* infection

Let us mention the new treatment rules recommended for the following patient groups [15]:

- In the presence of *H. pylori*-positive PUD, eradication of the microorganism is recommended.
- On detection of *H. pylori* infection by biopsy based methods in the absence of PUD, *H. pylori* treatment may be considered. The decision to treat *H. pylori* associated gastritis without duodenal or gastric ulcer is subject to the clinician's judgment and deliberation is undertaken with the patient and family, taking into account potential risks and benefits of treatment for the patient.
- In *H. pylori* infected children, whose next of kin suffer from gastric cancer, treatment can be offered.
- The "test - and-treat" strategy is not recommended for children. The main purpose of the tests is to diagnose the cause of the clinical symptoms.

Currently practiced therapeutic approach takes the following into account:

- *H. pylori* acquired resistance to antibiotics, which requires bacterial strain susceptibility testing to a certain class of antibiotics in geographic areas where resistance is seen in encountered in a percentage of patients;
- Success rate in eradication of infection is directly dependent on the dose and duration of medication administered. In practice however, this is less apparent because of lower compliance in long cures and because of adverse effects (vomiting, nausea, malaise) in high doses;
- Bismuth (Bi^{3+}) salts preparations are effective but difficult to accept by children because of their bad taste;
- Therapeutic management aims not at eradication of *H. pylori* infection only but also at resolution of the pathology is determines (gastritis, reflux, dyspepsia etc.) and therefore triple therapy may be associated with prokinetics and hygienic-dietary regime to spare digestion;
- Unwanted side effects of the antibiotics cure can be reduced by administration of probiotic preparations that restore normal intestinal flora.

The following treatments should be implemented [15]:

- First line eradication regimens are: triple therapy with a PPI + amoxicillin + imidazole, or PPI + amoxicillin + clarithromycin + amoxicillin or bismuth salts + imidazole or sequential therapy. Sequential therapy involves dual therapy with a PPI and amoxicillin for 5 days, successively followed by five days of triple therapy (a PPI with clarithromycin and metronidazole / tinidazole). In fact, this scheme may be considered as quadruple therapy provided in a sequential manner. It is speculated that the initial use of amoxicillin reduces bacterial load and provides protection against resistance to clarithromycin.
- Clarithromycin antibiotic susceptibility testing is recommended prior to clarithromycin triple therapy in areas / populations definable as clarithromycin highly resistant (> 20%) to *H. pylori*.
- The recommended period for triple therapy is 7-14 days. Costs, compliance and adverse effects should be taken into account.
- A reliable non-invasive test for eradication is recommended at least 4-8 weeks after treatment.

In cases of treatment failure, the following 3 options are recommended:

- EGD with culture and sensitivity tests, including alternative antibiotics if not performed prior to standard treatment.
- *Insitu* fluorescence hybridization (FISH) on paraffin-embedded biopsies, if clarithromycin susceptibility testing was not performed before standard therapy.
- Therapy changing by addition of an antibiotic, using various antibiotics, as well as addition of bismuth, and / or increase of the dose and / or treatment duration.

If not possible to perform a primary culture, the following regimens are suggested as second-line or rescue therapy [15]:

- Quadruple therapy consists of metronidazole + amoxicillin + PPI + bismuth. In most guidelines, quadruple therapy is the recommended second-line therapy, but this is a complicated regimen to administer. In addition, bismuth salts are not universally available.

- Triple therapy consists of PPI + levofloxacin (moxifloxacin) + amoxicillin. Regimen evaluation using fluoroquinolones, including levofloxacin, as second-line therapy in children is limited. In studies in adults, the treatment seems to be effective.

Although studies during ideal therapy duration for second-line treatment are not conclusive, a longer treatment duration is recommended, up to 14 days.

Other procedures

- Surgical procedures are rarely needed in treatment of patients with *H. pylori* infection. However, the ulcer, surgery may be required for certain complications unresponsive to medical treatment, including difficult to treat abdominal pain, gastric outlet obstruction, perforation and severe bleeding.

- Consultations pediatric gastroenterologists: For evaluation, endoscopy and biopsy to confirm *Helicobacter pylori* infection and rule out other causes for abdominal pain or bleeding;

- Surgeon - For intervention in patients with severe or intractable pain or bleeding or patients with intestinal perforation or obstruction of the gastro-intestinal tract;

- Radiologist - For patients requiring upper gastrointestinal imaging with contrast-enhanced studies.

Hygienic-dietary regime

A sparing digestive hygienic-dietary regime is recommended, including meals and snacks every 3-4 hours with correct chewing and avoidance of food aggressors. Foods such as fruit juices and certain dairy products may have a modest bacteriostatic effect on *H. pylori*. Active principles (sulforaphane and indole-3-carbinol) of the Brassicaceae family are also included here.

- Two randomized, placebo-controlled studies have evaluated the effect of probiotic food as an adjunct to standard triple therapy for eradication of *H. pylori* infection in children and have had conflicting results [58, 59].

- In a recent prospective study in adults, it was suggested that the addition of vitamin C to a regimen of *H. pylori* with amoxicillin, metronidazole, and bismuth can significantly increase the *H. pylori* eradication rate [60].

13. Medicines used in *H. pylori* eradication therapy [61-73]

Antibiotics, beta-lactamases

Beta-lactamases used to treat *H. pylori* infected patients are stable in an acidic environment, binding to proteins in bacterial cell walls, inducing direct lysis in the wall, and inhibiting cell wall synthesis.

Amoxicillin (Amoxil®, Polymox®, Trimox®, Wymox®)

Bacterially active against *Helicobacter pylori*. Available as GTT 50mg/ml; susp.125, 200, 250, or 400mg/5ml; caps 250 and 500 mg chewable tablets and 125, 200, 250, or 400mg.

Antibiotics, macrolides

Macrolides used to treat *H. pylori* infection are stable in the stomach, entering the bacterial cell, binding to receptors on the ribosomal subunits and inhibiting bacterial protein synthesis.

Clarithromycin (Biaxin®, Fromilid®)

This displays bactericidal activity against *H. pylori* antimicrobial spectrum similar to that of erythromycin but stable in acid and with fewer adverse gastrointestinal effects. Available as 125 or 250mg/5ml granules for suspension and 250 or 500 mg film-coated tablets.

Antibiotics, antiprotozoans

Used in the treatment of *H. pylori* infected patients, this antibiotic generates intracellular products affecting bacterial DNA.

Metronidazole (Flagyl®, Protostat®)

Metronidazole diffuses well into all tissues, is stable in an acidic environment, and provides bactericidal activity against *H. pylori*. Available as ex tempore 50 sau100mg/5ml suspension, 250 or 500mg tablets and 375 mg capsules.

Antibiotics, tetracyclines

Tetracyclines bind to ribosomal subunits and inhibit protein synthesis of susceptible bacteria. Use in paediatric patients should be limited in cases where other antibiotic regimens fail.

Tetracycline hydrochloridum (Achromycin®, Sumycin®, Terramycin®)

Bacteriostatic but may be bactericidal in high concentrations. Also available as 250 or 500mg tablets, 100, 250, or 500 mg capsules, and 125mg/5ml suspension.

H^2 receptor antagonists

H_2 receptors are located on acid-producing parietal cells. Blocking the action of the histamine suppresses gastric acid secretion.

Ranitidine (ranitidinum) or Famotidine (famotidinum)

H_2 antagonists prescribed for 8 weeks, when most *H. pylori* associated ulcers are cured. H_2 blockers have no antibacterial effect, therefore antibiotics should be used to eradicate *H.*

http://dx.doi.org/10.5772/58326

pylori. Available as 15mg/ml syrup, 75, 150, or 300 mg tablets, as well as effervescent tablets 150mg.

Proton Pump Inhibitors

This class of medicinal products includes acid inhibitors more potent than H_2 receptor antagonists; they block the secretion of gastric acid proton pump (Na + / H +-ATP-ase), the final common path of the secretion. This class is recommended as part of a regimen of medications in symptomatic patients with *H. pylori* infection. Similar to H_2-receptor blocking treatment, proton pump inhibitor (PPI) treatment only does not eliminate the *H. pylori* infection, but increases the bacteriostatic activity against *H. pylori*.

Examples of trade names depending on the active substance:

- Omeprazole: Omeprazole®, Prilosec®, Omez®, Omeran®, Ulto® (available within 10, 20 or 40 mg per tablet)
- Esomeprazole: Nexium®, Emanera®, Helide®, Esomeprazole Sandoz® (20 or 40 mg)
- Pantoprazole: Controlo®, Nolpaza® (20 or 40 mg per tablet)
- Lansoprazol: Prevacid®, Lanzul® 30mg

Proton Pump Inhibitors are potent gastric acid blockers. For best effectiveness, to be administered before the first meal of the day. Enteric film-coated granules in capsules, they ensure adequate bioavailability. For children unable to swallow whole capsules, the grains are opened and put in acid substances (e.g. apple juice), which is preferable to administer to the lower bioavailability suspension. Available as 10 or 20 mg SR capsules and granules for suspension *per os* 20 or 40 mg/package.

Lansoprazole (Prevacid®)

Potent gastric acid blocker. Best administered just before the first meal of the day. Enteric film-coated granules in capsules, ensuring adequate bioavailability. For children unable to swallow the intact capsules, granules are placed in acid substances (e.g., applesauce or apple juice), preferable to the administration of lower bioavailable suspension. Available as capsules with 15 or 30 mg retard release and 15 mg or 30mg/package granules for suspension *per os*.[75-85]

Bismuth

Bismuth subsalicylate and bismuth subcitrate have complementary effects with most antimicrobials. Bismuth disrupts enzymatic activity in bacterial cell walls. Bismuth is particularly effective in the lysis of the cell wall of the microorganism when close to the gastric epithelium and relatively inaccessible to most antimicrobial agents.

Bismuth subsalicylate (Pepto-Bismol®)

These lyse bacterial cell walls, prevent microorganism adhesion to epithelium and inhibit *urease*.

Available as 262 mg chewable tablets (bismuth subsalicylate) and 262mg or 525mg/15ml solution.

Bismuth subcitrate (De - Nol®) acts similarly. The patient should be warned against normal black stools during the treatment administration.

Patient care

In children with *H. pylori* and complications of the peptic ulcer disease (PUD), including bleeding, severe pain, perforation, or obstruction, care must include the following [86-106]:

- Attention to the airway, breathing and circulatory status
- Monitoring of fluid resuscitation, with consideration for transfusion
- Careful nasogastric lavage in stabilization of upper gastro-intestinal bleeding
- Antacid therapy with proton pump inhibitors (PPIs), maximum dosage
- Appropriate consultation with specialists in endoscopy or other procedures
- In children with stress-induced PUD, the treatment of the severe disease or traumatic injury
- additional outpatient care includes monitoring the patient's symptoms, assessment of patient tolerance to treatment regimen, and follow-up tests to confirm the effectiveness of the treatment. The tests should be conducted at least 6 weeks and preferably 3 months after treatment.

Outpatient treatment of patients

- Patients should avoid all irritating drugs, including anti-inflammatory drugs (NSAIDs), aspirin, and preparations with corticosteroid
- It is necessary for the treatment of iron deficiency anaemia.

Prophylactic measures

- The transmission mode of *H. pylori* infection is not fully understood.
- Data from epidemiological studies suggest that the following measures may be helpful to reduce transmission:
- Policies supporting improvement of living conditions, particularly in developing countries;
- For all patients with chronic symptoms of the gastro-intestinal tract, appropriate reference for definitive diagnosis and treatment, which may also help to prevent exposure of family members and close contacts.[103-111]
- *H. pylori* infection vaccines: several studies performed with *urease* -based vaccines have shown limited efficacy in humans. Vaccines based on recombinant CagA-VacA-0AP proteins display good immunogenicity of CagA - based cow - 0AP good immunogenicity and safety profile in phase I, but no subsequent efficacy studies have been reported. No further results from clinical trials on *H. pylori* vaccines have been reported in recent years. Currently, there is no authorised anti - *H. pylori* vaccine [74].

***H. pylori* Complications**

- PUD - perforation, gastrointestinal bleeding

- Iron deficiency anaemia
- Malignancies of:- The gastric mucosa associated to lymphoid tissue (MALT) - Adenocarcinoma of the gastric corpus, and the antrum
- Gastric outlet obstruction
- Increased sensitivity to enteric infections such as salmonella and giardiasis because of *H. pylori*-induced hypochlorhydria [92, 96]

14. Prospects study

1. Prospects for the eradication of *H. pylori* infection with multidrug therapy are good, with up to 95% reported efficacy rates.
2. Treatment is often unsuccessful because of lack of patient compliance and antibiotic resistance.
3. When cleaning is completed, long-term reinfection rates are low. Among children living in developing countries or among families with infected members, reinfection rates may be increased.
4. In this moment, the nature of *H. pylori* infection transmission is not fully understood. Therefore, the ability to implement appropriate preventive measures to control the infection is limited.
5. The theory concerning *H. pylori* person-to-person transmission, supported by data from epidemiological studies, may prove useful in promoting policies to improve the living and hygiene conditions and reduce crowdedness.
6. The true effect of educational authorities to reduce transmission of *H. pylori* in the patient's family (e.g., teaching children about proper hygiene and toilet practices) is unknown. However, such efforts may be part of a sensible approach to reducing the transmission of all infection pathogens in the infection of the gastrointestinal tract [109-111].

15. Conclusions

The infection with *H. pylori* is a common problem in pediatric practice and its origin is related with poor socio-econo-mic conditions. Only a small number of children with well-defined clinical syndromes are benefited at present from testing and treatment.

The first line eradication regimens are triple therapy with a PPI, amoxicillin and imidazole, or PPI, amoxicillin, clarithromycin and amoxicillin or bismuth salts and imidazole or sequential therapy.

Each country may need to be adapted the recommendations guidelines to national health care systems, because certain tests or treatment regimens may not be available and /or reimbursed by health insurance programs.

Author details

Florica Nicolescu*

Address all correspondence to: florica.nicolescu@gmail.com

Toxicology Department, "Carol Davila" University of Medicine and Pharmacy, Bucharest, Romania

References

[1] Blecker U. *Helicobacter pylori*-associated gastroduodenal disease in childhood. *South Med J*. Jun 1997;90(6):570-6; quiz 577.

[2] Warren JR, Marshall BJ. Unidentified curved bacilli on gastric epithelium in active chronic gastritis. *Lancet.* 1983;1:1273–5.

[3] Hill R, Pearman J, Worthy P, Caruso V, Goodwin S, Blincow E. *Campylobacter pyloridis* and gastritis in children. *Lancet.* 1986;1:387.

[4] Mutaz I Sultan, Carmen Cuffari, Pediatric *Helicobacter pylori* Infection, *emedicine.medscape.com/article/929452.*

[5] Goodwin CS, McCulloch RK, Armstrong JA, Wee SH. Unusual cellular fatty acid and distinctive ultrastructure in a new spiral bacterium (*Campylobacter pyloridis*) from the human gastric mucosa. *J Med Microbiol.* 1987;19:257–67.

[6] Peterson WL, Graham DY. *Helicobacter pylori.* In: Feldman M, Friedman, Sleisenger MH, Scharschmidt BF, editors. *Sleisenger and Fordtran's gastrointestinal and liver disease pathophysiology diagnosis management.* Philadelphia: WB Saunders Company; 2002. pp. 732–46.

[7] Phadnis SH, Paelow MH, Levy M, Ilver D, Caulkins CM, Conners JB, et al. Surface localization of *Helicobacter pylori* urease and heat shock protein homolog requires bacterial autolysis. *Infec Immun.* 1996;64:905–12.

[8] Opekun AR, Gilger MA, Denyes SM, Nirken MH, Philip SP, Osato MS, et al. *Helicobacter pylori* infection in children of Texas. *J Pediatr Gastroenterol Nutr.* 2000;31:405–10.

[9] Kate V, Ananthakrishanan N, Ratnakar C, Badrinath S. Anti-*H.pylori* IgG seroprevalence rates in asymptomatic children and adults form south India. *Indian J Med Microbiol.* 2001;19:20–5.

[10] Malaty HM, Haveman T, Graham DY, Fraley K. *Helicobacter pylori* infection in asymptomatic children: Impact of epidemiological factors on accuracy of diagnostic tests. *J Ped Gastroenterol Nutr.* 2002;35:59–63.

[11] Rosenberg JJ. *Helicobacter pylori*. *Pediatr Rev.* Feb 2010;31(2):85-6; discussion 86.

[12] Gold BJ. New approach to *Helicobacter pylori* infection in children. *Curr Gastroenterol Rep.* 2001;3:235–47.

[13] Cervantes DT, Fischbach LA, Goodman KJ, Phillips CV, Chen S, Broussard CS. Exposure to *Helicobacter pylori*-positive siblings and persistence of *Helicobacter pylori* infection in early childhood. *J Pediatr Gastroenterol Nutr.* May 2010;50(5):481-5.

[14] M Rowland, C Imrie, B Bourke, B Drumm, How should *Helicobacter pylori* infected children be managed?, Gut BMJ,1999;45:I36-I39 doi:10.1136/gut.45.2008.i36

[15] Koletzko S, Jones NL, Goodman KJ, et al. Evidence-based guidelines from ESPGHAN and NASPGHAN for *Helicobacter pylori* infection in children. *J Pediatr Gastroenterol Nutr.* Aug 2011;53(2):230-43

[16] Gold BD, Colletti RB, Abbott M, Czinn S, Elitsur Y, Hassall E, et al. *Helicobacter pylori* infection in children: Recommendation for diagnosis and treatment. *J Pediatr Gastroenterol Nutr.* 2000;31:490–7.

[17] Day AS, Sherman PM. Accuracy of office-based immunoassay for the diagnosis of *Helicobacter pylori* infection in children. *Helicobacter*. 2002;7:205–9.

[18] 54. Makristathis A, Hirschl AM, Lehours P, Megraud F. Diagnosis of *Helicobacter pylori* infection. Helicobacter. 2002;9:7–14.

[19] Bahu MG, da Silvaria TR, Maguilnick I, Ulbrich-Kulczynski J. Endoscopic nodular gastritis: An endoscopic indicator of high-grade bacterial colonization and severe gastritis in children with *Helicobacter pylori*. *J Pediatr Gastroenterol Nutr.* 2003;36:217–22.

[20] Konno M, Fujii N, Yokota S, et al. Five-year follow-up study of mother-to-child transmission of *Helicobacter pylori* infection detected by a random amplified polymorphic DNA fingerprinting method. *J Clin Microbiol*. 43(5):2246-50.

[21] Ahmed KS, Khan AA, Ahmed I, et al. Impact of household hygiene and water source on the prevalence and transmission of *Helicobacter pylori*: a South Indian perspective. *Singapore Med J.* Jun 2007;48(6):543-9.

[22] Grubel P, Huang L, Masubuchi N, Stutzenberger FJ, Cave DR. Detection of *Helicobacter pylori* DNA in houseflies (*Musca domestica*) on three continents. *Lancet*. Sep 5 1998;352(9130):788-9.

[23] Appelmelk BJ, Simoons-Smit I, Negrini R, et al. Potential role of molecular mimicry between *Helicobacter pylori* lipopolysaccharide and host Lewis blood group antigens in autoimmunity. *Infect Immun*. Jun 1996;64(6):2031-40.

[24] Figueiredo C, Machado JC, Yamaoka Y. Pathogenesis of *Helicobacter pylori* Infection. *Helicobacter*. 2005;10 Suppl 1:14-20.

[25] Rick JR, Goldman M, Semino-Mora C, et al. *In situ* expression of cagA and risk of gastroduodenal disease in *Helicobacter pylori*-infected children. *J Pediatr Gastroenterol Nutr*. Feb 2010;50(2):167-72.

[26] Baysoy G, Ertem D, Ademoglu E, et al. Gastric histopathology, iron status and iron deficiency anemia in children with *Helicobacter pylori* infection. *J Pediatr Gastroenterol Nutr*. Feb 2004;38(2):146-51.

[27] Williams MP, Pounder RE. *Helicobacter pylori*: from the benign to the malignant. *Am J Gastroenterol*. Nov 1999;94(11 Suppl):S11-6.

[28] Correa P, Haenszel W, Cuello C, Tannenbaum S, Archer M. A model for gastric cancer epidemiology. Lancet 1975; 2: 58-60.

[29] Correa P. A human model of gastric carcinogenesis. Cancer Research 1988; 48: 3554-3560.

[30] Correa P. Human gastric carcinogenesis: a multistep and multifactorial process. First American Cancer Society Award lecture on cancer epidemiology and prevention. Cancer Research 1992; 52: 6735-6740.

[31] Correa P, Piazuelo MB. The gastric precancerous cascade. Journal of Digestive Diseases 2012; 13(1): 2-9.

[32] Ashorn M, Rago T, Kokkonen J, et al. Symptomatic response to *Helicobacter pylori* eradication in children with recurrent abdominal pain: double blind randomized placebo-controlled trial. *J Clin Gastroenterol*. Sep 2004;38(8):646-50.

[33] Gold BD, Colletti RB, Abbott M, et al. *Helicobacter pylori* infection in children: recommendations for diagnosis and treatment. *J Pediatr Gastroenterol Nutr*. Nov 2000;31(5): 490-7.

[34] Spee LA, Madderom MB, Pijpers M, van Leeuwen Y, Berger MY. Association between *Helicobacter pylori* and gastrointestinal symptoms in children. *Pediatrics*. Mar 2010;125(3):e651-69.

[35] Yaghoobi M, Farrokhyar F, Yuan Y, Hunt RH. Is There an Increased Risk of GERD After *Helicobacter pylori* Eradication?: A Meta-Analysis. *Am J Gastroenterol*. Jan 19 2010.

[36] Moon A, Solomon A, Beneck D, Cunningham-Rundles S. Positive association between *Helicobacter pylori* and gastroesophageal reflux disease in children. *J Pediatr Gastroenterol Nutr*. Sep 2009;49(3):283-8.

[37] Franchini M, Veneri D. Helicobacter pylori-associated immune trombocitopenia, Platelets, 2006;17(2);71-7

[38] Takahashi M, Kimura H, Watanabe K Helicobacter pylori infection in patients with idiopathic short starure. Pediatrics International, 2002;44(3):277-80

[39] Capurso G, Lahner E, Marcheggiano A, Caruana P, Carnuccio A, Bordi C, Delle Fave G, Annibale B. Involvement of the corporal mucosa and related changes in gastric acid secretion characterize patients with iron deficiency anemy associated with Helicobacter pylori infection. Aliment Pharmacol Ther 2001; 15(11): 1753-1761.

[40] Pelicano R, Franceschi F, Saracco G, Fagoonee S, Roccarina D, Gasbarrini A. Helicobacters and extragastric diseases. Helicobacter 2009; 14(Suppl 1): 58-68.

[41] Arnold DM, Bernotas A, Nazi I, Stasi R, Kuwana M, Liu Y, Kelton JG, Crowther MA. Platelet count response to *H. pylori* treatment in patients with immune thrombocytopenic purpura with and without *H. pylori* infection: a systematic review. Haematologica 2009; 94(6): 850-856.

[42] Franceschi F, Navarese EP, Mollo R, Giupponi B, De Marco G, Merra G, Gasbarrini G, Silveri NG. Helicobacter pylori and atherosclerosis. A review of the literature. Recent Progr Med 2009; 100(2): 91-96.

[43] Rogha M, Nikvarz M, Poumoghaddas Z et al. Is Helicobacter pylori infection a risk factor for coronary heart disease? ARYA Atherosclerose 2012; 8(1): 5-8.

[44] Pirouz T, Zounubi L, Keivani H, Rakhshani N, Hormazdi M. Detection of Helicobacter pylori in paraffin-embedded specimens from patients with chronic liver diseases, using the amplification method. Digestive Diseases and Sciences 2009; 54(7): 1456-1459.

[45] Suerbaum S, Michetti P, *Helicobacter pylori* infection. N Engl Med 2002; 347: 1175-86

[46] Rothenbacher D, Bode G, Berg G, Gommel R, Gonser T, Alder G, et al. Prevalence and determinants of *Helicobacter pylori* infection in preschool children: A population based study from Germany. *Int J Epidemiol.* 1998; 27: 135–41.

[47] Opekun AR, Gilger MA, Denyes SM, Nirken MH, Philip SP, Osato MS, et al. *Helicobacter pylori* infection in children of Texas. *J Pediatr Gastroenterol Nutr.* 2000; 31: 405–10

[48] Wizla-Derambure N, Michaud L, Ategbo S, Vincent P, Ganga-Zandzou S, Turck D, et al. Familial and community environmental risk factors for *Helicobacter pylori* infection in children and adolescents. *J Pediatr Gastroenterol Nutr.* 2001; 33: 58–63.

[49] Mourad-Baars PE, Verspaget HW, Mertens BJ, Luisa Merain M. Low prevalence of *Helicobacter pylori* infection in young children in the Netherlands. *Eur J Gastroenterol Hepatol.* 2007; 19: 213–6.

[50] Kate V, Ananthakrishanan N, Ratnakar C, Badrinath S. Anti-*H. pylori* Ig G seroprevalence rates in asymptomatic children and adults form south India. *Indian J Med Microbiol.* 2001; 19: 20–5.

[51] Gold BJ. *Helicobacter pylori* infection in children. *Curr Prob Pediatr.* 2001; 31: 247–66.

[52] Rocha GA, Rocha AM, Silva LD, Samtos A, Bocewicz AC, Queiroz RM, et al. Transmission of *Helicobacter pylori* infection in families of preschool-aged children from Minas Gerais, Brazil. *Trop Med Int Health.* 2003; 8: 987–91.

[53] Malaty HM, Haveman T, Graham DY, Fraley K, *Helicobacter pylori* infection in asymptomatic children: Impact of epidemiological factors on accuracy of diagnostic tests. *J Ped Gastroenterol Nutr.* 2002; 35: 59–63.

[54] Ndip RN, Malange AE, Akoachere JF, MacKay WG, Titanji VP, Weaver LT. *Helicobacter pylori* antigens in faeces of asymptomatic children in the Buea and Limbe health districts of Cameroon: A pilot study. *Trop Med Int Health.* 2004; 9: 1036–40.

[55] Rajindrajith S et al, *Helicobacter pylori* Infection in Children, *Saudi J Gastroenterol*, 2009, 15 (2): 86-94.

[56] Sullivan PB, Thomas JE, Wight DG, et al. *Helicobacter pylori* in Gambian children with chronic diarrhoea and malnutrition. *Arch Dis Child.* Feb 1990;65(2):189-91.

[57] Bujanover Y, Konikoff F, Baratz M. Nodular gastritis and *Helicobacter pylori. J Pediatr Gastroenterol Nutr.* Jul 1990;11(1):41-4.

[58] Lionetti E, Miniello VL, Castellaneta SP, et al. *Lactobacillus reuteri* therapy to reduce side-effects during anti-*Helicobacter pylori* treatment in children: a randomized placebo controlled trial. *Aliment Pharmacol Ther.* Nov 15 2006;24(10):1461-8.

[59] Goldman CG, Barrado DA, Balcarce N, et al. Effect of a probiotic food as an adjuvant to triple therapy for eradication of *Helicobacter pylori* infection in children. *Nutrition.* Oct 2006;22(10):984-8.

[60] Zojaji H, Talaie R, Mirsattari D, et al. The efficacy of *Helicobacter pylori* eradication regimen with and without vitamin C supplementation. *Dig Liver Dis.* Sep 2009;41(9): 644-7.

[61] Ruggiero P. *Helicobacter pylori* infection: what's new. *Curr Opin Infect Dis.* Jun 2012;25(3):337-44.

[62] Bahremand S, Nematollahi LR, Fourutan H, et al. Evaluation of triple and quadruple *Helicobacter pylori* eradication therapies in Iranian children: a randomized clinical trial. *Eur J Gastroenterol Hepatol.* May 2006;18(5):511-4.

[63] Bhasin DK, Sharma BC, Ray P, et al. Comparison of seven and fourteen days of lansoprazole, clarithromycin, andamoxicillin therapy for eradication of *Helicobacter pylori*: a report from India.. *Helicobacter.* Jun 2000;5(2):84-7.

[64] Bonamico M, Strappini PM, Bonci E, et al. Evaluation of stool antigen test, PCR on ORAL samples and serology for the noninvasive detection of *Helicobacter pylori* infection in children. *Helicobacter*. Feb 2004;9(1):69-76.

[65] Booka M, Okuda M, Shin K, et al. Polymerase chain reaction--restriction fragment length polymorphism analysis of clarithromycin-resistant *Helicobacter pylori* infection in children using stool sample. *Helicobacter*. Jun 2005;10(3):205-13.

[66] Bourke B, Ceponis P, Chiba N, et al. Canadian *Helicobacter* Study Group Consensus Conference: Update on the approach to *Helicobacter pylori* infection in children and adolescents - an evidence - based evaluation. *Can J Gastroenterol*. Jul 2005;19(7): 399-408.

[67] Cammarota G, Cianci R, Cannizzaro O, et al. High-dose versus low-dose clarithromycin in 1-week triple therapy, including rabeprazole and levofloxacin, for *Helicobacter pylori* eradication. *J Clin Gastroenterol*. Feb 2004;38(2):110-4.

[68] Chan KL, Zhou H, Ng DK, Tam PK. A prospective study of a one-week nonbismuth quadruple therapy for childhood *Helicobacter pylori* infection. *J Pediatr Surg*. Jul 2001;36(7):1008-11.

[69] Chan KL, Zhou H, Ng DK, Tam PK. A prospective study of a one-week nonbismuth quadruple therapy for childhood *Helicobacter pylori* infection. *J Pediatr Surg*. Jul 2001;36(7):1008-11.

[70] Chong SK, Lou Q, Asnicar MA, et al. *Helicobacter pylori* infection in recurrent abdominal pain in childhood: comparison of diagnostic tests and therapy. *Pediatrics*. Aug 1995;96(2 Pt 1):211-5.

[71] Czinn SJ. *Helicobacter pylori* infection: detection, investigation, and management. *J Pediatr*. Mar 2005;146(3 Suppl):S21-6.

[72] Di Caro S, Franceschi F, Mariani A, et al. Second-line levofloxacin-based triple schemes for *Helicobacter pylori* eradication. *Dig Liver Dis*. Jul 2009;41(7):480-5.

[73] Drumm B. *Helicobacter pylori* in the pediatric patient. *Gastroenterol Clin North Am*. Mar 1993;22(1):169-82.

[74] Graham DY, Rakel RE, Fendrick AM, et al. Practical advice on eradicating *Helicobacter pylori* infection. *Postgrad Med*. Mar 1999;105(3):137-40, 145-8.

[75] El-Omar EM, Oien K, Murray LS, et al. Increased prevalence of precancerous changes in relatives of gastric cancer patients: critical role of *H. pylori*. *Gastroenterology*. Jan 2000;118(1):22-30.

[76] Ernst PB, Gold BD. *Helicobacter pylori* in childhood: new insights into the immunopathogenesis of gastric disease and implications for managing infection in children. *J Pediatr Gastroenterol Nutr*. May 1999;28(5):462-73.

[77] Farrell MK. Dr. Apley meets *Helicobacter pylori*. *J Pediatr Gastroenterol Nutr*. Feb 1993;16(2):118-9.

[78] Feydt-Schmidt A, Kindermann A, Konstantopoulos N, et al. Reinfection rate in children after successful *Helicobacter pylori* eradication. *Eur J Gastroenterol Hepatol*. Oct 2002;14(10):1119-23.

[79] Fiedorek SC, Casteel HB, Pumphrey CL, et al. The role of *Helicobacter pylori* in recurrent, functional abdominal pain in children. *Am J Gastroenterol*. Mar 1992;87(3):347-9.

[80] Francavilla R, Lionetti E, Castellaneta SP, et al. Improved efficacy of 10-Day sequential treatment for Helicobacter *pylori* eradication in children: a randomized trial. *Gastroenterology*. Nov 2005;129(5):1414-9.

[81] Gillen D, el-Omar EM, Wirz AA, et al. The acid response to gastrin distinguishes duodenal ulcer patients from *Helicobacter pylori*-infected healthy subjects. *Gastroenterology*. Jan 1998;114(1):50-7.

[82] Gisbert JP, Luna M, Gomez B, et al. Recurrence of *Helicobacter pylori* infection after several eradication therapies: long-term follow-up of 1000 patients. *Aliment Pharmacol Ther*. Mar 15 2006;23(6):713-9.

[83] Gisbert JP, Perez-Aisa A, Castro-Fernandez M, et al. *Helicobacter pylori* first-line treatment and rescue option containing levofloxacin in patients allergic to penicillin. *Dig Liver Dis*. Apr 2010;42(4):287-90.

[84] Glassman MS. *Helicobacter pylori* infection in children. A clinical overview. *Clin Pediatr (Phila)*. Aug 1992;31(8):481-7.

[85] Gormally S, Drumm B. *Helicobacter pylori* and gastrointestinal symptoms. *Arch Dis Child*. Mar 1994;70(3):165-6.

[86] Graham DY, Shiotani A. The time to eradicate gastric cancer is now. *Gut*. Jun 2005;54(6):735-8.

[87] Guo CY, Wu YB, Liu HL, et al. Clinical evaluation of four one-week triple therapy regimens in eradicating *Helicobacter pylori* infection. *World J Gastroenterol*. Mar 1 2004;10(5):747-9.

[88] Hardikar W, Feekery C, Smith A, et al. *Helicobacter pylori* and recurrent abdominal pain in children. *J Pediatr Gastroenterol Nutr*. Feb 1996;22(2):148-52.

[89] Heldenberg D, Wagner Y, Heldenberg E, et al. The role of *Helicobacter pylori* in children with recurrent abdominal pain. *Am J Gastroenterol*. Jun 1995;90(6):906-9.

[90] Horvitz G, Gold BD. Gastroduodenal diseases of childhood. *Curr Opin Gastroenterol*. Nov 2006;22(6):632-40.

[91] Huang FC, Chang MH, Hsu HY, et al. Long-term follow-up of duodenal ulcer in children before and after eradication of *Helicobacter pylori*. *J Pediatr Gastroenterol Nutr*. Jan 1999;28(1):76-80.

[92] Huebner ES, Surawicz CM. Probiotics in the prevention and treatment of gastrointestinal infections. *Gastroenterol Clin North Am*. June 2006;35:355-65.

[93] Israel DM, Hassall E. Treatment and long-term follow-up of *Helicobacter pylori*-associated duodenal ulcer disease in children. *J Pediatr*. Jul 1993;123(1):53-8..

[94] Judd RH. *Helicobacter pylori*, gastritis, and ulcers in pediatrics. *Adv Pediatr*. 1992;39:283-306.

[95] Khurana R, Fischbach L, Chiba N, et al. Meta-analysis: *Helicobacter pylori* eradication treatment efficacy in children. *Aliment Pharmacol Ther*. Mar 1 2007;25(5):523-36.

[96] Kimia A, Zahavi I, Shapiro R, et al. The role of *Helicobacter pylori* and gastritis in children with recurrent abdominal pain. *Isr Med Assoc J*. Feb 2000;2(2):126-8.

[97] Kiyota K, Habu Y, Sugano Y, et al. Comparison of 1-week and 2-week triple therapy with omeprazole, amoxicillin,and clarithromycin in peptic ulcer patients with *Helicobacter pylori* infection: results of a randomized controlled trial. *J Gastroenterol*. 1999;34 Suppl 11:76-9.

[98] Knippig C, Arand F, Leodolter A, et al. Prevalence of *H. pylori*-infection in family members of *H. pylori* positive and its influence on the reinfection rate after successful eradication therapy: a two-year follow-up. *Z Gastroenterol*. Jun 2002;40(6):383-7.

[99] Koivisto TT, Rautelin HI, Voutilainen ME, et al. First-line eradication therapy for *Helicobacter pylori* in primary health care based on antibiotic resistance: results of three eradication regimens. *Aliment Pharmacol Ther*. Mar 15 2005;21(6):773-82.

[100] Logan RP, Gummett PA, Schaufelberger HD, et al. Eradication of *Helicobacter pylori* with clarithromycin and omeprazole. *Gut*. Mar 1994;35(3):323-6.

[101] Long SS, Pickering LK, Prober CG, eds. *Helicobacter pylori*. In: *Principles and Practice of Pediatric Infectious Diseases*. New York, NY: Churchill Livingstone; 1997:1029-33.

[102] Moshkowitz M, Reif S, Brill S, et al. One-week triple therapy with omeprazole, clarithromycin, and nitroimidazole for *Helicobacter pylori* infection in children and adolescents. *Pediatrics*. Jul 1998;102(1):e14.

[103] Nista EC, Candelli M, Cremonini F, et al. Levofloxacin-based triple therapy vs. quadruple therapy in second-line *Helicobacter pylori* treatment: a randomized trial. *Aliment Pharmacol Ther*. Sep 15 2003;18(6):627-33.

[104] Paoluzi OA, Visconti E, Andrei F, et al. Ten and eight-day sequential therapy in comparison to standard triple therapy for eradicating *Helicobacter pylori* infection: a randomized controlled study on efficacy and tolerability. *J Clin Gastroenterol*. Apr 2010;44(4):261-6.

[105] Parsonnet J. *Helicobacter pylori*. *Infect Dis Clin North Am*. Mar 1998;12(1):185-97.

[106] Parsonnet J, Hansen S, Rodriguez L, et al. *Helicobacter pylori* infection and gastric lymphoma. *N Engl J Med*. May 5 1994;330(18):1267-71.

[107] Raguza D, Machado RS, Ogata SK, et al. Validation of a monoclonal stool antigen test for diagnosing *Helicobacter pylori* infection in young children. *J Pediatr Gastroenterol Nutr*. Apr 2010;50(4):400-3.

[108] Siberry GK, Iannone R, eds. Formulary: drug doses. In: *The Harriet Lane Handbook*. 15th ed. St Louis, MO: Mosby; 2000:622, 630, 645-6, 674-5, 772-3, 795, 837.

[109] Vinette KM, Gibney KM, Proujansky R, Fawcett PT. Comparison of PCR and clinical laboratory tests for diagnosing *H. pylori* infection in pediatric patients. *BMC Microbiol*. Jan 27 2004;4:5.

[110] Wewer V, Andersen LP, Paerregaard A, et al. Treatment of *Helicobacter pylori* in children with recurrent abdominal pain. *Helicobacter*. Sep 2001;6(3):244-8.

[111] Windle HJ, Kelleher D, Crabtree JE. Childhood *Helicobacter pylori* infection and growth impairment in developing countries: a vicious cycle?. *Pediatrics*. Mar 2007;119(3):e754-9.

Chapter 7

Helicobacter pylori Infection, Gastric Physiology and Micronutrient deficiency (Iron and Vitamin C) in Children in Developing Countries

Shafiqul Alam Sarker

Additional information is available at the end of the chapter

http://dx.doi.org/10.5772/58375

1. Introduction

At least half the world's population are infected by *Helicobacter pylori (H. pylori),* making it the most widespread infection in the world [1]. Although infection occurs worldwide, there are significant differences in the prevalence of infection both within and between countries [2-4]. The overall prevalence of *H. pylori* infection in developed countries is lower than that in developing countries [3, 5]. The increased infection rate in developing countries is likely due to poor sanitary and/or living conditions. In such communities the incidence of *H pylori* infection in infancy is also high [6, 7], and has also been associated with malnutrition and growth faltering [8]. Epidemiological data suggest the prevalence of *H. pylori* infection in children under 10 years resident in developed countries to be 0 to 5% compared to 13 to 60% in their developing country counterparts [9]. The age at which this bacterium is acquired seems to influence the possible pathologic outcome of the infection - people infected at an early age are likely to develop more intense inflammation that may be followed by atrophic gastritis with a higher risk of gastric ulcer, gastric cancer or both. Acquisition at an older age brings different gastric changes that are more likely to result in duodenal ulcer. Individuals infected with *H. pylori* have a 10 to 20% lifetime risk of developing peptic ulcers and a 1 to 2% risk of acquiring stomach cancer [10]

H. pylori infection also exerts diverse effects of gastric physiology - it may increase or reduce gastric acid secretion or result in no overall change in the acid output [11]. It is important to know why *H. pylori* infection produces different aberrations in gastric physiology, and consequently gastric or duodenal ulcer or gastric cancer. *H. pylori* infection has also been suggested to be associated with a variety of conditions outside of the alimentary tract. The list of the proposed 'extragastric' association continues to grow despite the fact that *H. pylori* is a non-invasive organism and as such the infections are essentially confined to the surface of gastric-type mucosa. In an initial overview of the non-gastrointestinal manifestations of *H. pylori* [12], some biological plausibility has been suggested that underlie its association with iron deficiency anemia (IDA); cross sectional studies have demonstrated a relatively strong association. [13]

In this chapter, we will review and update the consequence of *H. pylori* infection, its role on the gastric acid secretion and some other conditions, notably IDA and iron absorption in children. The relationship between *H. pylori* infection and vitamin C levels in the blood and gastric juice will also be reviewed.

2. Consequences of initial *H. pylori* infection in children

There are not enough studies on the natural history of gastric infections in childhood years. In older children and adolescents, and adults it appears that *H. pylori* infection and the accompanying gastritis are lifelong unless specific eradication therapies are employed. However, several epidemiological studies, using serology [14, [15] and breath tests ([16, 17] as indirect markers of gastric infection reported spontaneous clearance in the pre-school aged children. Current evidence suggests that the overwhelming majority of *H. pylori* infected children and adolescents develop a chronic-active, antral- predominant gastritis) [18]. There is a single report suggesting the potential for *H. pylori* colonization of stomach of children without mucosal inflammation in antrum or gastric fundus [19]. Although, infection with the Cag A-positive strain was associated with more pronounced changes in the gastric physiology, limited studies in children reported no association between Cag A status and the severity of gastritis [20].

Some studies reported pan-gastritis involving both body and antrum in children infected with *H. plyori* [21, 22]. However, a formal mapping study to delineate the extent and the severity of bacterial colonization of the stomach, as well as the accompanying host cells mucosal inflammatory response to infection is lacking. To date there are not enough studies in children evaluating the healing of mucosal inflammation following eradication therapy. There are indirect evidences to suggest that resolution of inflammatory response may occur more rapidly in children than had been reported for adults [23]. In France, Ganga-Zandzou and colleagues prospectively monitored the consequences of untreated *H. pylori* infection in a group of asymptomatic children [24]. Although the density of bacterial colonization was not changed, there was both marked antral nodularity and more severe mucosal inflammation in the antrum over the 2-year follow-up of the children. However, there is the lack for comparable studies in other pediatric population, e.g. among those residing in developing countries and a greater length of follow-up. Further studies are needed to delineate the inflammatory and immune responses during development in order to provide additional insights into the interactions between the *H. pylori* and the host in such populations.

http://dx.doi.org/10.5772/58375

2.1. *H. pylori* infection and gastric acid perturbation

Acid secretion by the gastric parietal cell is regulated by paracrine, endocrine, and neural pathways. The physiological stimuli for acid secretion include histamine, acetylcholine, and gastrin, each of which binds to receptors located on the basolateral plasma membranes of the cells. The antral region of stomach contains G cells which release hormone gastrin. When meal is ingested, the protein component stimulates G cell to release Gastrin, which travels through the bloodstream to parietal cells in the body region (fundus) to secret acid [25]. Gastrin directly does not stimulate parietal cells but stimulates the adjacent enterochromafin-like cell (ECL cells) to release histamine, which in turn stimulates the parietal cells. Stimulation of acid secretion typically involves an activation of a cAMP-dependent protein kinase cascade that triggers the translocation and insertion of the proton pump enzyme, H,K-ATPase, into the apical plasma membrane parietal cells [26]. As the acid accumulates and overcome the buffering effects of the food, the fall in intragastric pH inhibits further release of gastrin and thus prevents secretion of excessive amount of acids (negative feedback control).

Helicobacter pylori infection exerts diverse effects on gastric physiology. In acute *H pylori* infection transient hypochlorhydria in adults is well documented [27, 28]. However, the relationship between chronic *H. pylori* infection and gastric acid secretion is not fully understood. It may increase gastric acid secretion, reduce it or results no overall changes in acid output. [11]. These alterations in acid secretion depend on the degree and distribution of gastritis caused by the infection [29, 30]. In subjects with an antral predominant gastritis, without atrophy, acid secretion is normal or increased. This is the pattern of gastritis seen in patients who develops duodenal ulceration. When gastritis is body predominant, a situation leading to gastric atrophy, *H. pylori* infection lead to markedly reduced acid secretion or achlorhydria which is also seen in patients who develops non-cardiac gastric cancer. Finally, when gastritis is mixed antral or body, *H. pylori* may have no effect on acid secretion.

2.2. *H. pylori* infection and increased acid output (hyperchlorhydria)

H. pylori infection in the antral region of the stomach disrupts the negative feedback control of gastrin release, resulting inappropriately high and sustained levels of gastrin following meal [31, 32]. In those subjects, the gastritis is non-atrophic and, therefore, the increased gastrin release stimulates the healthy body region of stomach to secret excessive amounts of acid [33, 34]. The increased amount of acid output produced by this pattern of gastritis results in an increased duodenal acid loads damaging the duodenal mucosa, which may eventually result in ulcers formation [35]. Eradicating *H. pylori* infection in subjects with this type of gastritis leads to lowering of serum gastrin with concomitant reductions in acid output.

2.3. *H. pylori* infection and low acid output (hypochlorhydria)

In subjects with atrophic gastritis or body predominant gastritis, there also is increased gastrin release, but that is not accompanied with increased acid secretion. In such subjects, acid secretion is reduced or completely absent (achlorhydria) [36, 37]. The low acid secretion, despite increased gastrin levels, indicates markedly impaired ability of oxyntic mucosa to secret acid in response to gastrin. Following eradication of *H. pylori* infection in patients with this pattern of gastritis, there is recovery in acid secretion [36, 37]. However, the degree of recovery in acid outputs is variable – acid output resumes to normal level in some patients while very small increase occur in others [36]. The recovery in acid outputs following eradication of infection coincides with the disappearance of organism as well as resolution of inflammation of the body mucosa. However, there is little evidence of resolution of the atrophy of body mucosa. Capurso *et al.* (23) observed that both pangastritis and pangastritis-induced hypochlorhydria were more prevalent in adult patients with *H. pylori* who had anemia than in those who did not have anemia.

3. Role of *H. pylori* infection in gastric acid perturbation in children

There are only a few pediatric case reports on gastric acid secretion in *H. pylori* infection. Several studies in the pre-*H. pylori* era [38, 39] and very recently [40] studies observed the maximal acid output higher in children with duodenal ulcer than in the children without peptic-ulcer disease. However, no study has examined the relationship between gastric acid secretion and *H. pylori* infection in asymptomatic young children living in developing countries. The effect of *H. pylori* on gastric acid production can be examined by studying individuals with and without infection or, more directly by examining before and after eradication of *H. pylori* [41] In an attempt to see if *H. pylori* infection is associated with gastric acid perturbation in Bangladeshi children, basal gastric acid output (GAO-B) and stimulated gastric acid output (GAO-S) just before and after pentagastrin stimulation in age matched *H. pylori*-infected and non-infected children were measured. Experiments were repeated in infected children 8 weeks after completing a 2-week course of anti-*H. pylori* therapy to evaluate the influence of *H. pylori* on gastric acid secretion. Comparison of acid output between infected and non-infected children both before and after eradication therapy is shown in Table 1. Both the basal acid output (GAO-B) and the stimulated gastric acid outputs (GAO-S) were significantly lower in *H. pylori* infected children compared to *H. pylori* negative group. The mean GAO-B and GAO-S of the infected children were estimated to be 30% and 50% respectively of that of non-infected children. Successful eradication therapy was associated with a significant rise of both the basal and the stimulated acid output values reaching equivalence to those in the *H. pylori*-negative children. Improvement of GAO following anti- *H. pylori* therapy suggests a causal link of *H. pylori* infection and depressed GAO in this population. Whether the observed reversibility of acid secretion to normal level within a relatively short term period of eradication therapy was associated with recovery from corpus gastritis is not known as gastric biopsy for histological examination was not performed. It is also important to know the acid secretory status after a long term period of eradication in settings with possibilities of having re-infection by the organism as a consequence of poor hygiene and environmental contamination.

	Non-infected (n=30)	p	Infected before treatment (n=30)	p	Infected after treatment (n=28)
Basal Acid Output (BAO)	0.23 ± 0.30	0.06	0.62 ±0.9	NS	0.65 ± 0.65
Stimulated Acid Output	2.04 ±1.4	0.001	3.4 ±2.5	NS	3.3 ±2.1

Table 1. Comparison of acid outputs (mMol/h between infected and non-infected children along with effect of anti-*H. pylori* therapy

4. Potential mechanisms of *H. pylori*-induced hypochlorhydria

H pylori induced hypochlorhydria might be due to the bacterium releasing some substances that can directly inhibit acid secretion. Several candidate substances have been identified, which inhibits parietal cell function *in vitro*, but the evidence for involvement of these substances for the *in-vivo* effects remains weak. *H. pylori* infection also produces ammonia, which may uncouple the proton pump [42]. But the ammonia produced by *H. pylori* infection in hypochlorhdric subjects is relatively small [43]. Another problem in attributing the impairment of oxyntic mucosal function to the presence of *H. pylori* organisms is that density of colonization of the gastric mucosa with the organism is similar or lower in subjects with hypocholorhydria than in subjects with normal or high acid secretion [36]. Therefore, current knowledge precludes attributing impaired function of oxyntic mucosa as a direct effect of some bacterial factor.

An alternative explanation for the impaired acid secretory function is infection-induced inflammation of the oxyntic mucosa, since the severity of inflammation of the body mucosa is more marked in subjects with *H. pylori* associated hypochlorhydria than in subjects with *H. pylori* infection with normal or increased acid secretion [44]. This raises the possibility that a product of inflammatory response following infection might inhibit acid secretion.

The molecular mechanisms underlying *H. pylori*-induced hypochlorhydria is not completely understood. However, it has been shown that *H. pylori*–induced pro-inflammatory factors, such as interleukin-1β, may contribute to hypochlorhydria [26, 45].The increased production of this cytokines may be important because it is very potent inhibitor of acid secretion [46] and and may play a role in chronic *H. pylori*-induced hypochlorhydria. Polymorphisms in IL-1β gene cluster may control the extent and the duration of hypochlorhydria with initial *H. pylori infection* [47], which has been noted to be linked to increased risk for atrophy and consequently gastric cancer [48]. It is possible that inflammatory factors, such as IL-1β cause an inhibition of acid secretion from parietal cells via paracrine pathways. Using freshly isolated rabbit gastric glands and culture parietal cells, Fang and colleague observed that Vac-A toxin treatments inhibits gastric acid secretion by preventing the recruitment of gastric H, K-adenosine triphosphatase (H, K-ATPase), the parietal cell enzyme mediating acid secretion. [49]. This was the first evidence that *H. pylori* Vac-A toxin impairs gastric parietal cell physiology by disrupting the apical membrane cycloskeletal linkers of the gastric parietal cells. Studies in animal models as well as epidemiologic studies of *H. pylori* isolates from humans have suggested that VacA toxin enhances the ability of *H. pylori* to colonize in the stomach and contributes to the development of symptomatic diseases (15).

4.1. Potential consequences of *H. pylori* induced hypochlorhydria

H. pylori, by producing hypochlorhydria or impaired gastric barrier may contribute to childhood malnutrition in developing countries through malabsorption or increased susceptibility to enteric infections [50]. Several observations demonstrated a correlation between *H. pylori* and malabsorption of essential nutrients; epidemiological studies have shown an association between *H. pylori* infection and iron deficiency anemia, while the absorption of some vitamins such as vitamin B12, vitamin A, vitamin C, folic *acid* and Vitamin E may also be affected by the infection [51]. The main mechanism related to malabsorption of these components is the modified intragastric pH (hypo or achlorhydria) due to *H. pylori* infection. On the other hand, *H. pylori* eradication has been shown to improve serum level of iron and vitamin B12, and some effects on Vitamin A and Vitamin E absorption as well as late effects on ghrelin levels [51].

5. *H. pylori* infection and iron deficiency anemia

5.1. Iron deficiency and iron deficiency anemia

Iron deficiency (ID) and iron deficiency anemia (IDA) are major public health problems, especially in children and women of childbearing age in developing countries [52], and is considered one of the ten leading global risks factors in terms of its attributable disease burden [53]. It has been estimated that globally approximately 1.6 billion people, representing 25% of the total population are anemic [54]. ID is considered to account for 50% of identified anemia, and 800,000 deaths worldwide can be attributed to IDA. Deficiency of this trace element has adverse implications on health at all stages of life. When iron deficiency occurs during critical windows of brain development, the resultant cognitive deficits may be irreversible and unresponsive to subsequent improvements in the iron status [55]. In adults, ID and IDA can adversely impact physical work capacity and work productivity - variables that may have a detrimental impact on their economic potential [56].

5.2. *H. pylori* and iron deficiency anemia

Several reports have demonstrated an association between *H. pylori* infection and anemia, ID, and IDA, although the mechanisms of the interactions have not been well defined [13, 57-60]. A few case reports indicate that successful eradication of *H. pylori* results in improving iron status and anemia [61-63]. Other studies implicate *H. pylori* as a cause of IDA, refractory to oral iron treatment (refractory iron deficiency or sideropenic anemia); similarly eradication of *H. pylori* has resulted in improved iron status in children [58, 64-67]. Overall, these findings suggest that a substantial proportion of global ID and IDA might be attributed to *H. pylori* infection, leading to a recommendation by some for *H. pylori* eradication therapy in infected individuals with unexplained IDA [68]. However, methodological limitations, including small sample sizes and lacks of control groups, among others, do not allow conclusive interpretation of the results. No previous study has examined whether or not active *H. pylori* infection is causally linked to IDA in young children living in less developed countries. Although the mechanisms for *H. pylori*-associated IDA is not fully understood, *H. pylori*-induced chronic pan gastritis with resultant achlor-or hypo-chlorhydria [41, 69] and reduced ascorbic *acid* secretion in the *gastric* mucosa [70, 71] may lead to reduced iron absorption since they are essential for alimentary iron absorption; they not only convert ferric iron to the ferrous form, which maintains solubility at the alkaline pH of the duodenum, but also chelates with ferric chloride that is also stable at a pH >3. Uptake of iron by *H. pylori* is also suggested [72]. Whether *H. pylori* is a cause or associated with ID or IDA is not fully elucidated.

In Bangladesh, a randomized controlled community based study was conducted to determine whether or not *H. pylori* is a cause of IDA or a reason for treatment failure of iron supplementation in children with IDA [73]. The population consisted of 260 children, 2-5 years (200 *H. pylori* infected, detected by positive urea breath test [UBT], and 60 uninfected) with IDA. IDA was defined as a combination of low hemoglobin (Hb <110 g/L) and a low serum ferritin (SF <12 μg/L) plus elevated serum transferrin receptor (sTfR >8.3 mg/L) [74]. ID was defined as Hb <110 g/L and SF <12 μg/L, or sTfR >8.3 mg/L. They were randomly assigned to one of 4 regimens: (i)2-week course of anti-*H. pylori* (anti- *H. pylori*) triple therapy (amoxicillin 15mg/kg.dose and clarithromycin 7.5mg/kg.dose, both administered twice daily; and a single 20 mg dose of omeprazole per day) plus a 90-day course of oral ferrous sulfate in elixir (3 mg/kg elemental iron daily) (anti- *H. pylori* therapy plus iron);(ii) a 2-week's anti- *H. pylori* therapy plus placebo for iron for 90 days (anti- *H. pylori* alone);(iii) 2-week's course of placebo for anti- *H. pylori* therapy but ferrous sulfate (3 mg/kg for 90 days) (Fe alone); and (iv) 2-week's placebos for anti- *H. pylori* therapy and a 90-day course of placebo for iron (positive control). For precisely determining the role of *H. pylori* infection in the treatment failure of iron supplementation, the study included a fifth group of children with IDA but without *H. pylori* infection (negative control), who were treated with open iron therapy alone for 90 days. Iron status was reassessed after 90 days in all children; those with continued IDA/ID were given a 60-day course of ferrous sulfate.

The results of the study indicated that iron status, as reevaluated on day-90, improved in all groups. However, the improvement was significantly higher among 3 groups receiving iron (anti- *H. pylori* plus iron, iron alone or negative control receiving iron). A greater proportion of infected children receiving iron experienced correction of IDA than those receiving placebo or anti- *H. pylori* alone (68% for anti- *H. pylori* plus iron, 76%)for iron alone, 25% for placebo and 36% for anti- *H. pylori* alone, F=49, p <0.0001 (Figure 1). The results suggest no role of anti- *H. pylori* in IDA. Regarding ID, iron therapy had the most pronounced effect - correction occurred in 100% of children receiving iron compared to only 50% of children receiving anti- *H. pylori* alone or placebo. It is important to note that compared to placebo or iron therapy, anti- *H. pylori* therapy did not improve iron status or decrease IDA and ID prevalence. Therefore, the study concluded that *H. pylori* is neither causally linked with IDA nor is a reason for treatment failure of iron supplementation in children. The findings were in contrast with a randomized controlled trial by Choe and colleague who showed that treatment of the infection was associated with a more rapid response to oral iron compared with iron supplementation alone, and that *H. pylori* eradication led to enhanced iron metabolism even in those not receiving oral iron therapy, suggesting a causal relationship between *H. pylori* infection and IDA [62]. A recent meta-analysis of 12 case reports and series, 19 observational epidemiologic studies and 6 interventional trials, concluded *H. pylori* infection to be a major risk factor for iron deficiency or IDA especially in high-risk groups [75]. Several other meta-analyses of randomized controlled clinical trials suggested that treatment of *H. pylori* infection could be effective in improving anemia and iron statue in IDA patients infected by *H. pylori*, particularly in patients with moderate or severe anemia [76], [77], [78]. Although an association between the pathogenesis of IDA and *H. pylori* infection has been well recognized, a causal link is yet to be established.

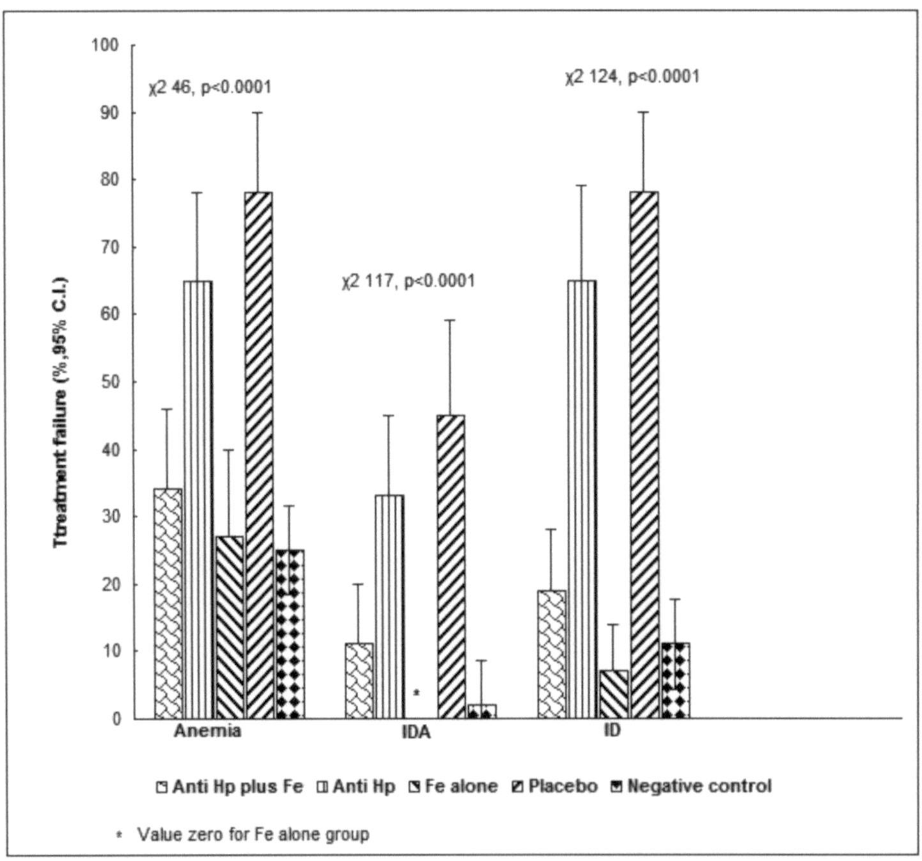

Figure 1. Treatment failure (%) of anemia, IDA, and ID in children receiving different therapies. *Value of zero for the Fe-alone group (Adapted from Sarker *et. al.* 2008)

http://dx.doi.org/10.5772/58375

5.3. *H. pylori* and iron absorption

Non-heme iron absorption requires an acidic milieu. Non-water-soluble iron compounds, e.g. ferrous and ferric pyrophosphate are often used in the fortification programs because they cause no unacceptable organoleptic changes in the fortified food. However, these compounds need gastric acid for their solubilization and absorption. Therefore, if gastric acid output is compromised as a consequence of *H. pylori* infection in a large proportion of the target population, the effect of food fortification programs using ferrous fumarate might be less than expected due to reduced absorption of iron from fortified foods. Keeping this in mind, a study was conducted in 12 Bangladeshi children to measure iron absorption from a non-water-soluble iron compound (ferrous fumarate) and from a water-soluble iron compound (ferrous sulfate) before and after treatment of their *H. pylori infections*. For comparison, 12 uninfected age matched children were studied in parallel; all children had IDA [79]. Iron absorption from ferrous fumarate was compared with that from a highly bioavailable, water-soluble iron compound (ferrous sulfate) in a randomized, crossover study using a double stable-isotope technique. Incorporation of ^{57}Fe and ^{58}Fe into erythrocytes 14 days after administration was used as an index of iron absorption [80]. The study noted geometric mean of iron absorption from ferrous sulfate and ferrous fumarate to be 19.7% and 5.3% respectively ($P < 0.0001$; $n = 12$) before treatment and 22.5% and 6.4% respectively after treatment ($P < 0.0001$; $n = 11$) of *H. pylori*-infected children (Table 2). The corresponding values for uninfected children were 15.6% and 5.4% ($P < 0.001$; $n = 12$). Geometric mean relative absorption (absorption of ferrous fumarate compared to ferrous sulfate) was 26.9% and 34.8% in *H. pylori*-infected and uninfected children respectively, and 28.3% in *H. pylori*-infected children after treatment. The results clearly indicate that iron absorption from ferrous fumarate was significantly lower than that from ferrous sulfate in both *H. pylori*-infected and uninfected Bangladeshi children and also that *H. pylori* infection, *per se,* does not influence iron absorption in young children. The efficacy of ferrous fumarate in iron fortification programs to prevent iron deficiency in young children should, therefore, be further evaluated. The results of iron absorption tests may rule out the possibility of *H. pylori* induced hypochlorhydria in interfering iron absorption in Bangladeshi children.

5.3.1. *Mechanism of IDA*

The interaction between *H. pylori* and iron metabolism, based on clinical, ferrokinetic and microbiological evidences has generated increasing interest. Iron is an essential micronutrient for virtually all organisms, and *H. pylorus is* no exception. *H. pylori* may cause iron deficiency anemia by competing with the host for the acquisition of alimentary iron. In the stomach, ingested food provides iron in heme and nonheme forms. The low pH and the digestive enzymes in the stomach release iron from ligands to the gastric lumen. *H. pylori* and the host both compete for the free iron by deploying mechanisms specifically devised to sequester and facilitate the acquisition of iron as well as other essential metals. *H. pylori* seems particularly adept at competing for iron [81]; it has been established that *H. pylori* competes for iron in murine hosts to an extent so as to cause iron deficiency when the dietary iron intake is poor [82]. In order to ensure a sufficient supply of iron from the environment, *H. pylori* cells display

	H. pylori -infected children before treatment (n=12)			*H. pylori* -infected children after treatment (n=11)			Uninfected children (n=12)		
	Ferrous fumarate	Ferrous sulfate	Relative absorption	Ferrous fumarate	Ferrous sulfate	Relative absorption	Ferrous fumarate	Ferrous sulfate	Relative absorption
		%			%			%	
Geometric mean	5.3	19.7	26.9	6.4	22.5	28.3	5.4	15.6	34.8
+1SD	13.5	32.9	49.0	12.9	33.0	47.7	12.7	30.1	64.3
-1SD	2.1	11.8	14.8	3.2	15.4	16.8	2.3	8.1	18.8
P[1]		<0.0001			<0.0001			<0.001	

[1]P value for iron absorption from ferrous fumarate compared with that from ferrous sulfate within each group.

Adapted from Sarker et al. 2004

Table 2. Fractional iron absorption from ferrous fumarate and ferrous sulfate in uninfected children with iron deficiency anemia (IDA) and in *Helicobacter pylori* infected children with IDA before and after treatment

a repertoire of high-affinity iron-uptake systems. It seems that *H. pylori* strains isolated from patients with IDA demonstrates enhanced iron-uptake activity and may be more adept at competing with the host for iron [83]. So far, little is known about how *H. pylori* cells acquire iron bound to host-binding proteins. *In-vitro* studies indicate that human lactoferrin (LF) supports full growth of *H. pylori* in media lacking other iron sources [72]. LF is released from neutrophil, which captures iron from transferrin in conditions with iron-poor state (hypoferrimia) and has been observed to be abundant in human stomach resection specimens from patients with superficial or atrophic gastritis [84], [84]. The iron uptake by *H. pylori* via a specific human LF receptor may thus play a major role in the virulence of *H. pylori* infection in its uptake of iron. A 70-kDa LF-binding protein from the outer membrane proteins of *H. pylori* was identified in bacterium grown in an iron-starved medium, implicating the protein in iron uptake [85]. Comparative binding experiments with bovine or human LF, and with transferrin of horse, bovine or human origin indicated that this protein is highly specific for human LF. By means of this LF-binding protein, *H. pylori* is able to by-pass the human hypoferremic defensive response -a phenomenon when total extracellular iron is reduced in the host limiting bacterial growth. Further *in vivo* studies demonstrated increased concentration of LF in the biopsy specimen [86] and in the gastric juice [86] of patients with *H. pylori*-related gastritis, and also that LF tissue levels correlate significantly with the degree of inflammation of the gastric mucosa. Two outer membrane proteins, FrpB1 and FrpB2 have also been implicated in hemoglobin binding [81]. In keeping with this, the ability of *H. pylori* to use hemoglobin as an iron source is well documented [87]. Several iron-repressible outer membrane proteins from *H. pylori*, including FrpB1, seem to be responsible for heme utilization [88]

5.4. *H. pylori* and vitamin C

Ascorbic acid is the reduced form of the vitamin, which can act as a potent antioxidant for neutralizing nitrite-derived mutagens protecting against gastric carcinogenesis [90]. Vitamin C is first absorbed and then is actively secreted, mainly in the antral mucosa, from plasma into gastric juice. Once there, it is able to react with nitrosating agents preventing N-nitroso compounds formation; however, vitamin C in the stomach interacts with iron improving its absorption. In children, *H. pylori* infection was associated with reduced gastric juice ascorbic acid concentration, and the effect was more pronounced in patients with the CagA positive strain [20]. In adults, *H. pylori* infection is also recognized to lower the concentration of vitamin C in gastric juice as evident from a study involving randomly chosen 25-74 years old men and women of north Glasgow, UK. Compared to the non-infected, the *H. pylori* infected had 20% lower concentration of vitamin C in their plasma. [91]. The mechanism whereby *H. pylori* infection lowers vitamin C concentration in gastric juice is unclear, but there are several possibilities. Infection has been associated with significant reduction of gastric juice vitamin C concentration due to chronic gastritis and/or *H pylori* oxidase activity [92]. Study in Korean children also demonstrated significant negative correlation between vitamin C level in gastric juice and the degree of active and chronic inflammation in the antral mucosa. Vitamin C levels in whole blood, plasma, and gastric juice and the gastric juice pH were also closely related to the severity of *H. pylori* infection and the histologic changes in the stomach in those children [93].*H. pylori* has been noted to potentiate the polymorphonuclear leukocyte oxidative burst [94], accompanied by a considerable production of reactive oxygen metabolites. Within the microcirculation of the gastric mucosa ascorbic acid may be consumed during scavenging of these reactive oxygen metabolites as vitamin C is the first line of defense against the oxygen free radical damage in the human body [95]. Low level of Vitamin C may be a consequence of an irreversible inactivation of the ingested vitamin C in the intestinal lumen prior to its absorption. Studies have demonstrated that *H. pylori* produces reductions in stomach vitamin C due to its degradation to dehydroascorbic acid (DHAA) - a metabolite that may be oxidized afterwards irreversibly to 2,3- Diketo- 1-gluconic acid. DHAA is unstable at high pH values, and thus hypochlorhydria or achlorhydria may reduce the stability even further and thus the bioavailability of this vitamin.

In developing countries, low intake of vitamin C-enriched food is associated with higher prevalence of *H. pylori* infection, and together will lead to significantly reduced systemic availability of this vitamin. Therefore, prolonged *H. pylori* infection, as it is frequent in developing countries, may impact absorption of several micronutrients including vitamin C. The impact of *H. pylori* infection on the prevalence of micronutrient malnutrition is not currently known, but it is known that there is a strong correlation of both high prevalence of *H. pylori* infection and micronutrient deficiency in developing regions. Various fortification programs are being carried out in developing regions using iron and/or zinc sources e.g. electrolytic iron, ferric pyrophosphate, and zinc oxide. They need secretion of an adequate amount of hydrochloric acid for optimal absorption. Higher prevalence of *H. pylori* infection is associated with low levels of vitamin C in serum and in gastric juice in children [20]; however, there is no consensus about the usefulness of vitamin C supplementation in the management of *H. pylori* infection. In review of the current literature, it may be concluded that high concentration of vitamin C in gastric juice might inactivate *H. pylori* urease [98], the key enzyme for survival of the pathogen and its colonization into acidic stomach. However, it is not certain if vitamin C will be useful in regions with high prevalence of iron and/or zinc deficiency as well as high *H. pylori* contamination rates.

6. Conclusion

The combination of micronutrient deficiency and more frequent enteric infections consequent to *H pylori*–induced hypochlorhydria is likely to have a profound impact on health of children in developing countries with high prevalence of *H pylori* and lower intake of reliable nutritional sources of bioavailable iron and ascorbic acid. Thus, prevention of *H pylori* infection could potentially have an important impact on iron deficiency anemia or other micronutrient deficiencies in the developing world.

Acknowledgements

I gratefully acknowledge Dr. Mohammed Abdus Salam, Director, Research & Clinial Administration and Strategy, icddr,b for his review and valuable comments.

Author details

Shafiqul Alam Sarker

Centre for Nutrition and Food Security (CNFS), Gastroenterology Unit, Dhaka Hospital, International Centre for Diarrhoeal Diseases Research, Bangladesh

References

[1] Pounder, R.E. and D. Ng, The prevalence of Helicobacter pylori infection in different countries. Aliment Pharmacol Ther, 1995. 9 Suppl 2: p. 33-9.

[2] Malaty, H.M., et al., Helicobacter pylori in Hispanics: comparison with blacks and whites of similar age and socioeconomic class. Gastroenterology, 1992. 103(3): p. 813-6.

[3] Mitchell, H.M., et al., Epidemiology of Helicobacter pylori in southern China: identification of early childhood as the critical period for acquisition. J Infect Dis, 1992. 166(1): p. 149-53.

[4] Goh, K.L., Prevalence of and risk factors for Helicobacter pylori infection in a multiracial dyspeptic Malaysian population undergoing endoscopy. J Gastroenterol Hepatol, 1997. 12(6): p. S29-35.

[5] Graham, D.Y., et al., Seroepidemiology of Helicobacter pylori infection in India. Comparison of developing and developed countries. Dig Dis Sci, 1991. 36(8): p. 1084-8.

[6] Kehrt, R., et al., Prevalence of Helicobacter pylori infection in Nicaraguan children with persistent diarrhea, diagnosed by the 13C-urea breath test. J Pediatr Gastroenterol Nutr, 1997. 25(1): p. 84-8.

[7] Sarker, S.A., et al., Prevalence of Helicobacter pylori infection in infants and family contacts in a poor Bangladesh community. Dig Dis Sci, 1995. 40(12): p. 2669-72.

[8] Thomas, J.E., et al., Early Helicobacter pylori colonisation: the association with growth faltering in The Gambia. Arch Dis Child, 2004. 89(12): p. 1149-54.

[9] HM., M., Epidemiology of Infection.. In: Mobley HLT, Mendz GL, Hazell SL, editors. Helicobacter pylori: Physiology and Genetics. Washington (DC): ASM Press; 2001. Chapter 2. Available from: http://www.ncbi.nlm.nih.gov/books/NBK2421/, 2001.

[10] Kusters, J.G., A.H. van Vliet, and E.J. Kuipers, Pathogenesis of Helicobacter pylori infection. Clin Microbiol Rev, 2006. 19(3): p. 449-90.

[11] McColl, K.E., E. el-Omar, and D. Gillen, Interactions between H. pylori infection, gastric acid secretion and anti-secretory therapy. Br Med Bull, 1998. 54(1): p. 121-38.

[12] Leontiadis, G.I., V.K. Sharma, and C.W. Howden, Non-gastrointestinal tract associations of Helicobacter pylori infection. Arch Intern Med, 1999. 159(9): p. 925-40.

[13] Yip, R., et al., Pervasive occult gastrointestinal bleeding in an Alaska native population with prevalent iron deficiency. Role of Helicobacter pylori gastritis. Jama, 1997. 277(14): p. 1135-9.

[14] Malaty, H.M., et al., Natural history of Helicobacter pylori infection in childhood: 12-year follow-up cohort study in a biracial community. Clin Infect Dis, 1999. 28(2): p. 279-82.

[15] Tindberg, Y., M. Blennow, and M. Granstrom, Clinical symptoms and social factors in a cohort of children spontaneously clearing Helicobacter pylori infection. Acta Paediatr, 1999. 88(6): p. 631-5.

[16] Perri, F., et al., Helicobacter pylori infection may undergo spontaneous eradication in children: a 2-year follow-up study. J Pediatr Gastroenterol Nutr, 1998. 27(2): p. 181-3.

[17] Sarker, S.A., et al., Helicobacter pylori: prevalence, transmission, and serum pepsinogen II concentrations in children of a poor periurban community in Bangladesh. Clin Infect Dis, 1997. 25(5): p. 990-5.

[18] Bahu Mda, G., et al., Endoscopic nodular gastritis: an endoscopic indicator of high-grade bacterial colonization and severe gastritis in children with Helicobacter pylori. J Pediatr Gastroenterol Nutr, 2003. 36(2): p. 217-22.

[19] Gottrand, F., et al., Normal gastric histology in Helicobacter pylori-infected children. J Pediatr Gastroenterol Nutr, 1997. 25(1): p. 74-8.

[20] Baysoy, G., et al., Gastric histopathology, iron status and iron deficiency anemia in children with Helicobacter pylori infection. J Pediatr Gastroenterol Nutr, 2004. 38(2): p. 146-51.

[21] Queiroz, D.M., et al., Differences in distribution and severity of Helicobacter pylori gastritis in children and adults with duodenal ulcer disease. J Pediatr Gastroenterol Nutr, 1991. 12(2): p. 178-81.

[22] Dohil, R., et al., Gastritis and gastropathy of childhood. J Pediatr Gastroenterol Nutr, 1999. 29(4): p. 378-94.

[23] Kato, S., et al., Long-term follow-up study of serum immunoglobulin G and immunoglobulin A antibodies after Helicobacter pylori eradication. Pediatrics, 1999. 104(2): p. e22.

[24] Ganga-Zandzou, P.S., et al., Natural outcome of Helicobacter pylori infection in asymptomatic children: a two-year follow-up study. Pediatrics, 1999. 104(2 Pt 1): p. 216-21.

[25] Blaser, M.J. and J.C. Atherton, Helicobacter pylori persistence: biology and disease. J Clin Invest, 2004. 113(3): p. 321-33.

[26] Yao, X. and J.G. Forte, Cell biology of acid secretion by the parietal cell. Annu Rev Physiol, 2003. 65: p. 103-31.

[27] Sobala, G.M., et al., Acute Helicobacter pylori infection: clinical features, local and systemic immune response, gastric mucosal histology, and gastric juice ascorbic acid concentrations. Gut, 1991. 32(11): p. 1415-8.

[28] Iijima, K., et al., Changes in gastric acid secretion assayed by endoscopic gastrin test before and after Helicobacter pylori eradication. Gut, 2000. 46(1): p. 20-6.

[29] McColl, K.E., E. el-Omar, and D. Gillen, Helicobacter pylori gastritis and gastric physiology. Gastroenterol Clin North Am, 2000. 29(3): p. 687-703, viii.

[30] Louw, J.A., et al., Distribution of Helicobacter pylori colonisation and associated gastric inflammatory changes: difference between patients with duodenal and gastric ulcers. J Clin Pathol, 1993. 46(8): p. 754-6.

[31] Levi, S., et al., Campylobacter pylori and duodenal ulcers: the gastrin link. Lancet, 1989. 1(8648): p. 1167-8.

[32] McColl, K.E., et al., Plasma gastrin, daytime intragastric pH, and nocturnal acid output before and at 1 and 7 months after eradication of Helicobacter pylori in duodenal ulcer subjects. Scand J Gastroenterol, 1991. 26(3): p. 339-46.

[33] el-Omar, E., et al., Eradicating Helicobacter pylori infection lowers gastrin mediated acid secretion by two thirds in patients with duodenal ulcer. Gut, 1993. 34(8): p. 1060-5.

[34] Harris, A.W., et al., Eradication of Helicobacter pylori in patients with duodenal ulcer lowers basal and peak acid outputs to gastrin releasing peptide and pentagastrin. Gut, 1996. 38(5): p. 663-7.

[35] Hamlet, A. and L. Olbe, The influence of Helicobacter pylori infection on postprandial duodenal acid load and duodenal bulb pH in humans. Gastroenterology, 1996. 111(2): p. 391-400.

[36] El-Omar, E.M., et al., Helicobacter pylori infection and chronic gastric acid hyposecretion. Gastroenterology, 1997. 113(1): p. 15-24.

[37] Gutierrez, O., et al., Cure of Helicobacter pylori infection improves gastric acid secretion in patients with corpus gastritis. Scand J Gastroenterol, 1997. 32(7): p. 664-8.

[38] Euler, A.R., et al., Basal and pentagstrin-stimulated gastric acid secretory rates in normal children and in those with peptic ulcer disease. J Pediatr, 1983. 103: p. 766-8.

[39] Christie, D.L. and M.E. Ament, Gastric acid hypersecretion in children with duodenal ulcer. Gastroenterology, 1976. 71(2): p. 242-4.

[40] Kato, S., et al., Effect of Helicobacter pylori infection on gastric acid secretion and meal-stimulated serum gastrin in children. Helicobacter, 2004. 9(2): p. 100-5.

[41] Sarker, S.A., et al., Influence of Helicobacter pylori infection on gastric acid secretion in pre-school Bangladeshi children. Helicobacter. 17(5): p. 333-9.

[42] Sachs, G., Gastritis, Helicobacter pylori, and proton pump inhibitors. Gastroenterology, 1997. 112(3): p. 1033-6.

[43] Gillen, D., et al., Helicobacter pylori infection potentiates the inhibition of gastric acid secretion by omeprazole. Gut, 1999. 44(4): p. 468-75.

[44] El-Omar, E.M., et al., Increased prevalence of precancerous changes in relatives of gastric cancer patients: critical role of H. pylori. Gastroenterology, 2000. 118(1): p. 22-30.

[45] Furuta, T., et al., Interleukin 1beta polymorphisms increase risk of hypochlorhydria and atrophic gastritis and reduce risk of duodenal ulcer recurrence in Japan. Gastroenterology, 2002. 123(1): p. 92-105.

[46] Wallace, J.L., et al., Secretagogue-specific effects of interleukin-1 on gastric acid secretion. Am J Physiol, 1991. 261(4 Pt 1): p. G559-64.

[47] Windle, H.J., D. Kelleher, and J.E. Crabtree, Childhood Helicobacter pylori infection and growth impairment in developing countries: a vicious cycle? Pediatrics, 2007. 119(3): p. e754-9.

[48] Furuta, T., et al., Effect of Helicobacter pylori infection on gastric juice pH. Scand J Gastroenterol, 1998. 33(4): p. 357-63.

[49] Wang, F., et al., Helicobacter pylori VacA disrupts apical membrane-cytoskeletal interactions in gastric parietal cells. J Biol Chem, 2008. 283(39): p. 26714-25.

[50] Gilman, R.H., et al., Decreased gastric acid secretion and bacterial colonization of the stomach in severely malnourished Bangladeshi children. Gastroenterology, 1988. 94(6): p. 1308-14.

[51] Vitale, G., et al., Nutritional aspects of Helicobacter pylori infection. Minerva Gastroenterol Dietol. 57(4): p. 369-77.

[52] McLean, E., et al., Worldwide prevalence of anaemia, WHO Vitamin and Mineral Nutrition Information System, 1993-2005. Public Health Nutr, 2008: p. 1-11.

[53] WHO, The World Health Report 2002: Reducing risks, promoting healthy life. 2002, Geneva: World Health Organization.

[54] McLean, E., et al., Worldwide prevalence of anaemia, WHO Vitamin and Mineral Nutrition Information System, 1993-2005. Public Health Nutr, 2009. 12(4): p. 444-54.

[55] Beard, J.L., Why iron deficiency is important in infant development. J Nutr, 2008. 138(12): p. 2534-6.

[56] WHO and UNICEF (2004) Focusing on anaemia; towards an integrated approach for effective anaemia control. Volume,

[57] Seo, J.K., J.S. Ko, and K.D. Choi, Serum ferritin and Helicobacter pylori infection in children: a sero-epidemiologic study in Korea. J Gastroenterol Hepatol, 2002. 17(7): p. 754-7.

[58] Kostaki, M., S. Fessatou, and T. Karpathios, Refractory iron-deficiency anaemia due to silent Helicobacter pylori gastritis in children. Eur J Pediatr, 2003. 162(3): p. 177-9.

[59] Marignani, M., et al., Reversal of long-standing iron deficiency anaemia after eradication of Helicobacter pylori infection. Scand J Gastroenterol, 1997. 32(6): p. 617-22.

[60] Cardenas, V.M., et al., Iron deficiency and Helicobacter pylori infection in the United States. Am J Epidemiol, 2006. 163(2): p. 127-34.

[61] Annibale, B., et al., Reversal of iron deficiency anemia after Helicobacter pylori eradication in patients with asymptomatic gastritis. Ann Intern Med, 1999. 131(9): p. 668-72.

[62] Choe, Y.H., et al., Randomized placebo-controlled trial of Helicobacter pylori eradication for iron-deficiency anemia in preadolescent children and adolescents. Helicobacter, 1999. 4(2): p. 135-9.

[63] Russo-Mancuso, G., et al., Iron deficiency anemia as the only sign of infection with Helicobacter pylori: a report of 9 pediatric cases. Int J Hematol, 2003. 78(5): p. 429-31.

[64] Hershko, C., et al., Role of autoimmune gastritis, Helicobacter pylori and celiac disease in refractory or unexplained iron deficiency anemia. Haematologica, 2005. 90(5): p. 585-95.

[65] Bergamschi, G., Role of autoimmune gastritis, Helicobacter pylori and celiac disease in refractory or unexplained iron deficiency anemia. Hematologica, 2005. 90: p. 577A.

[66] Barabino, A., et al., Unexplained refractory iron-deficiency anemia associated with Helicobacter pylori gastric infection in children: further clinical evidence. J Pediatr Gastroenterol Nutr, 1999. 28(1): p. 116-9.

[67] Ashorn, M., T. Ruuska, and A. Makipernaa, Helicobacter pylori and iron deficiency anaemia in children. Scand J Gastroenterol, 2001. 36(7): p. 701-5.

[68] Malfertheiner, P., et al., Current concepts in the management of Helicobacter pylori infection: the Maastricht III Consensus Report. Gut, 2007. 56(6): p. 772-81.

[69] Iijima, K., et al., Gastric acid secretion of normal Japanese subjects in relation to Helicobacter pylori infection, aging, and gender. Scand J Gastroenterol, 2004. 39(8): p. 709-16.

[70] Rokkas, T., et al., Helicobacter pylori infection and gastric juice vitamin C levels. Impact of eradication. Dig Dis Sci, 1995. 40(3): p. 615-21.

[71] Annibale, B., et al., Concomitant alterations in intragastric pH and ascorbic acid concentration in patients with Helicobacter pylori gastritis and associated iron deficiency anaemia. Gut, 2003. 52(4): p. 496-501.

[72] Husson, M.O., et al., Iron acquisition by Helicobacter pylori: importance of human lactoferrin. Infect Immun, 1993. 61(6): p. 2694-7.

[73] Sarker, S.A., et al., Causal relationship of Helicobacter pylori with iron-deficiency anemia or failure of iron supplementation in children. Gastroenterology, 2008. 135(5): p. 1534-42.

[74] Dallman, P., Laboratory diagnosis of iron deficiency in infancy and early childhood. Annales Nestle, 1995. 53: p. 18-24.

[75] Muhsen, K. and D. Cohen, Helicobacter pylori infection and iron stores: a systematic review and meta-analysis. Helicobacter, 2008. 13(5): p. 323-40.

[76] Qu, X.H., et al., Does Helicobacter pylori infection play a role in iron deficiency anemia? A meta-analysis. World J Gastroenterol. 16(7): p. 886-96.

[77] Huang, X., et al., Iron deficiency anaemia can be improved after eradication of Helicobacter pylori. Postgrad Med J. 86(1015): p. 272-8.

[78] Yuan, W., et al., Iron deficiency anemia in Helicobacter pylori infection: meta-analysis of randomized controlled trials. Scand J Gastroenterol. 45(6): p. 665-76.

[79] Sarker, S.A., et al., Helicobacter pylori infection, iron absorption, and gastric acid secretion in Bangladeshi children. Am J Clin Nutr, 2004. 80(1): p. 149-53.

[80] Kastenmayer, P., et al., A double stable isotope technique for measuring iron absorption in infants. Br J Nutr, 1994. 71(3): p. 411-24.

[81] Carrizo-Chavez, M.A., A. Cruz-Castaneda, and J. Olivares-Trejo Jde, The frpB1 gene of Helicobacter pylori is regulated by iron and encodes a membrane protein capable of binding haem and haemoglobin. FEBS Lett. 586(6): p. 875-9.

[82] Keenan, J.I., et al., The effect of Helicobacter pylori infection and dietary iron deficiency on host iron homeostasis: a study in mice. Helicobacter, 2004. 9(6): p. 643-50.

[83] Yokota, S., et al., Enhanced Fe ion-uptake activity in Helicobacter pylori strains isolated from patients with iron-deficiency anemia. Clin Infect Dis, 2008. 46(4): p. e31-3.

[84] Luqmani, Y.A., et al., Expression of lactoferrin in human stomach. Int J Cancer, 1991. 49(5): p. 684-7.

[85] Dhaenens, L., F. Szczebara, and M.O. Husson, Identification, characterization, and immunogenicity of the lactoferrin-binding protein from Helicobacter pylori. Infect Immun, 1997. 65(2): p. 514-8.

[86] Nakao, K., et al., Relation of lactoferrin levels in gastric mucosa with Helicobacter pylori infection and with the degree of gastric inflammation. Am J Gastroenterol, 1997. 92(6): p. 1005-11.

[87] Senkovich, O., et al., Unique host iron utilization mechanisms of Helicobacter pylori revealed with iron-deficient chemically defined media. Infect Immun. 78(5): p. 1841-9.

[88] Worst, D.J., B.R. Otto, and J. de Graaff, Iron-repressible outer membrane proteins of Helicobacter pylori involved in heme uptake. Infect Immun, 1995. 63(10): p. 4161-5.

[89] Block, G., Vitamin C and cancer prevention: the epidemiologic evidence. Am J Clin Nutr, 1991. 53(1 Suppl): p. 270S-282S.

[90] Zhang, Z.W., M. Abdullahi, and M.J. Farthing, Effect of physiological concentrations of vitamin C on gastric cancer cells and Helicobacter pylori. Gut, 2002. 50(2): p. 165-9.

[91] Woodward, M., H. Tunstall-Pedoe, and K. McColl, Helicobacter pylori infection reduces systemic availability of dietary vitamin C. Eur J Gastroenterol Hepatol, 2001. 13(3): p. 233-7.

[92] Odum, L. and L.P. Andersen, Investigation of Helicobacter pylori ascorbic acid oxidating activity. FEMS Immunol Med Microbiol, 1995. 10(3-4): p. 289-94.

[93] Park, J.H., et al., Correlation between Helicobacter pylori infection and vitamin C levels in whole blood, plasma, and gastric juice, and the pH of gastric juice in Korean children. J Pediatr Gastroenterol Nutr, 2003. 37(1): p. 53-62.

[94] Mooney, C., et al., Neutrophil activation by Helicobacter pylori. Gut, 1991. 32(8): p. 853-7.

[95] Frei, B., L. England, and B.N. Ames, Ascorbate is an outstanding antioxidant in human blood plasma. Proc Natl Acad Sci U S A, 1989. 86(16): p. 6377-81.

[96] Banerjee, S., et al., Effect of Helicobacter pylori and its eradication on gastric juice ascorbic acid. Gut, 1994. 35(3): p. 317-22.

[97] Jarosz, M., et al., Effects of high dose vitamin C treatment on Helicobacter pylori infection and total vitamin C concentration in gastric juice. Eur J Cancer Prev, 1998. 7(6): p. 449-54.

[98] Pal, J., M.G. Sanal, and G.J. Gopal, Vitamin-C as anti-Helicobacter pylori agent: More prophylactic than curative- Critical review. Indian J Pharmacol. 43(6): p. 624-7.

[99] Payne, S.M., Iron acquisition in microbial pathogenesis. Trends Microbiol, 1993. 1(2): p. 66-9.

[100] Bullen, J.J., C.G. Ward, and H.J. Rogers, The critical role of iron in some clinical infections. Eur J Clin Microbiol Infect Dis, 1991. 10(8): p. 613-7.

[101] Otto, B.R., A.M. Verweij-van Vught, and D.M. MacLaren, Transferrins and heme-compounds as iron sources for pathogenic bacteria. Crit Rev Microbiol, 1992. 18(3): p. 217-33.

[102] Ciacci, C., et al., Helicobacter pylori impairs iron absorption in infected individuals. Dig Liver Dis, 2004. 36(7): p. 455-60.

[103] Azab, S.F. and A.M. Esh, Serum hepcidin levels in Helicobacter pylori-infected children with iron-deficiency anemia: a case-control study. Ann Hematol. 92(11): p. 1477-83.

Section 5

Modern Methods of Bacterial DNA Recovering

Chapter 8

Helicobacter pylori and Liver – Detection of Bacteria in Liver Tissue from Patients with Hepatocellular Carcinoma Using Laser Capture Microdissection Technique (LCM)

Elizabeth Maria Afonso Rabelo-Gonçalves,
Bruna Maria Röesler and
José Murilo Robilotta Zeitune

Additional information is available at the end of the chapter

http://dx.doi.org/10.5772/57080

1. Introduction

Hepatocellular carcinoma (HCC) is the most common primary tumor of the liver in humans [1]. It is the fifth most common cancer in men (523,000 cases per year, 7.9% of all cancers) and the seventh among women (226,000 cases per year, 3.7% of all cancers) [2], with over a half of million new cases diagnosed annually. It is the second leading cause of the cancer related mortality in the world [3,4,5] and its prevalence differs according to geographic location, gender, age and ethnicity [6].

In general, the distribution of HCC cases presents great geographic variation, with higher incidence in Easter Asia and sub-Saharan Africa where infection with hepatitis B virus (HBV) is endemic with rates of over 20 per 100,000 individuals. Mediterranean countries such as Italy, Spain and Greece have intermediate rates of 10 to 20 per 100,000 individuals. The North and South America have a relatively low incidence (< 5 per 100,000 individuals) [4], although a rising incidence was observed in the USA, probably associated with the rise in hepatitis C virus (HCV) infection. Recent decreases in the incidence of HCC were reported among Chinese populations in Hong Kong, Shangai and Singapore; the incidence in Japan is also decreasing [3].

In Brazil, there are few reports on the prevalence of HCC [7]. It was suggested that the prevalence was considered low according to epidemiologic and retrospective studies [8]. In

1997, Brazilian researchers showed that HVB was the most common cause of liver disease in patients with HCC [9]. After that, another survey demonstrated that in Southeastern and Southern Brazil, HCV accounted for over 55% of cases. In the Northeast and North, HCV accounted for less than 50% and HBV accounted for 22-25% of cases; hepatitis B was more prevalent in the Northern than in the Southern regions [10].

The development of HCC has been attributed to several risk factors. In general, chronic viral infection with HBV and HCV is considered the major cause of HCC in 75-80% of cases [1], although HBV is globally considered the leading risk factor responsible for 50% of cases [11]. Furthermore, cirrhosis [12], exposure to the carcinogenic fungal aflatoxin B1 [13], inherited diseases [14], Wilson's disease [15] and heavy alcohol consumption [16] are also risk factors attributed to its development. Recently, upcoming risk factors for HCC include obesity, diabetes and related nonalcoholic fatty liver disease [3].

In 1994, researchers described the infectious agent *Helicobacter* (*H.*) *hepaticus* and its role in causing active hepatitis and associated liver tumors in mice [17]. Since then, several studies related to *H. hepaticus* experimental infection have demonstrated that this bacterium may induce a strong inflammatory change in the liver leading to HCC. Considering that *H. pylori* was classified as a class I carcinogen [18] and *Helicobacter* spp. DNA was detected in hepatic tissue from patients with different hepatobiliary diseases, it has been proposed that in humans, as in animals, *Helicobacter* spp. may also colonize and induce chronic hepatic diseases mainly HCC.

In fact, studies related to the possible association between *H. pylori* and hepatobiliary diseases have been developed since 1998, when Helicobacter DNA was identified in Chilean patients with chronic cholecystitis [19]. After that, a variety of researches have been conducted to verify the role of *H. pylori* in the development of HCC [20, 21, 22, 23, 24, 25, 26 e 27]. Considering the role of chronic inflammation and infection in the development of cancer, in the case of HCC, future studies should be performed to verify the role of *Helicobacter* infection in the liver pathophisiology [28]. However, whether this bacterium causes liver tumor or acts as a cofactor in the process of carcinogenesis needs to be confirmed.

The mechanism by which *H. pylori* colonizes the human liver is not totally enlightened. The *H. pylori* DNA detected in the liver tissue may result from bacterial translocation from the stomach into the blood through the portal system, especially in the later stages of chronic liver disease when portal hypertension occurs [1, 29, 30]. In addition, the bacteria may reach the liver by phagocytes and macrophages or circulating retrograde transfer from the duodenum [31]. However, the studies involving the growth of *H. pylori* from the HCC liver reinforce the bacterial colonization ruling out the possibility of retrograde contamination [32, 33]. Additionally, no other bacteria from the digestive tract are associated with human hepatocarcinogenesis [23, 34].

Several researchers have suggested that *H. pylori* may damage hepatocytes in vitro by a cytopathic effect in a liver and HCC cell lines [35, 36]. Furthermore, it was demonstrated in a HCC cell line (Huh7) that an inoculum of *H. pylori* was able to adhere and internalize into hepatocytes and this result was also dependent on virulence factors of bacteria [37]. Proteomic analysis of human hepatic cell line (HepG2) co-cultured with *H. pylori* have revealed that bacteria may exert the pathological effect on HepG2 cells by up-regulating the expression of some proteins enrolled in transcription regulation, signal transduction and metabolism [38].

In most pathology laboratories, archives of formalin-fixed paraffin-embedded (FFPE) tissues represent the only tissue specimens available for routine diagnostics. A major advantage of such archives is that long-term clinical data is often available [39]. Furthermore, another benefit of using FFPE tissues is that they are the easiest to store and transport [40]. Because of this, FFPE tissues have been used in PCR-based studies related to cancer research, genetics, infectious diseases and molecular epidemiology [41]. Additionally, the use of FFPE tissue also allows employing modern transcriptomic and epigenomic methods with nucleic acids [39].

However, isolating high-quality genomic DNA from FFPE sections remains a challenge for researchers. Formalin is the most commonly used tissue fixative worldwide because it offers the best compromise between cost, practicality and morphological fixative properties [39, 42]. However, the fixation of tissue in formalin leads to extensive protein-DNA cross-linking of all tissue components and nucleic acids isolated from these specimens are highly fragmented [43]. This is particularly troublesome when long DNA regions are amplified, old paraffin blocks are used or fixation time is over three days [41, 44]. Because of this, FFPE tissue requires special protocols in order to extract small amounts of DNA suitable for amplification [45]. Nevertheless, methods of DNA extraction from FFPE tissue are generally laborious and time consuming.

Although studies on the role of the *H. pylori* in the development of HCC were more frequent in the last decade [46], most of them presents a prospective nature. This probably occurs because the retrospective studies frequently employ FFPE liver tissue and DNA extraction is a limiting factor in this type of sample. However, several researchers have detected *H. pylori* and its virulence factors (vacA genes and 26 kDa) in paraffin embedded liver samples [21, 27, 34, 47, 48].

Laser capture microdissection (LCM) is a technique that has recently become available for isolation of individual or groups of cells from a heterogeneous tissue sections by microscopic visualization. The technique was first described in 1996 by researchers of the National Institutes of Health (NIH) in Bethesda, MD [49] and allows the isolation of cells reducing the interference from nontarget cell population. The method allows selection of unmixed starting material for DNA, RNA or protein extraction for further downstream analyses [50].

The LCM system is based on an inverted light microscope fitted with a laser device to facilitate the visualization and procurement of cells [51]. The PALM MicroBeam System (Carl Zeiss, MicroImaging GmbH, Göottingen, Germany) was used in this study and it is based on the Laser Microdissection and Pressure Catapulting technology. This system consists of an inverted microscope with a motorized stage and a pulsed "cold" nitrogen ultra-violet (UV) laser. The laser is focused through the objective lenses to a micron-sized spot diameter. The narrow laser focal spot allows the ablation of the material while the surrounding tissue remains fully intact. The microscope stage and UV laser are controlled by a PC, and a video camera allows for tissue sections to be displayed on the PC screen. Cells or regions of interest are then identified and manually delineated on the computer screen using the software program. The microscope is then instructed to collect delineated regions. The noncontact capture of homogeneous tissue samples or individual cells is achieved by means of catapulting using PALM's patented Laser Pressure Catapulting technology. With the same laser, the separated cells, or the selected tissue area, can be directly catapulted into the eppendorf cap containing a depressed lid [52, 53]. The Figure 1 shows the LCM technology employed in this study.

LCM has been used in a wide variety of applications, including pathology [54, 55], organ transplantation [56, 57], gene expression [52, 58] and molecular characterization of cancer cells [59, 60, 61]. LCM is compatible with most stains and tissue preservation techniques including frozen sections, FFPE tissues, cytology preparations and cultured cells [52, 62]. Because of its high precision and accuracy LCM has been successfully employed to isolation of bacterial cells in FFPE tissues including *H. pylori* [48, 61, 62, 64, 65].

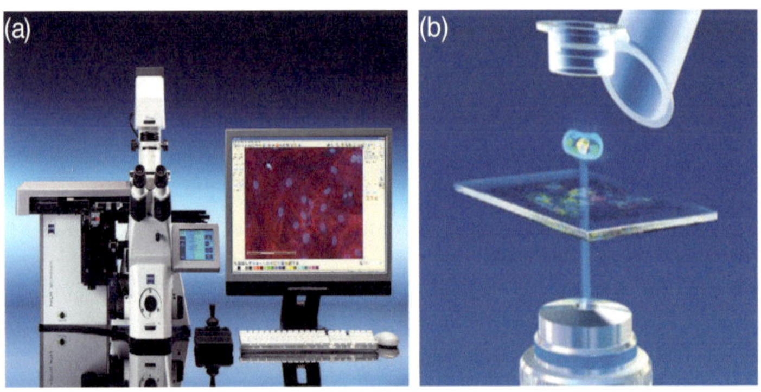

Figure 1. Images of LCM technology used in the study. In A is represented the complete PALM MicroBeam system. In B is illustrated the path of the laser beam passing through the objective lens to reach the tissue slice and the catapulting process for capturing the cells of interest into the Eppendorf cap. Source of the images: www.zeiss.de.

2. Clinical samples, methods and results

2.1. Clinical samples

This study was carried out utilizing six cases of FFPE liver tissue from patients with HCC from Department of Anatomic Pathology, Faculty of Medical Sciences, State University of Campinas (UNICAMP), Campinas, São Paulo, Brazil. The mean ages of patients was 56.0 years, with 4 male cases (66,6%) and 2 female cases (33,4%). All the fragments of liver were obtained during hepatic surgery (either transplantation or partial hepatectomy). These samples were *H. pylori* positive previously detected by polymerase chain reaction (PCR) with *H. pylori* specific 16S rRNA primers [27]. The selection criteria for the paraffin blocks included specimens archived for 5 years (2008 to 2012). The present study was approved by the Ethics Committee of the Faculty of Medical Sciences, UNICAMP (CEP 616/2009).

2.2. Methods

2.2.1. Tissue preparation for LCM

Six *H. pylori* positive samples were cut into 10µm-thick sections and mounted on 0.17mm PEN membrane-covered slides (Carl Zeiss, MicroImaging GmbH, Göttingen, Germany). After slicing, the sections were placed at 60°C for 30 minutes, then deparaffinized in 3 xylene baths (3x1min), rehydrated in decreasing alcohols (100%, 95% e 70%, each for 30 seconds) and washed for 30 seconds in tap water. Further, the routine staining with carbol fuchsin was performed [66]. At this step the sections have remained in the dye for at most 15 seconds. The stained sections were observed under the microscope for the identification of bacteria.

2.2.2. Bacterial microdissection

Stained bacteria were microdissected using a PALM MicroBeam system (Carl Zeiss, MicroImaging GmbH, Göttingen, Germany) (Figure 1A). The areas with target bacteria were traced around and microdissected together with the pieces of thin membrane by laser microbeam and then ejected into the Eppendorf tube cap by a single laser shot (Figure 1B). The tube was stored at -80°C until DNA extraction.

2.2.3. DNA extraction

After microdissection, the cap was inserted into an Eppendorf tube containing 100µl digestion buffer, prepared with 10mM Tris-HCl (pH 8.0), 1mM EDTA, 1% Tween 20 and 0.3% proteinase K. After that, samples remained in a water bath at 56°C for 3 hours and the tube was heated to 95°C for 5 min to inactivate proteinase K. The crude lysate was directly employed as template for PCR. All of these procedures were previously described with minor modifications [48].

2.2.4. PCR amplification

The samples were further amplified by PCR using *H. pylori* 16S rRNA primers. The sequence of the sense primer (JW21) was 5′-GCGACCTGCTGGAACATTAC-3′(position 691-710) and the antisense primer (JW22) was 5′-CGTTAGCTCCATTACTGGAGA-3′ (position 829-809) and they amplified a product of approximately 129bp [27]. Briefly, 1µl of DNA extracted was added to 25µl PCR mix containing deoxynucleoside triphosphates (dNTPs) at concentrations of 200 µM each, 2.0µl of 25mM MgCl2, 0.25 µl of GoTaq Hot Start Polymerase (Promega Corp., Madison, WI, USA), 4.0 µl of 5X GoTaq Flexi Buffer (supplied with the enzyme) and 20 pmol each primer (Life Technologies, Carlsbed, CA, USA). Amplification reactions included an initial 2-minute denaturation step at 94ºC, followed by 40 cycles of 30 seconds at 94ºC, 30 seconds at 55ºC and 45 seconds at 72ºC. A final extension step for 7 minutes at 72ºC was performed. The DNA extracted from *H. pylori* from FFPE gastric tissue was used as positive control and distilled water in place of the DNA samples was used as negative control for PCR assays.

2.2.5. Detection of PCR products

For analysis of the amplified products, 5µl of the amplicons were put on 1,5% agarose gels containing 1µg of ethidium bromide per ml. The amplicons were visualized by UV transillumination.

2.2.6. Sequence analysis

The 16S rRNA amplicons were further identified by sequence analysis using ABI Prism Dye Terminator sequencing kit with AmpliTaq DNA polymerase and the ABI 3500xL Sequencer (Applied Biosystems, Foster City, CA, USA). Sequence comparison was then carried out using the Blast program and GenBank databases.

2.3. Results

Analyzing the tissue sections stained with carbol fuchsin, we visualized microorganisms resembling *H. pylori* mainly in hepatic sinus from HCC samples. The number of cocci was greater than of bacilli (Figure 3).

Our PCR results showed that all six microdissected samples were positive for 16S rRNA gene (Figure 2) and showed 98% similarity to *H. pylori* 16S rRNA gene by sequence analysis (GeneBank accession number CP003419.1) (Figure 4).

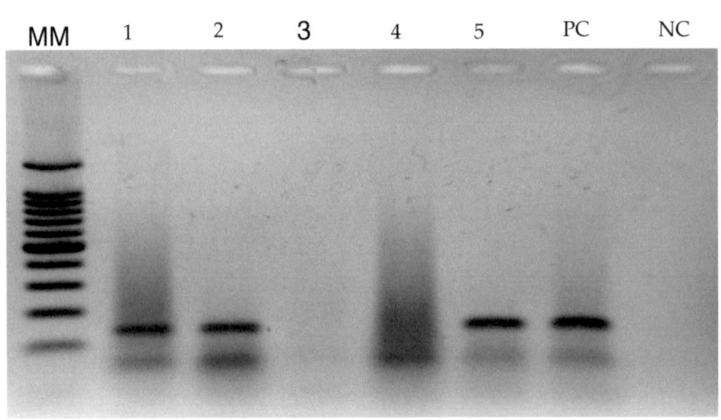

Figure 2. Results of amplification of *H. pylori* 16S rRNA gene. 1, 2 and 5 are positive samples; 3 and 4 are negative samples. MM: molecular marker, PC: positive control and NC: negative control.

http://dx.doi.org/10.5772/57080

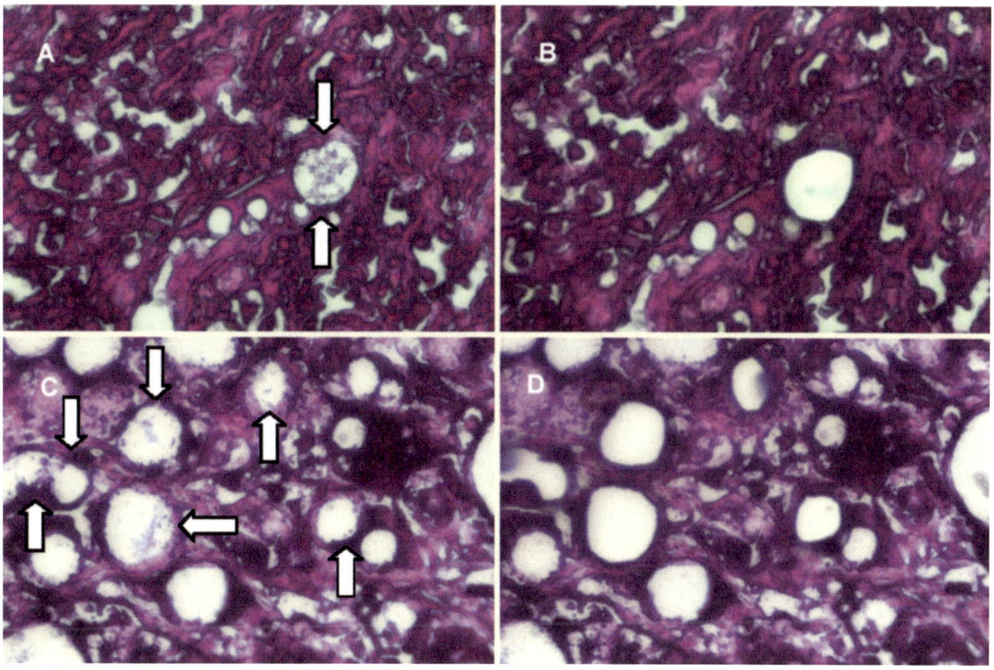

Figure 3. Optical microscopy of FFPE liver fragments of HCC patients with PCR-positive *H. pylori* 16S rRNA and stained with carbol fuchsin. In (A) and (C) bacteria are represented within sinusoid (arrows) before microdissection (magnification: 610X). In (B) and (D) the same samples are represented after bacterial microdissection (magnification: 610X).

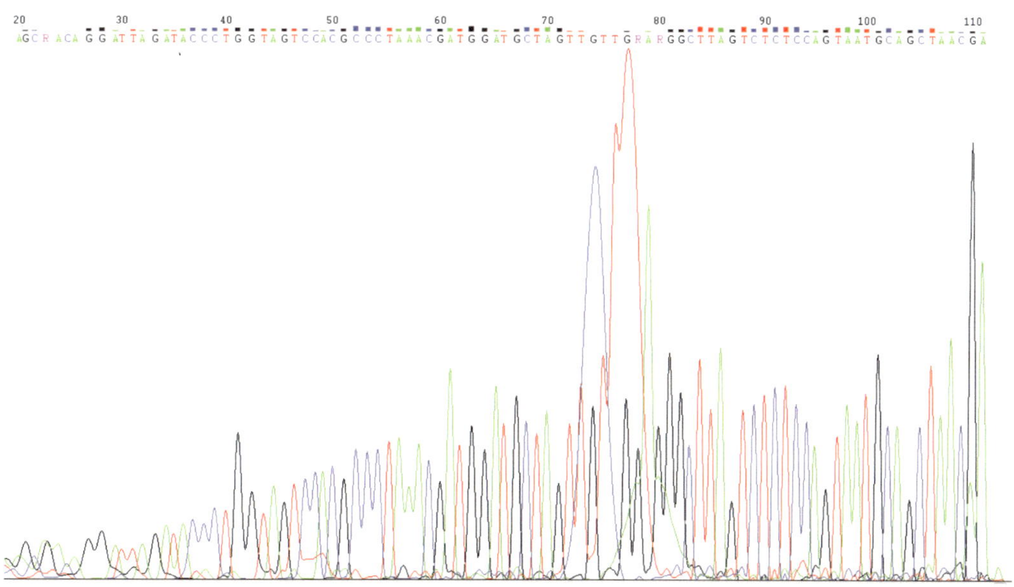

Figure 4. Electropherogram sequence of *H. pylori* 16S rRNA gene and alignment results of the BLAST databases.

3. Conclusion

The results described here confirm the identification of *H. pylori* in FFPE liver tissue from patients with HCC. Although specific primers were used for amplification of the *H. pylori* 16S rRNA gene, we cannot exclude the possibility of cross-reaction of these primers with other *Helicobacter* spp [65].

Considering the difficulty of DNA extraction from paraffin embedded samples, the use of LCM simplified the achievement of specific DNA because the DNA extraction process was reduced to a single digestion step of bacterial cells without further purification. Consequently, the crude lysate was used directly as template for PCR amplification. This is particularly advantageous when compared to traditional methods of DNA extraction that are generally laborious, toxic and time consuming [67].

Another advantage of using LCM is that it allowed the exact location of *H. pylori* in the liver, since bacteria were mainly found in the peritumoral tissue. Considering that our samples presented tumoral and peritumoral tissue in the same paraffin block, the technique was highly effective for obtaining a target bacterial population within a selected area in the HCC tissue. This is very important when we consider that the necrotic state and nuclease content of tissues may influence in recovering intact DNA specially when performing traditional methods for DNA extraction [68].

Furthermore, LCM was useful to reduce the interference from nontarget cell population considering that bacteria were found in small quantities in the liver tissue (Figure 3). In relation to nontarget cell population, it is important to consider that the major obstacle in the analysis of tumoral tissue is that it is composed by different cell types including stroma and inflammatory cells [69, 70, 71] and there is a potential dilution effect of the larger quantities of nontarget DNA found in whole tissue sections [64]. Thus, the employment of LCM was very efficient in isolating *H. pylori* despite of the reduced bacterial quantity in the HCC tissue.

In summary, we suggest that LCM can be extensively applied for identification of *H. pylori* in FFPE liver tissue. Further studies will be performed in order to amplify virulence genes of bacteria as well as to isolate *H. pylori* from other tissues using LCM technique.

Acknowledgements

This work was supported by grants from FAPESP (2009/09889-5) and FAEPEX 101/2011.

Author details

Elizabeth Maria Afonso Rabelo-Gonçalves*, Bruna Maria Röesler and José Murilo Robilotta Zeitune

*Address all correspondence to: elizabeth.goncalves@gc.unicamp.br

Department of Internal Medicine, Center of Diagnosis of Digestive Diseases, Faculty of Medical Sciences, State University of Campinas, Campinas, São Paulo, Brazil

References

[1] Tu QV, Okoli AS, Kovach Z, Mendz GL. Hepatocellular carcinoma: prevalence and molecular pathogenesis of *Helicobacter* spp. Future Microbiology 2009;4(10) 1283-1301.

[2] GLOBOCAN. International Agency for Research on Cancer (IARC). 2008. http://www-dep.iarc.fr. (accessed may 2013).

[3] El-Seragh HB. Epidemiology of viral hepatitis and hepatocellular carcinoma. Gastroenterology 2012;42(6) 1264-1273.

[4] Mittal S & El-Seragh HB. Epidemiology of hepatocellular carcinoma. Consider the population. Journal of Clinical Gastroenterology 2013;47 Suppl S2-6.

[5] World Health Organization. Mortality Database. WHO Statistical Information System. 2008. http://www.who.int/whosis (accessed may 2013).

[6] Hall AJ & Wild CP. Liver cancer in low and middle income countries. British Medical Journal 2003;326(7397) 994-995.

[7] Carvalho FM, Pereira TA, Gonçalves PL, Jarske RD, Pereira FEL, Louro ID. Hepatocellular carcinoma and liver cirrhosis TP53 mutation analysis reflects a moderate dietary exposure to aflatoxins in Espírito Santo State, Brazil. Molecular Biology Reports 2013; 40(8) 4883-4887.

[8] Bosch FX, Ribes J, Cléries R, Diaz M. Epidemiology of hepatocellular carcinoma. Clinical Liver Diseases 2005;9(2) 191-211.

[9] Gonçalves S, Pereira FF, Gayotto LC. Hepatocellular carcinoma in Brazil: report of a national survey (Florianopolis, SC, 1995). Revista do Instituto de Medicina Tropical de São Paulo 1997;39(3) 165-170.

[10] Carrilho FJ, Kikuchi L, Branco F, Gonçalves CS, Mattos AA. Brazilian HCC Study Group. Clinics 2010;65(12) 1285-1290.

[11] Parkin DM. The global health burden of infection-associated cancers in the year of 2002. International Journal of Cancer 2002;118(12) 3030-3044.

[12] Gao J, Xie L, Yang W, Zhang W, Gao S, Wang J, Xiang Y. Risk factors of hepatocellular carcinoma - current status and perspectives. Asian Pacific Journal of Cancer Prevention 2012;13(3) 743-750.

[13] Soman NR & Wogan GN. Activation of the c-Kis-ras oncogene in aflatoxin B1-induced hepatocellular carcinoma and adenoma in the rat: detection by denaturating gradient gel electrophoresis. Proceeding of the National Academy of Sciences 1993;90(5) 2045-2049.

[14] Taddei T, Mistry P, Schilsky ML. Inherited metabolic disease of the liver. Current Opinion in Gastroenterology 2008; 24(3) 278-286.

[15] Kumagi T, Horiike N, Abe M, Kurose K, Iuchi H, Masumoto T, Joko K, Akbar SF, Michitaka K, Onji M. Small hepatocellular carcinoma associated with Wilson's disease. Internal Medicine 2005;44(5) 493-443.

[16] La Vecchia C. Alcohol and liver cancer. European Journal of Cancer Prevention 2007;16(6) 497-495.

[17] Ward JM, Fox JG, Anver MR, Haines DC, George CV, Collins MJ Jr, Gorelick PL, Nagashima K, Gonda MA, Gilden RV. Chronic active hepatitis and associated liver tumors in mice caused by a persistent bacterial infection with a novel *Helicobacter species*. Journal of the National Cancer Institute 1994;86(16) 1222-1227.

[18] IARC: Working group on the evaluation of carcinogenic risks to human *Helicobacter pylori*. IARC Monography Evaluation Carcinogenic Risks Human 1994;61 177-240.

[19] Fox JG, Dewhirst FE, Shen Z, Feng Y, Taylor NS, Paster BJ, Ericson RL, Lau CN, Correa P, Araya JC, Roa I. Hepatic *Helicobacter species* identified in bile and gallbladder tissue from Chileans with chronic cholecystitis. Gastroenterology 1998;114(4) 755-763.

[20] Ponzetto A, Pellicano R, Leone N, Cutufia MA, Turrini F, Grigioni WF, D'Errico A, Mortimer P, Rizzetto M, Silengo L. *Helicobacter* infection and cirrhosis in hepatitis C virus carriage: is it an innocent bystander or a troublemaker? Medical Hypotheses 2000;54(2) 275-277.

[21] Dore MP, Realdi G, Mura D, Graham DY, Sepulveda AR. *Helicobacter* infection in patients with HCV-related chronic hepatitis, cirrhosis, and hepatocellular carcinoma. Digestive Diseases and Sciences. 2002;47(7) 1638-1643.

[22] Fan XG, Peng XN, Huang Y, Yakoob J, Wang ZM, Chen YP. *Helicobacter species* ribosomal DNA recovered from the liver tissue of Chinese patients with primary hepatocellular carcinoma. Clinical and Infectious Diseases 2002;35(12) 1555-1557.

[23] Verhoef C, Pot RG, de Man RA, Zondervan PE, Kuipers EJ, IJzermans JN, Kusters JG. Detection of identical *Helicobacter* DNA in the stomach and in the non-cirrhotic liver of patients with hepatocellular carcinoma. European Journal of Gastroenterology and Hepatology 2003;15(11) 1171-1174.

[24] Pellicano R, Mazzaferro V, Grigioni WF, Cutufia MA, Fagoonee S, Silengo L, Rizzetto M, Ponzetto A. *Helicobacter species* sequences in liver samples from patients with and without hepatocellular carcinoma. World Journal of Gastroenterology 2004;10(4) 598-601.

[25] Ito K, Nakamura M, Toda G, Negishi M, Torii A, Ohno T. Potential role of *Helicobacter pylori* in hepatocarcinogenesis. International Journal of Molecular Medicine 2004;13(2) 221-227.

[26] Rocha M, Avenaud P, Ménard A, Le Bail B, Balabaud C, Bioulac-Sage P, de Magalhães Queiroz DM, Mégraud F. Association of *Helicobacter species* with hepatitis C cirrhosis with or without hepatocellular carcinoma. Gut 2005;54(3) 396-401.

[27] Pirouz T, Zounubi L, Keivani H, Rakhshani N, Hormazdi M. Detection of *Helicobacter pylori* in paraffin-embedded specimens from patients with chronic liver diseases, using the amplification method. Digestive Diseases and Sciences 2009;54(7) 1456-1459.

[28] Gonciarz M, Wloch M, Gonciarz Z. *Helicobacter pylori* in liver diseases. Journal of Physiology and Pharmacology 2006;57(3) 155-161.

[29] Casafont F, Martin L, Pons-Romero F. Bacterial overgrowth in the small intestine in chronic liver disease. In: Blum HE, Bode JC, Bode Ch, Sartor RB(ed). Gut and the liver. London: Kluwer Academic Publishers; 1998. p 332-337.

[30] Tsunneyama K, Harada K, Kono N, Hiramatsu K, Zen Y, Sudo Y, Gershwin ME, Ikemoto M, Arai Y, Nakanuma Y. Scavenger cells with Gram-positive bacterial lipoteichoic acid infiltrate around the damaged interlobular bile ductus of primary biliary cirrhosis. Journal of Hepatology 2001;35(2) 156-163.

[31] Queiroz DMM & Santos A. Isolation of a *Helicobacter* strain from the human liver. Gastroenterology 2001;121(4) 1023-1024.

[32] Xuan SY, Qiang X, Zhou RR, Shi YX, Jiang WJ. *Helicobacter* infection in hepatocellular carcinoma tissue. World Journal of Gastroenterology 2006; 12(15) 2335-2340.

[33] Leelawat K, Suksumek N, Leelawat S, Lek-Uthai U. Detection of VacA gene specific for *Helicobacter pylori* in hepatocellular carcinoma and cholangiocarcinoma specimens of Thai patients. Southeast Asian Journal of Tropical Medicine and Public Health 2007;38(5) 881-885.

[34] Al-Soud AW, Stenram U, Ljungh A, Tranberg KG, Nilsson HO, Wadstrom T. DNA of *Helicobacter* spp. and common gut bacteria in primary liver carcinoma. Digestive and Liver Diseases 2008;40(2) 126-131.

[35] Taylor NS, Fox JG, Yan L. In vitro hepatotoxic factor in *Helicobacter hepaticus. H. pylori* and other *Helicobacter species*. Journal of Medical Microbiology 1995;42(1) 48-42.

[36] Chen R, Fan XG, Huang Y, Li N, Chen CH. In vitro cytotoxicity of Helicobacter pylori on hepatocarcinoma HepG2 cells. Al Zheng 2004; 23(1) 44-49.

[37] Ito K, Yamaoka Y, Ota H, El-Zimaity H, Graham DY. Adherence, internalization and persistence of *Helicobacter pylori* in hepatocytes. Digestive Diseases and Sciences 2008; 53(9) 2541-2549.

[38] Zhang Y, Fan XG, Chen R, Xiao ZQ, Feng XP, Tian XF, Chen ZH. Comparative proteome analysis of untreated and *Helicobacter pylori*-treated HepG2. World Journal of Gastroenterology 2005;11(22) 3485-3489.

[39] Frankel A. Formalin fixation in the '-omics' era: a primer for the surgeon-scientist. ANZ Journal of Surgery 2012;82(6) 395-402.

[40] Rivero ERC, Neves AC, Silva-Valenzuela MG, Sousa SOM, Nunes FD. Simple salting-out method for DNA extraction from formalin-fixed, paraffin-embedded tissues. Pathology Research and Practice 2006;202(7) 523-529.

[41] Greer CE, Wheeler CM, Manos MM. Sample preparation and PCR amplification form paraffin-embedded tissues. PCR Methods and Application Journal 1994;3(6) S113-S122.

[42] Klopfleisch R, Weiss AT, Gruber AD. Excavation of a buried treasure - DNA, mRNA, miRNA and protein analysis in formalin fixed, paraffin embedded tissues. Histology and Histopathology 2011;26(6) 797-810.

[43] Wu L, Pattern N, Yamashiro CT, Chui B. Extraction and amplification of DNA from formalin-fixed, paraffin-embedded tissues. Applied Immunohistochemistry and Molecular Morphology 2002; 10(3) 269-274.

[44] Karlsen F, Kalantari M, Chitemerere M, Johansson B, Hagmar B. Modifications of human and viral deoxyribonucleic acid by formaldehyde fixation. Laboratory Investigation 1994;71(4) 604-11.

[45] Muñoz-Cadavid C, Rudd S, Zaki SR, Patel M, Moser SA, Brandt ME, Gómez BL. Improving Molecular Detection of fungal DNA in formalin-fixed paraffin-embedded tissues: comparison of five tissue DNA extraction methods using parafungal PCR. Journal of Clinical Microbiology 2010;48(6) 2147-2153.

[46] Bulajic M, Panic N, Stimec B, Isaksson B, Jesenofsky R, Schneider-Brachert W, Löhr JM. PCR in *Helicobacter* spp. diagnostic in extragastric malignancies of digestive system. European Journal of Gastroenterology and Hepatology 2012; 24(2) 117-125.

[47] Nilsson HO, Mulchandani R, Tranberg KG, Stenram U, Wadström T. *Helicobacter species* identified in liver from patients with cholangiocarcinoma and hepatocellular carcinoma. Gastroenterology 2001;120(1) 323-324.

[48] Tian XF, Fan XG, Huang Y, Dai H, Ying RS. Procuration and identification of bacteria in paraffin-embedded liver tissues of hepatocellular carcinoma by laser-assisted microdissection technique. Acta Pathologica, Microbiologica et Imunologica Scandinavica 2008;116(1) 10-15.

[49] Emmer-Buck MR, Bonner RF, Smith PD, Chuaqui RF, Zhuang Z, Goldstein SR, Weiss RA, Liotta LA. Laser capture microdissection. Science 1996; 274(1274) 998-1001.

[50] Aaltonen KE, Ebbesson A, Wigerup C, Hedenfalk I. Laser capture microdissection (LCM) and whole genome amplification (WGA) of DNA from normal breast tissue - optimization for genome wide array analyses. BMC Research Notes 2011;4(3) 1-7.

[51] Liu A. Laser capture microdissection in the tissue biorepository. Journal of Biomolecular Techniques 2010; 21(3) 120-125.

[52] Esposito G. Complimentary techniques: laser capture microdissection - increasing specificity of gene expression profiling of cancer specimens. Advances in Experimental Medicine and Biology 2007; 593: 54-65.

[53] Sluka P, O'Donnell L, McLachlan R, Stanton PG. Application of laser-capture microdissection to analysis of gene expression in the testis. Progress in Histochemistry and Cytochemistry 2007; 42(2008) 173-201.

[54] Agar NS, Halliday GM, Barnetson RS, Jones A.M. A novel technique for the examination of skin biopsies by laser capture microdissection. Journal of Cutaneous Pathology 2003; 30(4) 265-270.

[55] Okuduku AF, Hahne JC, Von Deimling A, Wernert N. Laser-assisted microdissection, techniques and applications in pathology. International Journal of Molecular Medicine 2005; 15(5) 763-769.

[56] Kleheergher W, Rothämel T, Glöckner S, Lehmann U, Kreipe H. Laser-assisted microdisscetion and short tandem repeat PCR for the investigation of graft chimerism after solid organ transplantation. Pathobiology 2000;68(4-5)196-201.

[57] Lehmann U, Versmold A, Kreipe H. Combined laser-assisted microdissection and short tandem repeat analysis for detection of in situ microchimerism after solid organ transplantation. Methods in Molecular Biology 2005; 293: 113-123.

[58] Wang L, Zhu JS, Song MQ, Chen GQ, Chen JL. Comparison of gene expression profiles between primary tumor and metastatic lesions in gastric cancer patients using laser microdissection and cDNA microarray. World Journal of Gastroenterology 2006;12(43) 6949-6954.

[59] Jensen LH, Cruger DG, Lindebjerg J, Byriel L, Bruun-Petersen G, Jakobsen A. Laser microdissection and microsatellite analysis of colorectal adenocarcinomas. Anticancer Research 2006;26(3A) 2069-2074.

[60] Pai CY, Hsieh LL, Tsai CW, Chiou FS, Yang CH, Hsu BD. Allelic alterations at the STR markers in the buccal tissue cells of oral cancer patients and the oral epithelial cells of healthy betel quid-chewers: an evaluation of forensic applicability. Forensic Science International 2002;129(3) 158-67.

[61] Huang C, Yang L, Li Z, Yang J, Zhao J, Dehui X, Liu L, Wang Q, Song T. Detection of CCND1 amplification using laser capture microdissection coupled with real-time polymerase chain reaction in human esophageal squamous cell carcinoma. Cancer Genetics and Cytogenetics 2007;175(1) 19-25.

[62] Cheng L, Zhang S, MacLennan GT, Williamson SR, Davidson DD, Wang M, Jones TD, Lopez-Beltran A, Montironi R. Laser-assisted microdissection in translational re-

search: theory, technical considerations, and future applications. Applied Immunohistochemistry and Molecular Morphology 2013;21(1) 31-47.

[63] Ryan P, Kelly RG, Lee G, Collins JK, O'Sullivan GC, O'Conell J, Shanahan F. Bacterial DNA within granulomas of patients with Crohn's disease: detection by laser capture microdissection and PCR. American Journal of Gastroenterology 2004;99(8) 1539-1543.

[64] Klitgaard K, Molbak L, Jensen TK, Lindboe CF, Boye M. Laser capture microdissection of bacterial cells targeted by fluorescence in situ hybridization. BioTechniques 2005;39(6) 864-868.

[65] Rabelo-Gonçalves EM, Sgardioli IC, Lopes-Cendes I, Escanhoela CA, Almeida JR, Zeitune JM. Improved detection of *Helicobacter pylori* DNA in formalin-fixed paraffin-embedded (FFPE) tissue of patients with hepatocellular carcinoma using laser capture microdissection (LCM). *Helicobacter* 2013;18(3) 244-245.

[66] Rocha GA, Queiroz DMM, Mendes EN, Lage AP, Barbosa A. Simple carbolfuchsin staining for showing C. pylori and other spiral bacteria in gastric mucosa. Journal of Clinical Pathology 1989;42(9) 1004-1005.

[67] Steinau M, Patel SS, Unger ER. Efficient DNA extraction for HPV genotyping in formalin-fixed, paraffin-embedded tissues. Jounal of Molecular Diagnostic 2011;13(4) 377-381.

[68] Goelz SE, Hamilton SR, Vogelstein B. Purification of DNA from formaldeyde fixed and paraffin-embedded tissues. Biochemical and Biophysical Research Communications 1985;130(1) 118-126.

[69] Hanahan D, Weinberg RA. The hallmarks of cancer. Cell 2000;100(1) 57-70.

[70] Cheng L, Zhang S, Wang M, Davidson DD, Morton MJ, Huang J, Zheng S, Jones TD, Beck SD, Foster RS. Molecular genetic evidence supporting the neoplastic nature of stromal cells in 'fibrosis' after chemotherapy for testicular germ cell tumours. Journal of Pathology 2007;213(1) 65-71.

[71] Hanahan D, Weinberg R.A. Hallmarks of cancer: the next generation. Cell 2011; 144(5) 646-674.

Section 6

Eradication Therapy of H. pylori Infection: New Strategies

Chapter 9

Helicobacter pylori Infection — Challenges of Antimicrobial Chemotherapy and Emergence of Alternative Treatments

Amidou Samie, Nicoline F. Tanih and
Roland N. Ndip

Additional information is available at the end of the chapter

http://dx.doi.org/10.5772/57462

1. Introduction

Classified as a class one carcinogen, *Helicobacter pylori* is a gram-negative coccobacillus (0.5 μm wide by 2 - 4 μm long), microaerophilic, flagellated organism that has chronically infected more than 50% of the world's population [1, 2, 3, 4]. Significant evidence exist that links the bacterium to the pathogenesis and development of certain diseases such as gastric ulcers, chronic gastritis and stomach cancers, although most of the people harboring this organism are asymptomatic [5, 6]. The prevalence of infection caused by this organism increases with advancing age and is reported to be higher in developing countries and among low socio-economic populations, probably owing to conditions that favor the infection such as poor hygiene, crowded living conditions, and inadequate or no sanitation. The prevalence of this infection in human varies with geographical location and socio-demographic characteristics of the population; however does not parallel the incidence of morbidity caused by the infection [7, 8]. Studies have highlighted inconsistencies in the prevalence rates for *Helicobacter* and disease. In industrialized countries there is generally a low prevalence of *H. pylori* infection and yet a relatively high prevalence of gastric cancer. On the other hand, some countries with high *Helicobacter* prevalence rates have low gastric cancer prevalence [9].

Over the years, different treatment regimens have been proposed for eradication of *H. pylori*. Eradication of the organism has proven to be the first therapeutic approach and constitutes a reliable long-term prophylaxis of peptic ulcer relapse, accelerating ulcer healing and reducing the rate of ulcer complications [10]. Successful regimens generally require two or more antibiotics coupled with a proton pump inhibitor [11]. A proton pump inhibitor (PPI) or bismuth compounds and two antibiotics most commonly clarithromycin and metronidazole and/or amoxicillin [12]. However, problems related to poor patient compliance, undesirable side effect and resistance are presenting with numerous challenges as far as treatment failure is concern. Antibiotic resistance is a growing global concern both in the developing and in developed countries. Resistance to this organism has been delineated worldwide [13]. Many *H. pylori* strains have been reported to show resistance to the limited range of antibiotics used in its treatment *in vitro.* Of particular interest, resistance to metronidazole and clarithromycin has increased recently with more than 90% resistance reported against metronidazole and up to 36% against clarithromycin depending on regions [14, 15]. Emerging resistance of the bacterium to tetracycline, fluoroquinolones, and rifampicins, which are alternative antibiotics with known anti-*H. pylori* activity, have also been reported [14].

The emerging resistance to these antibiotics limits their use in the treatment of these infections [6, 16, 17]. Resistance to the antibiotics commonly used for treatment has been associated with mutations in specific genes which have been shown to be associated with these antibiotics. Clarithromycin resistance for example has been associated with point mutations in the peptidyl transferase-encoding region of 23S *rRNA* which affects the binding of macrolides to the bacterial ribosome, while *rdxA* and *frxA* are genes whose mutation has been associated with metronidazole resistance. Other genes such as the P-glycoprotein (P-gp) as well as mutations of *GyrA, GyrB,* and *16SrRNA* in *H. pylori* have also been associated with resistance fluoroquinolone and tetracycline respectively [18, 19].

With the problem of resistance to currently recommended antibiotics; there is the need to seek alternative compounds from other sources with proven antimicrobial activity to overcome the problem. This has encourage the search of active agents from natural products, with the ultimate aim of discovering potentially useful active ingredients that can serve as template for the synthesis of new antimicrobial drugs [20]. These include medicinal plants, honey and probiotics which have been variously described to be associated with increase success rates in the eradication of *H. pylori* both *in vitro* and *in vivo* [21, 22, 23, 24]. Several plants have been investigated for their anti-*H. pylori* activity. Some of these plants with proven activity include *Combretum molle, Calophyllum brasiliense, Sclerocarya birrea, Garcinia kola, Alepidea amatymbica, Bridelia. Micrantha, Peltophorum africanum, Cyrtocarpa procera Kunth* and some *Strychnos species* [25, 26, 27]. The antimicrobial activity of honey is now well documented [28, 29]. Manyi-Loh and co-workers investigated the anti-*H. pylori* activity of three South African honeys; Pure honey, citrus blossom and gold crest and found that all honey varieties demonstrated varying levels of anti-*H. pylori* activity [24]. Evidence exists that probiotics may inhibit growth of *H. pylori,* stimulate an immunological response and reduce inflammatory effect of infection by bacteria increasing the rate of *H. pylori* eradication [21]. Some probiotics that have been tested either singly or in combination include *Lactobacillus acidophilus, Lactobacillus rhamnosus, Lactobacillus bulgaricus, Lactobacillus casei, Streptococcus thermophilus, Bifidobacterium infantis* and *Bifidobacterium breve* [30]. In this communication, we provide information on the prevalence, epidemiology and antimicrobial chemotherapy and challenges in treatment of *H. pylori* in an effort to continuously highlight the clinical and epidemiological significance.

http://dx.doi.org/10.5772/57462

2. *Helicobacter pylori* infections, disease and prevalence

Helicobacter pylori (H. pylori) inhabit various areas of the human stomach [17]. The ability of this organism to convert the stomach acidic environment, a bactericidal barrier with protection against many infections, makes the environment suitable for its survival [4, 31]. Infection starts in the gastric antrum and spreads to the corpus, after extensive mucosal damage. Upon invasion, mucosa damage is caused that is eventually worsened by the acid produced in the stomach and this may lead to complications (ulcers and cancers) [16, 14]. Half of the world's population is infected by this gastric organism [32]. Since its discovery in 1983 by Marshall and Warren, infection with *H. pylori* has been shown to be strongly associated with chronic gastritis, peptic ulcer and gastric cancer using technologies available at the time and others (fibre endoscopy, silver staining of histological sections and culture techniques for microaerophilic bacteria). These authors proved beyond reasonable doubts that made an indisputable link between the bacteria and the diseases mentioned [3, 33].

Confirmed is the fact that this organism causes of 90% of all duodenal ulcers, 75% of all gastric ulcers and two forms of stomach cancer; adenocarcinoma and mucosa-associated lymphoid tissue (MALT) lymphoma [34]. The evidence of its association with gastric cancer, led to its classification as a class 1 carcinogen by the International Agency for Research on Cancer and the World Health Organization [35]. *H. pylori* is the first bacterium, and the second infectious organism after hepatitis B virus to be classified a carcinogen. A majority of *H. pylori*-infected individuals of (80–90%) have clinically asymptomatic gastritis, 10–15% develop peptic ulcer, and 1–2% gastric malignancies [36, 37]. Until the discovery of Marshall and Warren, diet, stress and life-style factors were considered major causes of gastritis and peptic ulcer, and the stomach, a sterile environment [38, 39].

Clinical outcome of long-term infection is variable and is considered to relate to bacterial virulence factors along with host genotype, physiology and environmental factors [40, 41, 42, 43]. The cytotoxin-associated gene, *cagA*, a marker for the cag pathogenicity island (PAI), is present in many but not all *H. pylori* strains. Its presence is associated with more severe clinical outcomes [44, 45]. *H. pylori* infection confers around a two-fold increase in the risk of developing gastric cancer particularly with strains expressing the cytotoxin-associated gene A antigen (*cagA*) [46]. The *vacA* gene is far from the cag PAI. At least some forms of *vacA* protein generate vacuoles in epithelial cells, disrupt tight junctions between epithelial tissues, interfere with antigen processing, etc. [47]. The *vacA* gene is present in all *H. pylori* strains and contains two importantly variable regions, s and m [40].

Geographic differences in predominant *H. pylori* genotypes, based either on virulence associated genes such as *vacA* and *cagA* or "housekeeping genes" have been delineated [40, 48]. Several other *H. pylori* genes that are related to the risk of disease have been identified some of which include, *iceA* and several other housekeeping genes" such as *ureA, ureC, ureAB, flaA, flaB, atpA, efp, mutY, ppa, trpC, ureI, yphC* etc, which may not be directly linked to disease [49, 50]. The cytotoxin-associated gene, *cagA*, a marker for the cag pathogenicity island (PAI), is present in many but not all *H. pylori* strains. Its presence is associated with more severe clinical outcomes [44, 45].

H. pylori is the principal species of the genus *Helicobacter* and a common human pathogen that is responsible for a variety of gastro–duodenal pathologies with high prevalence reported both in the developed and developing world since its discovery in 1983 by Marshall and Warren [51, 52]. Different studies worldwide have demonstrated the presence of this organism in their population. Substantial morbidity and mortality have been reported to be associated with *H. pylori* infection [15, 17, 42]. Fallen prevalence values has been observed in most developed countries; with rates from 25–50% in developed countries to 70–90% in the second and third world countries, this however varies [2, 7, 16, 53]. With improvements in treatments modalities, gastrointestinal pathology related to *H. pylori* is still ever present and remains a major burden on Western health systems. Populations like African American, Hispanic, Asian and Native American have experienced increased prevalence and infection rates are similar in males and females [54].

Rate of acquisition, rate of loss of infection and the length of persistence period all seem to determine the prevalence of this highly inflicting pathogen [7]. The prevalence of *H. pylori* infection has also been reported to vary widely by geographic area, age, socioeconomic status and even between ethnic groups of the same region [8, 15]. All these factors including environmental factors all play a role in the acquisition and transmission of *H. pylori* and further influence the wide variation in prevalence observed in the different population [55]. For example, variation exist the prevalence between more affluent urban populations and rural population. A lack of proper sensitization, drinking water and basic hygiene as well as poor diet and overcrowding all play a role in determining the overall prevalence of infection [2]. Although there is geographical and socio–demographic variation in the prevalence of human infection, prevalence does not parallel the incidence of morbidity caused by the infection [2, 16, 56]. Astoundingly high prevalence of *H. pylori* infection is observed in developing countries which does not commensurate the low prevalence of gastric cancer compared to the developed nations with a relatively low prevalence and yet a high prevalence of gastric cancer. For example, in Africa, the prevalence of infection is very high but the incidence of gastric carcinoma and other *H. pylori*-associated morbidities is relatively low. An anomality termed the African enigma' [6, 42]. Apparently, coinfection with other organisms is known to modulate the *H. pylori* immune reaction and has been proposed to explain the "African enigma" [57]. The organism is ubiquitous with childhood acquisition seemingly being the role and may last for years or decades however, it is difficult to ascertain when infection occurs clinically hence seroprevalence data are the source of information of *H. pylori* rates both in geographically and demographically diverse populations [2, 52, 58, 59, 60]. Retrospective sero-epidemiological studies have shown a cohort effect consistent with the hypothesis that infection is mainly acquired in early childhood [59, 61]. Seroprevalence values of (61%–100%) have been described from various studies conducted in Africa and these values vary among countries and between different racial groups present within each country [2, 42, 53]. Sero-prevalence studies in the western world have depicted rates not as high as those elaborated in Africa. Most individuals harbour specific antibodies for most of their lives especially in Africa [42].

In a rural village of Linqu Country, Shandong Province, China, a study of 98 children found that nearly 70 percent of those aged 5-6 years were infected with *H. pylori*, a rate equivalent to that reported for adults in that area, suggesting that most infection takes place early in childhood [61]. Generally, 50% of all children are infected by the age of 10 years, with prevalence rising to 80% in adults [7]. In their study of Kenyan school children, Nabwera and co-workers observed high prevalence among their subjects who were only aged 3–5 years, indicating that most children in the study area were infected before they reached their third birthday [62]. The highest rates of *H. pylori* prevalence have been reported in Eastern Europe, Asia, and many developing countries and developing populations in developed countries (for example, Native Americans) [63].

3. Repository of infection and transmission

Accurately assessing the incidence or route of transmission of *H. pylori* has been difficult because of the inaccuracy and cost of detecting (non-invasively) *H. pylori* [59]. Studies with regards to environmental factors and animal reservoirs as possible sources of infection have been examined. DNA has been extracted from food, animals and water sources suggesting they could be reservoirs of this organism [37]. However, there is no definitive evidence that they are natural or primary vehicles of transmission. Various studies have remarked a variety of factors such as bacterial host, genetic and environmental factors to determine the causative links to *H. pylori* infection, but knowledge of reservoirs and transmission still remains elusive [61]. Some routes of transmission have been described this include iatrogenic, oral-oral or faecal-oral routes [64, 65].

The host range of *H. pylori* is narrow and is found almost exclusively in humans and some non-human primates [66]. Humans been the only known reservoir of infection, hence the possibility of picking the infection from siblings, parents predominates via gastro-oral route [67]. Using specific culture approaches the organism has been isolated from vomitus [68, 69]. Perhaps the most important transmission route is faecal-oral transmission. Typically, isolation of this organism from faeces is not common though its isolation from faeces is established [61]. Sexual transmission of these organisms has not been observed [70].

Oral-oral transmission is regarded as a plausible route [39]. It has been shown to be potentiated by specific eating habits, such as the premastication of food by mothers before feeding children in some African countries. In Burkina Faso, premastication of food was common amongst families with high sero-positivity *H. pylori* status for both mother and child [71]. The importance of this cannot be over emphasized considering that childhood appears to be the critical period during which *H. pylori* is acquired, especially in areas of over-crowding and socio-economic deprivation [3, 24]. Possibility of dental plaque been a route of transmission has been proposed but this has failed in other studies though [72, 73]. In a recent study in South Africa, it was deduced that the oral cavity is unlikely to contribute to the spread of this organism as oral cavities were found not to favour prolonged colonization by the organism [53, 74]. Repeated use of gastric tubes from one patient to another by enodoscopists without proper sterilization may be a possible means of transmission. *H. pylori* infection has been shown to follow socio- other studies [73]. Gastroenterologists are occupationally at risk, however has proven the least common form of transmission [75].

4. *Helicobacter pylori* treatment

The need for an adequate prophylactic or therapeutic measures for *H. pylori* is very important being a serious, chronic, progressive and transmissible infection associated with significant morbidity and mortality especially in the developing world [76]. Over the years, several treatment regimens have been proposed for the eradication of *H. pylori*. However, development of a successful treatment for *H. pylori* infection has been fraught with difficulties; owing to its location within the stomach (that is, the mucus lining the surface epithelium, deep within the mucus secreting glands of the antrum, attached to cells and even within the cells) providing a great challenge to therapeutic measures [77]. The hostile environment in the gastric mucosa poses additional challenges reasons being the antibiotic therapy need to be active at pH values below neutral [24]. In addition, the ever existing presence of emerging resistant strains presents a formidable challenge which is at the verge of frustrating every attempt to a solution provision [78]. Infection with *H. pylori* will persist for life and may result in severe gastro duodenal complications without the intervention of antimicrobial therapy (treatment) [52, 79]. Complete eradication of the organism from the gut or stomach is the ultimate goal to treatment. A negative test for the bacterium four weeks or longer after treatment defines eradication [80].

There has been evolution with regards to treatment regimen for *H. pylori* infection since the early 1990s, when monotherapy was first recommended. However, employment of single agent is unacceptable because of extremely low eradication rates. *H. pylori* infections are treated with antibiotics, H2 blockers which reduces stomach acidicity and a proton pump inhibitor (PPI) that protects the stomach lining (bismuth compounds). This triple drug regimen involving; two antibiotics, bismuth salt and a proton pump inhibitor (PPI) or H2 blockers has been used as a standard treatment [13, 77, 81]. Bismuth compounds (colloidal bismuth sub citrate and bismuth subsalicylate) act by reducing intracellular ATP levels and interfere with the activity of urease enzyme, a key enzyme of *H. pylori* [77]. They also induce the formation of an ulcer-specific coagulum, preventing acid back diffusion and inhibit protein and cell wall synthesis as well as membrane function [82, 83]. Detachment of *H. pylori* from the gastric epithelium and a reduction in capsular polysaccharide production is the enabling function of bismuth compounds [77]. Typically, two types of acid reducers exist and include a proton pump inhibitor (PPI) and H2 blockers. H2 blockers include cimetidine, ranitidine, famotidine and nizatidine and this function by blocking histamine, which stimulates acid secretion. The PPI (omeprazole, lansoprazole, rabeprazole, pantoprazole and esomeprazole) on its part suppresses acid production by halting the mechanism that pumps the acid into the stomach [84]. PPI also increases antibiotic stability and efficacy [85].

The most commonly used antibiotics include metronidazole (MET), clarithromycin (CLR), amoxicillin (AMOX) and tetracycline (TET) all of which *H. pylori* is susceptible too except in cases of drug resistance [13, 86, 87]. Clarithromycin (500 mg twice a day [b.i.d.]) and amoxicillin (1 g b.i.d.) plus PPI for 7 days (treatment 1) are the most commonly used treatment combination the world over. Other regimens employed for 7-day include clarithromycin (500 mg b.i.d.) and metronidazole (500 mg b.i.d.) (treatment 2) and a double dose of PPI plus or amoxicillin (1 g b.i.d.) and metronidazole (500 mg b.i.d.) (treatment 3) a double dose of PPI plus [88]. Efficacy of the agents range from 85% - 95%. Susceptibility of *H. pylori* to these drugs has been reported to change with time, ethnicity, ulcer status, geographical location and test method [14]. Consequently, antibiotic recommended for patients may soon differ across regions of the world because different areas have begun to show resistance to particular antibiotics. These factors therefore have to be considered in making a prescription for the eradication of the infection.

5. Challenges to *Helibacter pylori* treatment regimens

The recommended regimens for *H. pylori* treatment and eradication pose a number of difficulties to patients such as poor compliance; coping with unpleasant adverse effects do little to encourage patient cooperation [15, 78]. Apart from patient non-compliance, antibiotic resistance is the major cause of treatment failure leaving clinicians with a limited list of drugs to choose from [14, 15, 89]. This can seriously affect attempts to eradicate the bacterium. Bacterial resistance to antimicrobials could be either primary (that is, present before therapy) or secondary (that is, develop as the result of failed therapy [77]. In different countries primary resistance in *H. pylori* has been reported in MET (6-95%), CLR (0-17%), and TET (0-6%) [90, 91]. Fairly recently, resistance to amoxicillin has been reported in many countries across the globe especially countries in Africa like Cameroon, Nigeria and South Africa where stringent control of drugs is lacking [17]. On the other hand metronidazole-containing regimens have recently been shown to have limited effectiveness owing to the alarming increase in the prevalence of resistance to this drug. Resistance to this antibiotic varies from 10% to 90% in different countries [92]. For example, Studies by Boyanova and colleagues reported a resistance rate of 28.6% for metronidazole against clinical isolates of *H. pylori* circulating in Sofia, Bulgaria [17, 90]. In our study in South Africa we reported a rate of 95.5% resistant. In Cameroon, studies have documented a very high resistance to metronidazole. Studies in Australia showed a resistance level of 36% of *H. pylori* isolates against metronidazole [93]. High resistance to metronidazole is attributed to the frequent and uncontrolled use of nitroimidazole derivatives for the treatment of protozoan infections and gynecological problems [17]. Clarithromycin resistance is referred to as the corner stone for treatment failure and is increasing worldwide [94]. A prevalence rate of 12.9% was recorded for Clarithromycin resistance in the U.S and rates as high as 24% were some European countries [91]. Resistance to clarithromycin frequently develops after treatment failure and more recently due to its increasing use in the treatment of upper respiratory tract infection [92]. Increasing prevalence of resistance to antimicrobial jeopardizes the success of therapeutic regimens aimed at the eradication of the infection making it sensitivity testing imperative prior to appropriate antibiotic selection [95].

Also, current antimicrobial susceptibility profiles of the isolates within the region should be known as this will act as a guide to clinician [96].

Resistance mechanisms to the commonly used antibiotics have been elaborated. Selection pressure may progressively increase resistance with the use of these antibiotics [88]. Plasmid associated resistance is rare. Drug efflux proteins can contribute to natural insensitivity to antibiotics and to emerging antibiotic resistance as is the case of many bacteria [97].

5.1. Metronidazole resistance mechanisms

Resistance to metronidazole (Mtz) has shown to limit the effectiveness of Mtz containing regimens [98, 99]. Mtz, a synthetic nitroimidazole is a prodrug and becomes active when reduced in the cytosol of the microorganism to a toxic metabolite. Unstable Mtz radicals react rapidly with proteins, RNA and DNA, eventually resulting in cell death [88, 99, 100]. Most Mtz sensitivity in *H. pylori* accounted for by NADPH nitroreductase a non-oxygen sensitive encoded by the *rdxA* gene reduces Mtz by a two-electron transfer step into a toxic metabolite that cannot be retransformed to its parent by molecular oxygen [99]. Resistance to Mtz is associated with mutation somewhere in the *rdxA* coding sequence [101]. Mutation of a second reductase NAD (P) H flavin oxidoreductase encoded by *frxA* could also confer low-level Mtz sensitivity in some strains [102]. Such resistance has been linked mostly to genetic mutations in the *rdxA* and *frxA* genes of the bacterium [100]. Based on gene sequencing and other reports concluded that most Mtz resistance in *H. pylori* depend on *rdxA* inactivation, of which mutations in *frxA* can enhance resistance, and that genes conferring Mtz resistance without *rdxA* inactivation are rare or nonexistent in *H. pylori* populations [100].

5.2. Resistance mechanisms to clarithromycin

Clarithromycin is part of the combination therapy used as the first-line therapy against *H. pylori*. Resistance to clarithromycin therefore is important ingredient for treatment failure. Clarithromycin acts by binding to the peptidyl transferase region of *23SrRNA* and inhibits bacterial protein synthesis just like other macrolides Clarithromycin resistance has been linked to mutation in the *23S rRNA* gene [103]. Several reports have demonstrated that more than 90% of macrolide resistance in *H. pylori* is mediated by either of two transition mutations Adenine to Guanine (A→G) at adjacent positions 2142 and 2143 in the bacterium's 23SrRNA gene [103]. A transversion mutation (A→C) at position 2143 has been reported to be the cause of resistance in 7% of the resistant isolates. Other mutation observed in clarithromycin resistant *H. pylori* isolates include A2515G and T2717C, A2116G, G2141A, A2144T, T2182C, G2224A, C2245T

5.3. Amoxicillin resistance mechanisms

H. pylori resistance to amoxicillin is not common. Deloney and schiller, showed that amoxicillin resistance in *H. pylori* could develop because of amino acid substitutions in the penicillin binding proteins (pbp) leading to structural alterations in the protein or interference with peptidoglycan synthesis [104]. Resistance to amoxicillin and related drugs is usually as a result of decreased permeability to the drug; increased efflux of the drug from the bacterial cell, modification of the PBPs that diminish the affinity of the drug for the protein, and the presence of β-lactamases that inactivate the antibiotic by hydrolyzing its ring structure [105]. Amoxicillin-resistant *H. pylori* strains harbour mutations on the pbp-1a gene with amino acid substitution Ser-414→Arg appears to be involved, leading to a blockage of penicillin transport. Resistance to amoxicillin may also result from the production of β -lactamases by the bacterium [106]. Colonization of the stomach with β -lactam- resistant bacteria of other species may lead to the transfer of amoxicillin resistance to *H. pylori* [17]. Mutations in *hopB* and *hopC* genes of the outer membrane have also been associated with resistance in amoxicillin [107].

5.4. Tetracycline resistance mechanism

Tetracyclines are often used as a second line therapy when *H. pylori* infections are not cured by the first line drug regimen. Tetracycline is a protein synthesis inhibitor. This is achieved by disrupting codon-anticodon interaction on the ribosome. It binds to the 30S ribosomal subunit, preventing attachment of aminoacyl-tRNA to the acceptor site [108]. Thus bacterial peptide synthesis is stopped leading to cell death. Resistance to tetracycline has been linked to mutation in 16SrRNA-encoding genes that affect the binding site of tetracycline. The change in a nucleotide triplet (AGA-926 to 928→TTC), cognate of the positions 965 to 967 in *Escherichia coli*, has been associated with resistance to these compounds maybe because of the absence of the h1 loop; the binding site of tetracyclines. Strains resistant to tetracycline and no mutation in position 926 to 928 have also been described [14, 86, 109].

5.5. Resistant Mechanism to Fluoroquinolone

Fluoroquinolones have proven their worth in the treatment of most infections. In the management of *H. pylori* infection, they are used as salvage therapy when all other therapies cannot help (Chisholm and Owen, 2009). Their mode of action is based on inhibition of A and B subunits of the gene encoding DNA gyrase (*gyrA* or *gyrB)* in the bacterial cell [110], automatically interfering with DNA replication. Resistance to quinolones is associated mutations in *gyrA* at positions 87 and 91 [105, 111].

5.6. Resistance associated to plasmid and Efflux mechanisms

Approximately half of *H. pylori* strains possess a plasmid with size ranging 1.8-63 kbp though the standard strain NCTC 11637 is plasmid free [112]. Plasmid size and number may vary appreciably amongst strains with a gross majority of strains possessing just one plasmid. *H. pylori* plasmids have also been associated with drug resistance though in their study indicated resistance was unlikely to be attributed to plasmid coded determinants [52, 113]. Drug efflux mechanism could be responsible for the observed resistance in *H. pylori* as well. Organisms get protected from possible toxic effects of metabolite accumulation or external compounds using the efflux mechanism. Compound efflux which is mediated through specific pumps could result in decreased susceptibility for a variety of antibiotic [114, 115]. Some families of multidrug efflux transporters have been described these include small multidrug resistance

(SMR) proteins, multidrug and toxic compound extrusion (MATE) proteins, the major facilitator superfamily (MFS), the ATP-binding cassette (ABC) superfamilies, and the resistance-nodulation-cell division (RND) family (helfF, hefC, and hefI) [116]. These active multidrug efflux mechanism and therefore compound efflux needs to be taken into account when determining resistance mechanisms in this organism. The therapy used for salvage of *H. pylori* has as one of its medications rifampicin and rifabutin [105]. Due to their irreversible blockage of DNA-dependent RNA polymerase; they are bactericidal. The β-subunit of the polymerase encoded by *rpoB* gene is inhibited by these medications and annuls protein synthesis of the bacteria [35, 117]. Resistance of *H. pylori* to these medications has been attributed to point mutations in the *rpoB* gene at positions 530, 540 and 545 [118].

6. Substitutes to circumvent challenges to treatment regimens

Due to the shortcoming presented by antibiotics with regards to treatment of *H. pylori*; Research towards development of new antimicrobial agents/ in a bid to scavenge for possible alternatives to overcome the problem of antibiotic resistance in this bacterial pathogen has been encouraged, such as research with plant extract and other natural products that possess antimicrobial potential like honey and probiotics with or without antibiotic both *in-vitro* and *in-vivo* to test for the antimicrobial activity [22, 24, 29, 119, 120].

6.1. Plants as a potential source of *H. pylori* treatment

Plant and plant products have repeated shown awesome hope in the treatment of recalcitrant infection. Medicinal plants usage all over the world preface the introduction of antibiotics and other modern drugs. It is estimated that plant materials are present in or have provided the models for about 50% of Western drugs [121]. Herbal medicines remain a normal part of life for most people worldwide especially amongst Africans and Asians and remains a component of healthcare in most countries worldwide especially Africa [121, 122]. WHO (World Health Organization) estimates 3.5 million people in developing countries rely on plant-based medicine for their primary healthcare and their usage has offered great benefit [122, 123, 124]. Research on herbal product has great significance for plants components could provide lead products for the development of new drugs hence leading to improvement of therapeutic results [124].

The demand to use natural products such as plants based products for the management of intractable infections has increased over the years [22]. Great attention has been directed to the screening of medicinal plants all over the world as a means to identify cheap sources of new drugs against *H. pylori,* a human gastric pathogen with high morbidity rate [2]. Scientific literature is rich on plant based studies on anti-*H. pylori* activity. A number of plants belonging to various families as well as compounds have been screened in the search for their anti-*H. pylori* potential worldwide. For example, Garlic (*Allium sativum L*) particularly allium vegetables have been shown exhibit a broad range of antibiotic spectrum against both Gram–positive and Gram negative bacteria including susceptibility to *H. pylori* antibiotic resistant strains [125]. Zeyrek and Oguz demonstrated *in vitro* anti-*H. pylori* activity of capsaicin at a concentration of 50μg/ml against metronidazole resistant and metronidazole-susceptible clinical isolates [126]. This plant also known as hot pepper is consumed as a flavoring spice and is reputed for its pharmacological, physiological and antimicrobial effects [127]. There is lower ulcer prevalence in people consuming higher amount of pepper compared to controls [128]. Studies by Zhang and colleagues in the Linqu County of Shandong Province, China, suggested that dietary consumption of cranberry (*Vaccitnium macrocarpon)* juice may reduce *H. pylori* infections in adults, which remains an important public health issue worldwide [129]. More plants which have been tested and proven to exhibit anti- *H. pylori* activity from their different continents in the world are listed (Table 1).

Analysis of tested plant extract revealed the presence of varying numbers of components depending on different solvent combination used for extraction. For example, 52 compounds were identified from acetone extract of *S. birrea* (which has been reported with anti- *H. pylori* activity) with n-octacosane being the most abundant (41.68%). Other compounds such as pyrrolidine, terpinen-4-ol, n-eicosane, cyclopentane, n-triacontane, aromadendrene and α-gujunene were delineated in *S. birrea*. Terpinen-4-ol and pyrrolidine however demonstrated strong antimicrobial activity against *H. pylori* at all concentrations tested. The identified compounds Terpinen-4-ol could be considered for further evaluation as therapeutic or prophylactic agents in the treatment of *H. pylori*-related infections [130]. Other compounds including quinones, flavones, flavonoid, flavonols, tannins, coumarins, traces of alkaloid, gallotannins, steroids (including β-sitosterol), phenolics and polyphenols, Terpenoids and essential oils Alkaloids, lectins and polypeptides have been isolated from most plants and found to exhibit profound antimicrobial activities in-vitro against an array of organisms although most of these compounds have not been tested against *H. pylori* [131].

The stem bark of the South American trumpet tree (*Tecoma ipe* Mart) has been reported as an important source of active quinone compound against *H. pylori* furanonaphthoquinone was isolated from this plant and has proven activity against *H. pylori* with (MIC 0.1μg/mL). idebenone, duroquinone, menadione, juglone and coenzyme Q1 are other quinines that have been reported with anti- *H. pylori* at low concentration of 0.8 to 3.2 μg /mL [132]. Anti-*H. pylori* activity of a number of flavonoids has been reported. In Turkey for example, *Cistus laurifolius* flower buds which is used traditionally in folk medicine to treat gastric ailments have been shown to possess significant anti-*H. pylori* activity with the flavonoid; quercetin 3-methyl ether (isorhamnetin) as the active component [133]. Inhibition of urease is recorded as the mechanism of action of some flavonoids as hesperidin [134]. Antimicrobial activity of coumarins isolated from the roots of *Ferulago campestris* against *H. pylori* isolates in Italy [135]. Kawase and others, found that a number of hydroxycoumarins;7- hydroxy-4-methylcoumarin, 6, 7-dihydroxy-4-methylcoumarin, 6-hydroxy-7-methoxy-4-methylcoumarin and 5, 7- dihydroxycyclopentanocoumarin showed comparable anti-*H. pylori* activity with metronidazole [136]. Generally, data about specific antibiotic properties of coumarins against *H. pylori* are scarce.

Continent and Species		Parts Used	Reference
Africa	Country		
Combretum molle (*Combretaceae*)	South Africa	Stem bark	[172]
*Bridelia micrantha (*Hochst, Baill., *Euphorbiaceae*).	South Africa	Stem bark	[173]
Lippia javanica	South Africa	Leaves	[174]
Hydonora africana	South Africa	check	[175]
Sclerocarya birrea (Anacardiaceae)	South Africa	Stem bark	[130]
Garcinia kola Heckel (Guttiferae)	South Africa	Seeds	[176]
Peltophorum africanum (Sond, Fabaceae)	South Africa	Stem bark	[23]
Ageratum conyzoides (Linn)	Cameroon	Whole plant	[176]
Lycopodium cernuum (Linn) Pic. Serm	Cameroon	check	[17]
Enantia chlorantha Oliver (Annonaceae)	Cameroon	Stem bark	[177] [178]
Eucalyptus camaldulensis Dehnh.	Nigeria	Leaves	[179]
Eucalyptus torelliana F. Muell. (Myrtaceae),	Nigeria	Stem bark	[179]
Europe			
South America/ North America			
*Byrsonima intermedia A. Juss. (Malpighiaceae***)**	Brazil	Leaves	[180]
Croton cajucara Benth. (Euphorbiaceae)	Brazil	Stem bark	[181]
Piper carpunya *Ruiz & Pav. (syn Piper lenticellosum C.D.C.) (Piperaceae)*	Ecuador	Leaves	[182]
Calophyllum brasiliense (Camb.)	Brazil	Stem bark	[25]
Artemisia douglasiana Besser (Asteraceae)	Argentina	Leaves	[183]
Alchornea triplinervia	Brazil	Leaves	[184]
Hancornia speciosa Gomez (Apocynaceae).	Brazil	Bark	[185]
Olea europaea L. (Oleaceae)	Mexico	Leaves/stem	[186]
Tagetes lucida Cav. (Asteraceae)	Mexico	Leaf/stem	[186]
Amphipterygium adstringens (Schltdl.) Standl. (Anacardiaceae)	Mexico	Bark	[186]
Priva grandiflora (Ortega) Moldenke (Verbenaceae)	Mexico	Aerial parts	[186]
Eupatorium petiolare Moc. ex DC. (Asteraceae)	Mexico	Aerial parts	[186]
Monarda austromontana Epling (Lamiaceae)	Mexico	Aerial parts	[186]
Gnaphalium canescens DC. (Asteraceae)	Mexico	Aerial parts	[186]
Larrea tridentata (Sessé & Moc. ex DC.) Coville (Zygophyllaceae)	Mexico	Aerial parts	[186]

Continent and Species		Parts Used	Reference
Tithonia diversifolia (Hemsl.) A.G. Asteraceae)	Mexico	Aerial parts	[186]
Grindelia inuloides Willd. (Asteraceae)	Mexico	Aerial parts	[186]
Buddleja perfoliata Kunth (Loganiaceae)	Mexico	Aerial parts	[186]
Heterotheca inuloides Cass. (Asteraceae)	Mexico	Aerial parts	[186]
Mirabilis jalapa L. (Nyctaginaceae)	Mexico	Aerial parts	[186]
Cyrtocarpa procera Kunth (Anacardiaceae)	Mexico	Bark	[186]
Teloxys graveolens (Willd.)W.A.Weber (Chenopodiaceae)	Mexico	Aerial parts	[186]
Annona cherimola Mill. (Annonaceae)	Mexico	Leaf/stem	[186]
Menthaxpiperita L. (Lamiaceae)	Mexico	Leaf/stem	[186]
Cuphea aequipetala Cav. (Lythraceae)	Mexico	Aerial parts	[186]
Ludwigia repens J. R. Forst. (Onagraceae)	Mexico	Aerial parts	[186]
Artemisia ludoviciana Nutt. subsp. *mexicana* (Willd. Ex Spreng.) Fernald (Asteraceae)	Mexico	Leaf/stem	[186]
Qualea parviflora Mart.	Brazil	bark	[187]
Calophyllum brasiliense	Brazil	stem bark	[25]
North America			
Cyrtocarpa procera Kunth (Anacardiaceae)	Mexico	Bark	[27]
Amphipterygium adstringens (Schltdl.) Standl. (Anacardiaceae)	Mexico	Bark	[186]
Casimiroa tetrameria		Leaves	[188]
ASIA			
Wasabia japonica	Japan	Leaves	[189]
Impatiens balsamina L	Asia	Root/stem/leaf, seed, and pod	[190]
Rhizopus oligosporus	Asia	fenugreek extracts	[191]
Plumbago zeylanica L	China	Leaves	[192]
Glycyrrhiza aspera	Iran	n/a	[193]
Juglans regia	Iran	n/a	[193]
Ligustrum vulgare	Iran	n/a	[193]
Thymus kotschyanus	Iran	n/a	[193]
Trachyspermum copticum	Iran	n/a	[193]
Xanthium brasilicum	Iran	n/a	[193]

Continent and Species		Parts Used	Reference
Bacopa monniera			[194]
Carthamus tinctorous L.(Asteraceae)	Khorasan	Flowers	[195]
Satureja hortensis L.(Lamiaceae)	Mashhad-Khorasan	Leaves	[195]
Artemisia dracunculus L. (Asteraceae)	Mashhad-Khorasan	Leaves	[195]
Citrus sinensis L (Rutaceae)	North of Iran	Peel of fruit	[195]
Punica granatum L. (Punicaceae)	Saveh- Markazi	Peel of fruit	[195]
Apium petroselinum L (Apiaceae)	Neishabur-Khorasan	Seeds	[195]
Carum bulbocastanum	Iran	Fruit	[196]
Carum carvi	Iran	Fruit	[196]
Mentha longifolia	Iran	Aerial	[196]
Saliva limbata	Iran	Aerial	[196]
Saliva sclarea	Iran	Aerial	[196]
Ziziphora clinopodioides	Iran	Aerial	[196]
Glycyrrhiza glabra	Iran	Root	[196]
Thymus caramanicus	Iran	Aerial	[196]
Xanthium brasilicum	Iran	Aerial	[196]
Trachyspermum copticum	Iran	Fruits	[196]
Acacia nilotica (L.)) (Fabaceae)	Pakistan	Leaves, flowers	[197]
Calotropis procera (Aiton)(Apocynaceae)	Pakistan	Leaves, flowers	[197]
Adhatoda vasica Nees (Zygophyllaceae)	Pakistan	Whole plant	[197]
Fagoniaar abica L(Acanthaceae	Pakistan	Whole plant	[197]
Casuarina equisetifolia L. (Casuarinaceae)	Pakistan	fruits	[197]
AUSTRALIA			
Pistacia (Mastic, Kurdica, Mutica and Cabolica)	Sydney	gums	[198]
Others			
Allium sativum L	USA	Leaves	[125]
Capsaicin		Pepper fruits	[126]
Vaccitnium macrocarpon, C		Cranberry	[129]
Prunus mume	Japan	Juice	[199]

Table 1. Anti-*H. pylori* medicinal plants occurring in more than one country worldwide

6.2. Honey as a control measure of *H. Pylori* infections

Honey has been used in folk-medicine in many countries since antiquity [137]. It is mentioned for healing purposes in the Bible, the Koran, and the Torah. Research related to honey has revealed the promising effects of honey as an alternative source of *H. pylori* treatment [138]. Its beneficial qualities have been endorsed to its antimicrobial, antioxidant, anti-inflammatory properties added to its phytocomponents [139]. Documentations now exist with proven ability of Honey to inhibit microbial growth, and honey has been successfully used on infections that do not respond to standard antiseptic and antibiotic therapy [28, 137]. In addition, In New Zealand and Saudi Arabia it was observed that concentrations of honey at approximating 20% v/v can inhibit the growth of *H. pylori* in vitro, grounded with the fact that Medihoney™ and manuka honeys have *in vivo* activity against ulcers, infected wounds and burns are significant findings which merits further and extensive investigations [138]. Honey obtained from different floral sources and different geographical region seem to vary in their antimicrobial potency due to inherent differences in their chemical composition which is greatly influenced by the prevailing climatic conditions and soil characteristics in the different geographical areas influencing the plants as well the type of honey composition produced by the foraging bees [140, 141]. Undoubtedly, several factors like floral source used to collect nectar, seasonal and environmental factors, as well as processing and storage conditions might influence the chemical composition of honey [142].

Honey is becoming acceptable as a reputable and effective therapeutic agent by practitioners of conventional medicine and by the general public [139] Honey can be used as an antiseptic for wounds, burns and ulcers, improving the assimilation of calcium and magnesium and decreasing acidity [29, 143]. Stimulation of inflammatory- cytokine production by monocytes and hydrogen peroxide produced as a result of injury or infection is likely the mechanism by which wounds are healed with the use of honey [137, 144]. Motivated by these findings, scientist sought out to investigate the activities of honeys further. Previously, the activity of honey has been reported to differ with types [145]. The presence of hydrogen peroxide, osmotic effect of honey, its naturally low pH, phenolic acids, lysosomes and flavanoids in honey are all thought to help inhibit bacterial growth when honey is applied to a wound. Its low content of water facilitates wound healing by hygroscopic absorption of water molecules on wound surfaces and by soothing of the wound [137]. Honey does not only contain sugars but also an abundance of minerals, vitamins, enzymes and amino acids [6, 137].

Anti- *H. pylori* activities of honey have been investigated with various honey types in different parts of the world. Honey with proven anti- *H. pylori* activity is listed on (Table 2). Different variety of honeys (crude) and solvent extracted honey have been shown to possess potential compounds with therapeutic activity which could be exploited further as lead molecules in the treatment of *H. pylori* infections [24]. Chemical analysis of the chloroform extract of the pure honey led to the identification of 24 volatile compounds belonging to known chemical families present in honey. Astoundingly, thiophene and N-methyl-D3-aziridine were identified as novel compounds [146].

Honey type	Country	References
Goldcrest honey	South Africa	[146]
Pure honey	South Africa	[146]
Citrus blossom	South Africa	[146]
Goldcrest	South Africa	[146]
Black forest	Germany	[137]
Langnese	Germany	[137]
Langnese Natural Bee Honey	Germany	[137]
Blossom Bee Honey	Switzerland	[137]
Al-Shifa Natural Honey	Iran	[137]
Al-Nada Clove Honey	Oman	[137]
Al-Nada Chestnut Honey	Oman	[137]
Manuka honey	Zealand,	[137]
Capillano	Australia	[137]

Table 2. Honey with Anti-*H. pylori* activity worldwide.

6.3. Use of probiotics in the treatment and management of *H. pylori* infections

According to an expert consultation conducted by the Food and Agriculture Organization and the World Health Organization, probiotics are "live microorganisms which when administered in adequate amounts confer a health benefit to the host." The regular intake of probiotic microorganisms has been demonstrated to prevent several disorders including diarrhea and inflammatory bowel disease [147]. Other advantages of the use of probiotics include the inhibition of enteric pathogens such as *Salmonella, Shigella* and *Citrobacter*, the decreasing of the luminal pH through the production of lactic acid or through competition with gut pathogens for host surface receptors [148]. The usefulness of probiotics on the eradication of *H. pylori* remains controversial. It has been suggested that the use of probiotic might have a positive impact on *Helicobacter* eradication. However, some studies have demonstrated that there was no change while some have shown an increase in the eradication rate of the bacteria from about 60% to 83% [21, 149]. *In vivo* models demonstrated that pre-treatment with a probiotic can prevent *H. pylori* infection and/or that administration of probiotics markedly reduced an existing infection [150]. Probiotics are often administered as supplemental treatment for the eradication of *H. pylori*. In this regard, a meta-analysis of 14randomized clinical trials was conducted by [151]. This study evaluated the role of supplemental probiotics in *H. pylori* eradication therapy and showed that the cure rates for standard antibiotic treatment when used alone and eradication co-therapy with probiotics, were 74.8% and 83.6%, respectively. The analysis further showed that the combined treatment, had not only increased the eradication rate, but had also decreased the occurrence of adverse effects due to antibiotics, like diarrhea. Several probiotics have been shown to have a beneficial effect on *H. pylori* infection [150, 151]. However, the exact mechanisms of action have not been clearly elucidated yet [152].

It is believed that probiotics may play an important role in the eradication and possibly the prevention of *H. pylori* infection and could serve as adjunctive treatment. Several probiotics have been shown to have beneficial effects on the treatment and eradication of *H. pylori* the majority of these probiotics known as the lactic acid-producing bacteria. Among these *Bifidobacterium* is one of the favorite genera, particularly in studies focused on the prevention of gastrointestinal infection and is often used in fermented dairy products or food supplements [153]. Some studies have been done in vitro (in test tubes or petri dishes) showing bifidobacterial activity against *H. pylori*. Examples include *Bifidobacterium lactis* which has been demonstrated to have an enhancing activity on the phagocytic capacity of polymorpho-nuclear cells [154]. *Bifidobacterium* spp have been shown to have positive effects of *H. pylori* infections. These are generally administered in dairy products such as yogurt and milk. Clinical trial studies have shown that probiotics-containing yogurt can offer benefits to restore *Bifidobacterium* spp/*E. coli* ratio in children and suppress the *H. pylori* load with increment of serum IgA but with reduction in IL-6 in *H. pylori*-infected children [155]. The Lactobacillus group constitutes an important source of probiotics that have been demonstrated to have a positive effect on *H. pylori* treatment. Strains with this ability include *Lactobacillus acidophilus, L. casei, L. johnsonii, L. salivarius* some of which are used as dairy starters [156]. Most studies have shown that lactobacilli or their cell-free cultures can inhibit or even kill *H. pylori* by preventing its adhesion to mammalian epithelial cells and preventing interleukin-8 release [157].

Fungal organisms particularly some strains of yeast have been used as probiotic as well.The best studied example is S. boulardii which is a live yeast that has been used extensively as a probiotic and often marketed as a dietary supplement [158]. It is a non-pathogenic yeast that has been prescribed for prophylaxis and treatment of diarrheal diseases caused by bacteria (Reference). Several clinical trials and experimental studies strongly suggest that *Saccharomyces boulardii* has a biotherapeutic capacity for the prevention and treatment of several gastrointestinal diseases including *H. pylori* infections [159]. *S. boulardii* mediates responses resembling the protective effects of the normal healthy gut flora. In a study conducted in Turkey, *S. boulardii* improved anti-*H. pylori* antibiotherapy-associated diarrhea, epigastric discomfort, and treatment tolerability. However, *S. boulardii* had no significant effect on the rate of *H. pylori* eradication in that study [160]. Importantly, *S. boulardii* has demonstrated clinical and experimental effectiveness in gastrointestinal diseases with a predominant inflammatory component, indicating that this probiotic might interfere with cellular signaling pathways common in many inflammatory conditions [161]. In another study by Cremonini probiotic supplementation significantly lowered the incidence of diarrhea and taste disturbance during *H. pylori* eradication compared to the placebo group.

Generally, probiotics can be administered as single microbial species. However, in some cases a combination of several types of probiotic species might yield a much more satisfactory result. In a study by Dylag and colleagues, the combination of *Lactobacillus, Bifidobacterium, Saccharomyces boulardi* and the treatment with *Escherichia coli* Nissle were found to be beneficial in inducing and maintaining remission of disease activity of gut inflammation and moderately severe ulcerative colitis [162]. Preparations containing certain Lactobacillus, Bifidobacterium strains or Saccaromyces boulardii could enhance by 5-10% the rate of successful eradication of *H. pylori* and reduce the incidence and severity of the side effects [163]. Instead of considering the probiotics alone, they have been considered in some studies as a safe adjuvant when added to triple eradication therapy against the symptoms induced by the major gastric pathogen, *Helicobacter pylori.*

Several mechanisms by which probiotic bacteria inhibit *H. pylori* have been proposed and include immunological mechanisms, antimicrobial substances, competition for adhesion, and the production of mucosal barrier [164]. Proposed mechanisms underlying the beneficial interaction between probiotics and *H. pylori,* and the modulation of the colonization of the gastric mucosa by this pathogen, include the production of lactic acid with *H. pylori* inhibition because of decreasing gastric pH; the direct killing of *H. pylori* through secreted metabolites with antimicrobial properties, including bacteriocins, autolysins, and organic acids; the interference with *H. pylori* adhesion to epithelial cells, both through the secretion of antimicrobial molecules and through direct competition for adhesion; and the ability to reduce *H. pylori*-induced gastritis through the stabilization of the mucosal barrier, the secretion of mucins, and the modulation of the host immune response to the infection [149]. Infection by *H. pylori,* often induce and inflammatory response which in turn exacerbate the disease through the increase production of inflammatory cytokines such as IL8 and TNF alpha. The subsequent inflammatory processes as well as the bacterial infection generally persist for decades resulting in mucosal damage, gastritis, and finally gastric neoplasm further potentiated by the failure of macrophages to eliminate *H. pylori* [165, 166]. One of the mechanisms by which, probiotics reduce *H. pylori* infections is through the production of conjugated linoleic acids. Conjugated linoleic acids (CLA) produced by *Lactobacillus acidophilus* for example was reported to decrease the activation of nuclear factor-kappa B. In fact strains of probiotic bacteria are known to convert linoleic acid to conjugated linoleic acid which has an immunomodulatory activity [167]. A study conducted by Hwang and colleagues showed that conjugated linoleic acid decreased the expressions of IL-8mRNA/protein as well as that of TNF-a mRNA [168]. This in turn, reduces the inflammation and therefore increases the cure rate of *H. pylori* infection. Some probiotics such as *L. acidophilus* induce a Th1-polarizing response characterized by high expression of interferon beta (IFN-β) and interleukin 12 (IL-12) [169]. This anti-inflammatory effect is contrary to the inflammatory response induced by *H. pylori* and therefore might reduce the effect of the infection on the host and increase the eradication of the pathogen although *H. pylori* contain a pathogenic feature known as vac A which can block the effect of the probiotic [170]. Studies by Yang and colleagues showed that higher doses of *L. acidophilus* pre-treatment reduced *H. pylori*-induced inflammation through the inactivation of the Smad7 and NFκB pathways by reversing the effect of *H. pylori* infection which often induces Smad7, NFκB, IL-8, and TNF-a production [171].

Helicobacter pylori treatment has evolved tremendously over the past decade. The use of different antibiotics has resulted to antibiotic resistance which has led to the adaptation of new ways of controlling the organism. The use of medicinal plants has proven its worth. However, much still need to be done, while very few clinical trials have been conducted over the last

http://dx.doi.org/10.5772/57462

decade. Clinical trials for the use of medicinal plants for the control of *H. pylori* infections are still awaited. The application of probiotics remains controversial although the tendency would be that these organisms are helpful in increasing the eradication rate as well as the reduction of the side effects of the infection.

Author details

Amidou Samie[1*], Nicoline F. Tanih[1] and Roland N. Ndip[2,3]

*Address all correspondence to: samie.amidou@univen.ac.za; samieamidou@yahoo.com

1 Department of Microbiology, University of Venda, Thohoyandou, South Africa1

2 Department of Microbiology and Parasitology, University of Buea, Cameroon

3 Department of Biochemistry and Microbiology, University of Fort Hare, South Africa

References

[1] Aguemon BD, Struelens MJ, Masougbodji A & Ouendo EM. Prevalence and risk factors for *Helicobacter pylori* infection in urban and rural Beninese population. Clinical Microbiology and Infection 2005 11 611–617.

[2] Ndip RN, Malange AE, Akoachere JFT, Mackay WG, Titanji VPK and Weaver LT. *Helicobacter pylori* antigens in faeces of asymptomatic children in the Buea and Limbe health districts of Cameroon: a pilot study. Tropical Medicine and International Health 2004 9 1036-1040.

[3] Ahmed K, Farzana R, Walter M, Godfrey L & Martin H. Histopathological profile of gastritis in adult patients seen at a referral hospital in Kenya. World Journal of Gastroenterology 2007 14 4117–4121.

[4] Tanih NF, Clarke AM, Mkwetshana N, Green E, Ndip LM and Ndip RN (2008). *Helicobacter pylori* infection in Africa: Pathology and microbiological diagnosis. African Journal of Biotechnology 2008 7 4653-4662.

[5] MacKay WG, Williams CL, McMillan M, Ndip RN, ShepherdAJ & Weaver LT. Evaluation of protocol using gene capture and PCR for detection of *Helicobacter pylori* DNA in feces. Journal of Clinical Microbiology 2003 41 4589–4592.

[6] Tanih NF, Dube C, Green E, Mkwetshana N, Clarke AM, Ndip LM & Ndip RN. *Helicobacter pylori* prevalence in Africa: drug resistance and alternative approaches to treatment. Annals of Tropical Medicine and Parasitology 2009 103(3) 189-204.

[7] Segal I, Ally R & Mitchell H. *Helicobacter pylori*: an African perspective. Quarterly Journal of Medicine 2001 94 561–565.

[8] Malcolm *et al*., 2004 Malcolm CA, MacKay WG, Shepherd A & Weaver LT. *Helicobacter pylori* in children is strongly associated with poverty. Scottish Medical Journal 2004 49(4)136-8.

[9] Lunet N and Barros H (2003). *Helicobacter pylori* infection and gastric cancer: facing the enigmas. International Journal of Cancer 2003 106 953–960 (2003)

[10] Yuen B, Zbinden R, Fried M, Bauerfeind P, Bernardi M. Cultural recovery and determination of antimicrobial susceptibility in *Heliocobacter pylori* by using commercial transport and isolation media. *Infection* 2005 33 77–81.

[11] Hung IF, Chan P, Leung S, Chan FS, Hsu A, But D, Seto WK, Wong SY, Chan CK, Gu Q, Tong TS, Cheung TK, Chu KM, Wong BC. Clarithromycin-amoxycillin-containing triple therapy: a valid empirical first-line treatment for Helicobacter pylori eradication in Hong Kong? Helicobacter 2009 14(6):505-11.

[12] Malfertheiner P, Megraud F, O'Morain CA, Atherton J, Axon AT, Bazzoli F, Gensini GF, Gisbert JP, Graham DY, Rokkas T, El-Omar EM & Kuipers EJ. Management of *Helicobacter pylori* infection--the Maastricht IV/ Florence Consensus Report. European *Helicobacter* Study Group. *Gut 2012* 61(5) 646-64.

[13] Alarcon T, Domingo D & Lopez-Brea M (1999). Antibiotic resistance problems with *Helicobacter pylori*. International Journal of Antimicrobial Agents 1999 12 19–26.

[14] Megraud F. *Helicobacter pylori* antibiotic resistance: prevalence, importance and advances in testing. Gut 2004 53 1374–1384.

[15] Tanih NF, Okeleye BI, Naidoo N, Green E, Mkwetshana N, Clarke AM, Ndip LM, Ndip RN (2010a). *Helicobacter pylori* prevalence in dyspeptic patients in the Eastern Cape Province of South Africa: ethnicity and disease status. South African Medical Journal 2010a 100 734-737.

[16] Asrat D, Nilsson I, Mengistu Y, Ashenafi S, Ayenew K, Al-Soud AW, Wadström T & Kassa E (2004). Prevalence of *Helicobacter pylori vacA* and *cagA* genotypes in Ethiopian dyspeptic patients. Journal of Clinical. Microbiology 2004 42 (6) 2682–2684.

[17] Ndip RN, Malange TAE, Ojongokpoko JEA, Luma HN, Malongue A, Akoachere JFK, Ndip LM, MacMillan M & Weaver LT. *Helicobacter pylori* isolates recovered from gastric biopsies of patients with gastro–duodenal pathologies in Cameroon: current status of antibiogram. Tropical Medicine and International Health 2008 13 848-854.

[18] Tanih NF & Ndip RN (2013). Molecular Detection of Antibiotic Resistance in South African Isolates of *Helicobacter pylori*. Gastroenterology Research and Practice 2013 259457. doi: 10.1155/2013/259457.

[19] Secka O, Berg DE, Antonio M, Corrah T, Tapgun M, Walton R, Thomas V, Galano JJ, Sancho J, Adegbola RA, Thomas JE. Antimicrobial susceptibility and resistance pat-

terns among Helicobacter pylori strains from The Gambia, West Africa. Antimicrobial Agents and Chemotherapy 2013 57(3) 1231-7.

[20] Aibinu IE, Odunayo RA, Adenipeku T, Adelowotan T & Odugbemi T. *In vitro* antimicrobial activity of crude extracts from plants *Bryophyllum pinnatum* and *kalanchoe crenata*. African Journal of Traditional, Complementary and Alternative Medicines 2002 4(3) 338-344.

[21] Navarro-Rodriguez T, Silva FM, Barbuti RC, Mattar R, Moraes-Filho JP, de Oliveira MN, Bogsan CS, Chinzon D & Eisig JN. Association of a probiotic to a *Helicobacter pylori* eradication regimen does not increase efficacy or decreases the adverse effects of the treatment: a prospective, randomized, double-blind, placebo-controlled study. BMC Gastroenterology 2013 26 13:56.

[22] Njume C, Afolayan AJ & Ndip RN. Diversity of plants used in the treatment of *Helicobacter pylori* associated morbidities in the Nkonkobe municipality of the Eastern Cape province of South Africa. Journal of Medicinal Plant Research 2011a 5(14) 3146 -3151.

[23] Okeleye BI, Samie A, Bessong PO, Mkwetshana NF, Green E, Clarke AM & Ndip RN. Crude ethyl acetate extract of the stem bark of *Peltophorum africanum* (Sond, Fabaceae) possessing in- vitro inhibitory and bactericidal activity against clinical isolates of *Helicobacter pylori*. Journal of Medicinal Plant Research 2010 4(14) 1432-1440.

[24] Manyi-Loh CE, Clarke AM, Mkwetshana NF & Ndip RN. Treatment of *Helicobacter pylori* infections: Mitigating factors and prospective natural remedies. African Journal of Biotechnology 2010a. 9:2032-2042.

[25] Souza MC, Beserra AM, Martins DC, Real VV, Santos RA, Rao VS, Silva RM & Martin DT. *In vitro* and *in vivo* anti-*Helicobacter pylori* activity of *Calophyllum brasiliense Camb*. Journal of Ethnopharmacology 2009 123(3) 452-8.

[26] Okeleye BI, Bessong PO, Ndip RN. Preliminary phytochemical screening and in vitro anti-helicobacter pylori activity of extracts of the stem bark of *Bridelia micrantha* (Hochst., Baill., Euphorbiaceae). Molecules 2011 16(8):6193-205.

[27] Escobedo-Hinojosa WI, Del Carpio JD, Palacios-Espinosa JF & Romero I. Contribution to the ethnopharmacological and anti-*Helicobacter pylori* knowledge of *Cyrtocarpa procera Kunth* (Anacardiaceae). Journal of Ethnopharmacology 2012 30 143(1):363-71.

[28] George NM & Cutting KF. Antibacterial honey (Medihoney™): in-vitro activity against clinical isolates of MRSA, VRE and other multiresistant Gram negative organisms, including *Pseudomonas aeruginosa*. Wounds 2007 19 231–236.

[29] Ndip RN, Malange- Takang AE, Echakachi CM, Malongue A, Akoachere JFK, Ndip LM, & Luma HN. *In-vitro* antimicrobial activity of selected honeys on clinical isolates of *Helicobacter pylori*. African Health Science 2007a 7 228-231.

[30] Ahmad K, Fatemeh F, Mehri N, Maryam S. Probiotics for the Treatment of Pediatric *Helicobacter pylori* Infection: A Randomized Double Blind Clinical Trial. Iran Journal of Pediatrics 2013 23(1) 79-84.

[31] Schreiber S, Bücker R, Groll C, Azevedo-Vethacke M, Garten D, Scheid P, Friedrich S, Gatermann S, Josenhans C & Suerbaum S. Rapid lose of motility of *Helicobacter pylori* in the gastric lumen *in vivo*. Infection and Immunity 2005 73(3) 1584-1589.

[32] Atherton JC. The pathogenesis of *Helicobacter pylori*-induced gastro-duodenal diseases. Annual Reviews of Pathology 2006 1 63-96.

[33] Permin H & Anderson PL. Inflammation, immunity and vaccines for *Helicobacter* infection. Helicobacter 2005 10 21-30.

[34] Jones KR, Cha JH & Merrell DS. Who's winning the war? Molecular mechanisms of antibiotic resistance in *Helicobacter pylori*. Current Drug Therapy 2008 3 190-203.

[35] Mégraud F & Lehours P. *Helicobacter pylori* detection and antimicrobial susceptibility testing. Clinical Microbiology Reviews 2007 20 280-283.

[36] Wu MS, Chow LP, Lin JT & Chiou SH. Proteomic Identification of Biomarkers Related to *Helicobacter pylori*-associated Gastro duodenal disease: challenges and opportunities. Journal of Gastroenterology and Hepatology 2008 23(11) 1657-61. doi: 10.1111/j.1440-1746.2008.05659.x.

[37] Dube C, Tanih NF and Ndip RN. *Helicobacter pylori* in water sources: a global environmental health concern. Reviews on Environmental Health 2009 24(1) 1-14.

[38] Marshall MJ & Warren RJ (1983). Unidentified curved bacilli on gastric epithelium in active chronic gastritis. Lancet 1983. I:1273-1275.

[39] Khalifa MM, Sharaf RR & Aziz RK. *Helicobacter pylori*: a poor man's gut pathogen? Gut Pathogens 2010 2 1-12.

[40] Van Doorn LJ, Figueiredo C, Mégraud F, Pena S, Midolo P, Queiroz DM, Carneiro F, Vanderborght B, Pegado MD, Sanna R, De Boer W, Schneeberger PM, Correa P, Ng EK, Atherton J, Blaser MJ, Quint WG. Geographic distribution of *vacA* allelic types of *Helicobacter pylori*. Gastroenterology 1999 116 823-830.

[41] Wang J, van Doorn LJ, Robinson PA, Ji X, Wang D, Wang Y, Ge L, Telford JL and Crabtree JE. Regional variation among *vacA* alleles of *Helicobacter pylori* in China. Journal of Clinical Microbiology 2003. 41:1942-1945.

[42] Holcombe C. *Helicobacter pylori*: the African enigma. Gut 1992 33 429–431.

[43] El-Omar EM, Carrington M, Cho WH, McColl KE, Bream JH, Young HA *et al.*. Interleukin-1 polymorphisms associated with increased risk of gastric cancer. Nature 2000 404 398-402.

[44] Ando T, Peek RM, Pride D, Levine SM, Takata T, Lee YC, Kusuyami K *et al.* (2002). Polymorphisms of *Helicobacter pylori* HP 0638 reflect geographic origin and correlate with *cagA* status. Journal of Clinical Microbiology 2002 40 239-246.

[45] Chattopadhyay S, Patra R, Ramamurthy T, Chowdhury A, Santra A, Dhali GK, Bhattacharya SK, Berg DE, Nair GB & Mukhopadhyay AK. Multiplex PCR assay for rapid detection and genotyping of *Helicobacter pylori* from gastric biopsy specimens. Journal of Clinical Microbiology 2004 42 2821-2824.

[46] Enroth H, Kraaz W, Engstrand L, Nyrén O & Rohan T. *Helicobacter pylori* Strain Types and Risk of Gastric Cancer: A Case-Control Study. Cancer Epidemiology Biomarkers and Prevention 2000 9 981-90.

[47] Cover TL & Blanke SR. *Helicobacter pylori vacA*, a paradigm for toxin multifunctionality. Nature Reviews Microbiology 2005 3(4) 320-32.

[48] Bravo LE, van Doorn LJ, Realpe JL & Correa P. Virulence associated genotypes of *Helicobacter pylori*: do they explain the African enigma. American Journal of Gastroenterology 2002 97 2839-2842.

[49] Atherton JC. The clinical relevance of strain types of *Helicobacter pylori*. Gut 1997 40(6) 701-3.

[50] Blaser MJ & Berg DE. *Helicobacter pylori* genetic diversity and risk of human disease. Journal of Clinical Investigation 2001 107 767-773.

[51] Abdurasheed A, Lawal OO, Abioye-kuteyi EA & Lamikanra A. Antimicrobial susceptibility of *Helicobacter pylori* isolates of dyspeptic Nigerian patients. Journal of Tropical Gastroenterology 2005 26 85–88.

[52] Kusters JG, van Vliet AHM & Kuipers EJ. Pathogenesis of *Helicobacter pylori* infection. Clinical Microbiology Reviews 2006 19(3) 449-490.

[53] Dube C, Tanih NF, Clarke AM, Mkwetshana N, Green E, Ndip RN. *H. pylori* infection and transmission in Africa: household hygiene and water sources are plausible factors exacerbating spread. African Journal of Biotechnology 2009b 8(22) 6028-6035.

[54] Dehesa M, Dooley CP, Cohen H, Fitzgibbons PL, Perez-perez GI & Blaser MJ). High Prevalence of *Helicobacter pylori* infection and histologic gastritis in asymptomatic hispanics. Journal of Clinical Microbiology 1991 29(6) 1128-1131.

[55] Dube C, Nkosi TC, Clarke AM, Mkwetshana N, Green E, Ndip RN. *Helicobacter pylori* antigenemia in an asymptomatic population of the Eastern Cape Province of South Africa: Public health implications. Reviews on Environmental Health 2009b 24(3): 249 - 255

[56] Mukhopadhyay AK, Kersulyte D, Jeong JY, Datta S, Ito Y, Chowdhury A, Chowdhury S, Santra A, Bhattacharya SK, Azuma T, Nair GB, Berg DE. Distinctiveness of gen-

otypes of Helicobacter pylori in Calcutta, India. Journal of Bacteriology 2000 182(11) 3219-27.

[57] Fritz LE, Slavik T, Delport W, Olivier B & Merwe WS. Incidence of *Helicobacter felis* and the effect of coinfection with *Helicobacter pylori* on the gastric mucosa in the African population. Journal Clinical Microbiology 2006 44(5) 1692-1696.

[58] Shi R, Xu S, Zhang H, Ding Y, Sun G, Huang X, Chen X, Li X, Yan Z & Zhang G. Prevalence and risk factors for *Helicobacter pylori* infection in Chinese populations. Helicobacter 2008 13(2) 157-65.

[59] Logan RPH, Walker MM. Epidemiology and diagnosis of *Helicobacter pylori* infection. In: ABC of Upper Gastrointestinal Tract. Logan, R.P.H., Harris, A, Misiewicz, J.J., Baron, J.H. (eds).BMJ books 2002. London pp.16-18.

[60] Kidd M, Louw JA & Marks IN. *Helicobacter pylori* in Africa: observations on an 'enigma within an enigma'. Journal Gastroenterology and Hepatology 1999a. 14(9) 851-8.

[61] Thomas JE, Dale A, Bunn JE, Harding M, Coward WA, Cole TJ & Weaver LT. Early *Helicobacter pylori* colonisation: the association with growth faltering in the Gambia. Archives of Disease of Childhood 2004 89(12) 1149-1154.

[62] Nabwera HM, Nguyen-Van –Tam JS, Logan RF & Logan RP. Prevalence of *Helicobacter pylori* in Kenyan school children aged 3-15 years and risk factors for infection. European Journal of Gastroenterology and Hepatology 2000 12(5) 483-487.

[63] Tkachenko MA, Zhannat NZ, Erman LV, Blashenkova EL, Isachenko SV, Isachenko OB, Graham DY & Malaty HM. Dramatic changes in the prevalence of *Helicobacter pylori* infection during childhood: a 10-year follow-up study in Russia. Journal of Pediatric Gastroenterology and Nutrition 200745 (4) 428-432.

[64] Janzon A, Sjöling A, Lothigius A, Ahmed D, Qadri F & Svennerholm AM. Failure to detect *Helicobacter pylori* in drinking and environmental water in Dhaka, Bangladesh, using highly sensitive real-time PCR assays. Applied and Environmental Microbiology 2009 75 (10) 3039-3044

[65] Tanih NF, McMillan M, Naidoo N, Ndip LM, Weaver LT &, Ndip RN. Prevalence of *Helicobacter pylori vacA, cagA* and *iceA* genotypes in South African patients with upper gastrointestinal diseases. Acta Tropica 2010c 116(1) 68-73

[66] Hannula M & Hänninen M. Phylogenetic analysis of *Helicobacter species* based on partial gyrB gene sequences. International Journal of Systematic and Evolutionary Biology 2007 57 (3) 444-449.

[67] Brown LM. *Helicobacter pylori*: Epidemiology and routes of transmission. Epidemiological Reviews 2000 22(2) 283-297.

[68] Leung WK, Siu KLK, Kwok CKL *et al*. Isolation of *Helicobacter pylori* from vomitus in children and its implication in gastro-oral transmission. American Journal Gastroenterology 1999 94 2881- 2884.

[69] Ndip RN, MacKay WG, Farthing MJG & Weaver LT. Culturing Helicobacter *pylori* from clinical specimens: review of microbiologic methods. Journal of Pediatric Gastroenterology and Nutrition 2003 36 616–622.

[70] Perez-Perez GL, Witskin SS, Decker MD & Blaser MJ. Seroprevalence of *Helicobacter pylori* infection in couples. Journal of Clinical Microbiology 1991 29 642–644.

[71] Aditya HG, Ominguez KL, Kalish M, Rivera- Hernandez D, Donohoe M, Brooks J & Mitchell D. Practice of feeding premasticated food to infants: A potential risk factor for HIV transmission. Pediatrics 2009 124 (2) 658-666.

[72] Desai HG, Gill HH, Shankaran K et al. (1991). Dental plaque: a permanent reservoir of *Helicobacter pylori*. Scandinavian Journal of Gastroenterology 1991. 26:1205-1208.

[73] Bernander S, Dalen J, Gastrin B et al. (2003). Absence of *Helicobacter pylori* in dental plaques in *Helicobacter pylori* positive dyspeptic patients. European Journal of Clinical Microbiology and Infectious Disease 2003 12 282-285.

[74] Olivier BJ, Bond RP, van Zyl WB, Delport M, Slavik T, Ziady C, sive Droste JT, Lastovica A & van der Merwe SW. Absence of *Helicobacter pylori* within the oral cavities of members of a healthy South African Community. Journal of Clinical Microbiology 2006 44(2) 635-636.

[75] Kikuchi S. & Dore MP. Epidemiology of *Helicobacter pylori* infection. Helicobacter 2005 10 1-10.

[76] Scarpignato C. Towards the ideal regimen for *Helicobacter pylori* eradication: the search continues. Digestive and Liver Disease 2004 36 243-247.

[77] Romano M & Cuomo A. Eradication of *Helicobacter pylori:* A clinical update. Medscape General Medicine and Gastroenterology 2004 6(1) 19.

[78] Hardin FJ & Wright RA. *Helicobacter pylori*: review and update. Archives of Hospital Physician 2002 38(5) 23-31.

[79] Lee YC Liou JM, Wu MS, Wu CY & Lin JT. Eradication of *Helicobacter pylori* to prevent gastro duodenal diseases: Hitting more than one bird with the same stone. Therapeutic Advances in Gastroenterology 2008 1(2) 111-120.

[80] Harris A & Misiewicz JJ. Management of *Helicobacter pylori* infection. In: *ABC of Upper Gastrointestinal Tract*. Logan RDH, Harris A, Misiewicz JJ, Baron JH. (eds). BMJ books London 2002 pp. 22-24.

[81] Manyi-Loh CE, Clarke AM, Munzhelele T, Green E, Mkwetshana NF & Ndip RN. Selected South African honeys and their extracts possess *in vitro* anti-*Helicobacter pylori* activity. Archive of Medical Research 2010b. 41:324-331.

[82] Meurer L & Bower D. (2002). Management of *Helicobacter pylori* infection. American Family Physician 2002 65 (7) 1327-36, 1339.

[83] Bland MV, Ismail S, Heinemann JA & Keenan J. The action of bismuth against *Helicobacter pylori* mimics but is not caused by intracellular iron deprivation. Antimicrobial Agents and Chemotherapy 2004 48 (6) 1983-1988.

[84] Gendull JH, Friedman SL & McQuaid KR. Identification of *Helicobacter pylori*. In: *Current Diagnosis and Treatment in Gastroenterology*. Gendull JH, Friedman SL, and McQuaid K R.(eds). Google books 2003 Pp. 328-335.

[85] Erah PO, Goddard AF, Barrett DA, Shaw PN & Spiller RC. The stability of amoxicillin, clarithromycin and metronidazole in gastric juice: relevance to the treatment of *Helicobacter pylori* infection. Journal of Antimicrobial Chemotherapy 1997 39:5-12.

[86] Cameron EAB, Powell KU, Baldwin L, Jones P, Bell GD & Williams SGJ. *Helicobacter pylori*: antibiotic resistance and eradication rates in Suffolk, UK, 1991-2001. Journal of Medical Microbiology 2004 53 535-538.

[87] Bonacorsi C, Raddi MSG, Iracilda ZC, Sannomiya M and Vilegas W. Anti-*Helicobacter pylori* activity and immunostimulatory effect of extracts from *Byrsonima crassa* Nied. (Malpighiaceae). Complementary and Alternative Medicine 2009 9 1472-6882.

[88] Njume C, Afolayan AJ & Ndip RN. An overview of antimicrobial resistance and the future of medicinal plants in the treatment of *Helicobacter pylori* infections. African Journal of Pharmacy and Pharmacology 2009 3 685-699.

[89] Glocker E, Berning M, Gerrits MM, Kusters JG & Kist M. Real-time PCR screening for *16S rRNA* mutations associated with resistance to tetracycline in *Helicobacter pylori*. Antimicrobial Agents and Chemotherapy 2005 49 3166–3170.

[90] Boyanova L, Stancheva I, Spassova Z, Katzarov N, Mitov I & Koumanova R. Antimicrobial resistance; primary and combined resistance to four antimicrobial agents in *Helicobacter pylori* in Sofia, Bulgaria. Journal of Medical Microbiology 2000 49 415-418.

[91] Huynh HQ, Couper RTL, Tran CD, Moore L, Kelso R and Butler RN. Nacetylcysteine, a novel treatment for *Helicobacter pylori* infection. Digestive Diseases and Sciences 2004 49 (11/12) 1853-1861.

[92] Wu J & Sung J (1999). Treatment of *Helicobacter pylori* infection. Hong Kong Medical Journal 1999 5 (2) 145-9.

[93] Mollison LC, Stingemore N, Wake RA, Cullen DJ & McGechie DB. Antibiotic resistance in *Helicobacter pylori*. Medical Journal of Australia 2000 173 521-523.

[94] De Francisco V, Margiotta M, Zullo A, Hassan C, Giorgio F, Burattini O, Stoppino G, Cea U, Pace A, Zotti M, Morini S, Panella C and Ierardi E (2007). Prevalence of primary clarithromycin resistance in *Helicobacter pylori* strains over a 15 year period in Italy. Journal of Antimicrobial Chemotherapy 2007 59 783-785.

[95] Destura RV, Labio ED, Barrett LJ, Alcantara CS, Gloria VI, Daez MLO & Guerrant RL. Laboratory diagnosis and susceptibility profile of *Helicobacter pylori* infection in the Philippines. Annals of Clinical Microbiology and Antimicrobial 2004 3 25-30.

[96] Sherif M, Mohran Z, Fathy H, Rockabrand DM, Rozmajzl PJ & Frenck RW. Universal high-level primary metronidazole resistance in *Helicobacter pylori* isolated from children in Egypt. Journal of Clinical Microbiology 2004 42 (10) 4832-4834.

[97] Bina JE, Alm RA, Uria-Nickelsen M, Thomas SR, Trust TJ & Hancock REW. *Helicobacter pylori* uptake and efflux: Basis for intrinsic susceptibility to antibiotics *in-vitro*. Antimicrobial Agents and Chemotherapy 2000 44 248-254.

[98] Al-Qurashi AR, El-Morsy F, Al-Quorain AA. Evolution of metronidazole and tetracycline susceptibility pattern in *Helicobacter pylori* at a hospital in Saudi Arabia. *International Journal of Antimicrobial Agents* 2001 17: 233–6.

[99] Buta N, Tanih NF & Ndip RN. Increasing trend of metronidazole resistance in the treatment of *Helicobacter pylori* infection: A global challenge. African Journal of Biotechnology 2010 9(8) 1115-1121.

[100] Jeong JY, Mukhopadhyay AK, Akada JK, Dailidiene D, Hoffman PS & Berg DE. Roles of *frxA* and *rdxA* nitroreductases of *Helicobacter pylori* in susceptibility and resistance to metronidazole. Journal of Bacteriology 2001 183 5155–5162.

[101] Jenks PJ, Ferrero RL, Labigne A. The role of the rdxA gene in the evolution of metronidazole resistance in Helicobacter pylori. Journal of Antimicrobial Chemotherapy 1999 43(6):753-8.

[102] Kwon DH, Hulten K, Kato M, Kim JJ, Lee M, El-zaatari FAK, Osato MS & Graham DY. DNA sequence analysis of *rdxA* and *frxA* from 12 pairs of metronidazole-sensitive and -resistant clinical *Helicobacter pylori* isolates. Antimicrobial Agents and Chemotherapy 2001 45(9) 2609–2615.

[103] Ahmad N, Zakaria WR, Abdullah SA & Mohamed R. Characterisation of clarithromycin resistance in Malaysian isolates of *Helicobacter pylori*. World Journal of Gastroenterology 2009 15(25):3161-3165.

[104] Deloney CR & Schiller NL. Characterization of an *in-vitro* selected amoxicillin resistant strain of *Helicobacter pylori*. Antimicrobial Agents and Chemotherapy 2000 44 3363–3373.

[105] Jones KR, Cha JH, Merrell DS. Who's Winning the War? Molecular Mechanisms of Antibiotic Resistance in Helicobacter pylori. Current Drug and therapeutics 2008 3(3):190-203.

[106] Rimbara E, Noguchi N, Kawai T and Sasatsu M. Correlation between substitution in Penicillins-binding protein and amoxicillin resistance in *Helicobacter pylori*. Microbiology and Immunology 2007 51(10) 939-944.

[107] Matteo MJ, Granados G, Olmos M, Wonaga A. and Catalano M. *Helicobacter pylori* amoxicillin heteroresistance due to point mutations in *pbp1*A in isogenic isolates. Journal of Antimicrobial Chemotherapy 2008 61(3) 474-477.

[108] Wu JY, Kim JJ, Reddy R, Wang WM, Graham DY & Kwon DH. Tetracycline-resistant clinical *Helicobacter pylori* isolates with and without mutations in 16SrRNA-encoding genes. Antimicrobial Agents and Chemotherapy 2005 49(2) 578-583.

[109] Dzierzanowska FK, Rozynek R, Celinska CD, Jarosz M, Pawlowska J, Szadkowski A, Budzysnska A, Nowak J, Romanozuk W, Prosiecki R, Jozwiak P. & Dzierzanowska D. Antimicrobial resistance of *Helicobacter pylori* in Poland. A multicenter study. International Journal of Antimicrobial Agents 2005 26 230-234.

[110] Wang YH, Wang JP, Gorvel YT, Chu J, Wu J, and Lei HY. *Helicobacter pylori* impairs murine dendritic cell responses to infection. PLoS One 2010.doi:. doi: 10.1371/journal.pone.0010844.

[111] Tanih NF, Ndip RN. The acetone extract of Sclerocarya birrea (Anacardiaceae) possesses antiproliferative and apoptotic potential against human breast cancer cell lines (MCF-7). Scientific World Journal. 2013

[112] Dharmalingam S, Rao UA, Jayaraman G & Thyagarajan SP. Relationship of plasmid profile with the antibiotic sensitivity pattern of *Helicobacter pylori* isolates from peptic ulcer disease patients in Chennai. Indian Journal of Medical Microbiology 2003 21(4) 257-261.

[113] Owen RJ, Bell GD, Desai M, Moreno M, Gant PW, Jones PH & Linton D. Biotype and molecular fingerprints of metronidazole resistant strains of *Helicobacter pylori* from antral gastric mucosa. Journal of Medical Microbiology 1993 38 6-12.

[114] Borges-Walmsley MI & Walmsley AR. The structure and function of drug pumps. Trends in Microbiology 2001 9 71–79.

[115] Kutschke A & Boudewijn LM de J. Compound efflux in *Helicobacter pylori*. Antimicrobial Agents and Chemotherapy 2005 49(7) 3009–3010.

[116] van Amsterdam K, Bart A, & van der Ende A. *Helicobacter pylori* Tol C efflux pump confers resistance to metronidazole. Antimicrobial Agents and Chemotherapy 2005 49(4) 1477–1482.

[117] Chisholm SA & Owen RJ. Frameshift mutations in *frxA* occur frequently and do not provide a reliable marker for metronidazole resistance in UK isolates of *Helicobacter pylori*. Journal of Medical Microbiology 2004 53 135–140.

[118] Glocker E, Bogdan C & Kist M. Characterization of rifampicin-resistant clinical *Helicobacter pylori* isolates from Germany. Journal of Antimicrobial Chemotherapy 2007 59 874-879

[119] Chaudhuri S, Chowdhury A, Datta S, Mukhopadhyay AK, Chattopadhyay S, Saha DR, Dhali G, Santra A, Nair GB, Bhattacharya S & Berg DE. Anti-*Helicobacter pylori*

therapy in India: differences in eradication efficiency associated with particular alleles of vacuolating cytotoxin (vacA) gene. Journal of Gastroenterology and Hepatology 2003 18 190-195.

[120] Tanih NF, Dube C, Green E, Mkwetshana N, Clarke AM, Ndip LM, Ndip RN. An African perspective on *Helicobacter pylori* prevalence, drug resistance and alternative approaches to treatment. Annals of Tropical Medicine and Parasitology 2009 103(3) 189-204.

[121] Bharati AC, Sahu AN. Ethnobotany, phytochemistry and pharmacology of *Biophytum sensitivum* DC. Pharmacognosy reviews 2012 6(11):68-73.

[122] Anesini C & Perez C. Screening of plants used in Argentine folk medicine for antimicrobial activity. Journal of Ethnopharmacology 1993 39 119–128.

[123] World Health Organization (1987). Report of the Second Meeting of Directors of WHO Collaborating Centres for Traditional Medicine. Document WHO/TRM/88.1. Geneva: WHO.

[124] Klos M, van de Venter M, Milne PJ, Traore HN, Meyer D, Oosthuizen V. *In vitro* anti-HIV activity of five selected South African medicinal plant extracts. Journal of Ethnopharmacology 2009 124(2) 182-8.

[125] Sivam GP. Protection against *Helicobacter pylori* and other bacterial infection by garlic. Journal of Nutrition 2001 131 (3s) 1106S-8S.

[126] Zeyrek FY & Oguz E (2005). *In vitro* activity of capsaicin against *Helicobacter pylori*. Annals of Microbiology 2005 55 (2) 125-127.

[127] Molina-Torres J, Garcia-chavez A & Ramirez-chavez E. Antimicrobial properties of alkamides present in flavouring plants traditionally used in Masoamerica: affinin and capsaicin. Journal of Ethnopharmacology 1999 64 241-248.

[128] Cichewicz RH & Thorpe PA. The antimicrobial properties of chile peppers (*Capsicum* species) and their uses in Mayan medicine. Journal of Ethnopharmacology 1996 52 61-70.

[129] Zhang L, Ma J, Pan K, Go VLW, Chen J & You WC. Efficacy of cranberry juice on *Helicobacter pylori* infection: a double-blind, randomized placebo controlled trial. *Helicobacter*.2005 10 (2):139-145.

[130] Njume C, Afolayan AJ, Green E & Ndip RN. Volatile compounds in the stem bark of *Sclerocarya birrea* (Anacardiaceae) possess potent antimicrobial activity against drug-resistant *Helicobacter pylori*. International Journal of Antimicrobial Agents 2011c 38 (4) 319 – 24.

[131] Ojewole JA, Mawoza T, Chiwororo WD, Owira PM. Sclerocarya birrea (A. Rich) Hochst. ['Marula'] (Anacardiaceae): a review of its phytochemistry, pharmacology and toxicology and its ethnomedicinal uses. Phytotherapy Research 2010 24(5) 633-9.

[132] Inatsu S, Ohsaki A, Nagata K. Idebenone acts against growth of *Helicobacter pylori* by inhibiting its respiration. Antimicrobial Agents Chemotherapy 2006 50(6):2237-9.

[133] Ustün O, Ozçelik B, Akyön Y, Abbasoglu U, Yesilada E. Flavonoids with anti-*Helicobacter pylori* activity from *Cistus laurifolius* leaves. Journal of Ethnopharmacology 2006 108(3) 457-61.

[134] Bylka W, Szaufer-Hajrych M, Matawska I and Goslinska O. Antimicrobial activity of isocytisoside and extracts of *Aquilegia vulgaris* L., Letters in Applied Microbiology 2004 39(1): 93-97.

[135] Basile A, Sorbo S, Spadaro V, Bruno M, Maggio A, Faraone N, Rosselli S. Antimicrobial and antioxidant activities of coumarins from the roots of *Ferulago campestris* (Apiaceae). Molecules 2009 14(3) 939-52.

[136] Kawase M, Tanaka T, Sohara Y, Tani S, Sakagami H, Hauer H, Chatterjee SS. Structural requirements of hydroxylated coumarins for in vitro anti-Helicobacter pylori activity. In Vivo. 2003 17(5):509-12.

[137] Nzeako BC & Al-Namaani F. The antibacterial activity of honey on *Helicobacter pylori*. Sultan Qaboos University Medical Journal 2006 (2) 71-76.

[138] Davis C. The use of Australian honey in moist wound management. Publication No. W05/159. Kingston, Australia: Rural Industries Research and Development Corporation 2005.

[139] Meda A, Lamien EC, Millogo J, Romito M, Nacoulma OG. Ethnopharmacological communication therapeutic uses of honey and honeybee larvae in central Burkina Faso. Journal of Ethnopharmacology 2004 95 103-107.

[140] Castro-Várquez LM, Díaz-Maroto MC, de Tores C & Pérez-Coello MS. Effects of geographical origins on the chemical and sensory characteristics of chestnut honeys. Food Research International 2010 43 2335-2340.

[141] Baltrusaitytė V, Venskutonis PR & Ceksterytė V. Radical scavenging activity of different floral origin honey and bee bread phenolic extracts. Food Chemistry 2007 101:502-514.

[142] Yao L, Datta N, Tomás-Barberán FA, Ferreres F, Martos I & Singanusong R. Flavonoids, phenolic acids and abscisic acid in Australian and New Zealand *Leptospermum* honeys. Food Chemistry 2003 81:159-168.

[143] Zaghloul AA, El-Shattaw HH, Kassem AA, Ibrahim EA, Reddy IK & Khan MA. Honey, a prospective antibiotic: extraction, formulation, and stability. Pharmazie 2001 56 643-647.

[144] Tonks AJ, Cooper RA, Jones KP, Blair S, Parton J & Tonks A. Honey stimulates inflammatory cytokine production from monocytes. Cytokine 2003 242-7.

[145] Basualdo C, Sgroy V, Finda MS & Marioli JM. Comparison of the antibacterial activity of honey from different provenance against bacteria usually isolated from skin wounds. Veterinary Microbiology 2007 124 375–381.

[146] Manyi –Loh CE, Clarke AM & Ndip RN. Identification of volatile compounds in solvent extracts of honeys produced in South Africa. African Journal of Agricultural Research 2011 6 (18) 4327 – 4334.

[147] Guarner F, Khan AG, Garisch J, Eliakim R, Gangl A, Thomson A, et al. World Gastroenterology Organisation Global Guidelines: probiotics and prebiotics October 2011. Journal of Clinical Gastroenterology 2012 46468–81.

[148] De Keersmaecker SC, Verhoeven TL, Desair J, Marchal K, Vanderleyden J, Nagy I. Strong antimicrobial activity of Lactobacillus rhamnosus GG against *Salmonella typhimurium* is due to accumulation of lactic acid. FEMS Microbiology Letters 2006 259 89-96.

[149] Dajani AI, Abu Hammour AM, Yang DH, Chung PC, Nounou MA, Yuan KY, Zakaria MA, Schi HS. Do probiotics improve eradication response to *Helicobacter pylori* on standard triple or sequential therapy? Saudi Journal of Gastroenterology 2013 19(3) 113-20. doi: 10.4103/1319-3767.111953.

[150] Hamilton-Miller JM. The role of probiotics in the treatment and prevention of *Helicobacter pylori* infection. International journal of antimicrobial agents 2003 22:360–6.

[151] Tong JL, Ran ZH, Shen J, Zhang CX, Xiao SD (2007). Meta-analysis: The effect of supplementation with probiotics on eradication rates and adverse events during *Helicobacter pylori* eradication therapy. Alimentary Pharmacology & Therapeutics's 2007 25 155–68.

[152] Chen LS, Ma Y, Maubois JL, He SH, Chen LJ, Li HM. Screening for the potential probiotic yeast strains from raw milk to assimilate cholesterol. *Dairy Science and Technology 2010* 90 537–548.

[153] Gomi A, Harima-Mizusawa N, Shibahara-Sone H, Kano M, Miyazaki K, Ishikawa F. Effect of *Bifidobacterium* bifidum BF-1 on gastric protection and mucin production in an acute gastric injury rat model. Journal of Dairy Science 2013 96(2) 832-7.

[154] Arunachalam K, Gill HS, Chandra RK. Enhancement of natural immune function by dietary consumption of *Bifidobacterium lactis* (HN019). European Journal of Clinical Nutrition 2000 54(3) 263-7.

[155] Yang YJ, and Sheu BS. Probiotics-Containing Yogurts Suppress *Helicobacter pylori* Load and Modify Immune Response and Intestinal Microbiota in the *Helicobacter pylori*-Infected Children. Helicobacter 2012 17: 297–304

[156] Vlasova AN, Chattha KS, Kandasamy S, Liu Z, Esseili M, Shao L, Rajashekara G, Saif LJ. Lactobacilli and Bifidobacteria Promote Immune Homeostasis by Modulating In-

nate Immune Responses to Human Rotavirus in Neonatal Gnotobiotic Pigs. PLoS One 2013 8(10):e76962.

[157] O'Connor A, Molina-Infante J, Gisbert JP, O'Morain C. Treatment of *Helicobacter pylori* Infection. *Helicobacter* 2013 Suppl 1:58-65.

[158] McFarland LV. Review Systematic review and meta-analysis of *Saccharomyces boulardii* in adult patients. World Journal of Gastroenterology 2010 16(18): 2202-22.

[159] Hickson M. Probiotics in the prevention of antibiotic-associated diarrhoea and *Clostridium difficile* infection. *Therapeutic Advances in Gastroenterology* 2011 4(3) 185–197.

[160] Cindoruk M, Erkan G, Karakan T, Dursun A, Unal S. Efficacy and safety of *Saccharomyces boulardii* in the 14-day triple anti-*Helicobacter pylori* therapy: a prospective randomized placebo-controlled double-blind study. *Helicobacter 2007* 12 309–316.

[161] Kelesidis T and Pothoulakis C. Efficacy and safety of the probiotic *Saccharomyces boulardii* for the prevention and therapy of gastrointestinal disorders. Therapeutic Advances in Gastroenterology 2012 5(2) 111–125.

[162] Dylag K, Hubalewska-Mazgaj M, Surmiak M, Szmyd J, Brzozowski T. Probiotics in the mechanism of protection against gut inflammation and therapy of gastrointestinal disorders. Current Pharmaceutical Design 2013 Jun 10. [Epub ahead of print]

[163] Buzás GM. [Probiotics in gastroenterology -- from a different angle]. Orvosi hetilap 2013 154(8) 294-304.

[164] Lesbros-Pantoflickova D, Corthésy-Theulaz I, and Blum AL. *Helicobacter pylori* and Probiotics. Journal of Nutrition 2007 137 (3) 812S-818S.

[165] Wilson KT, Crabtree JE. Immunology of *Helicobacter pylori*: insights into the failure of the immune response and perspectives on vaccine studies, Gastroenterology 2007 133: 288–308.

[166] Backert S, Clyne M. Pathogenesis of *Helicobacter pylori* infection. Helicobacter 2011 Suppl 1:19-25.

[167] Belury MA. Dietary conjugated linoleic acid in health: physiological effects and mechanisms of action, Annual Review of Nutrition 2002 22 505–531.

[168] Hwang SW, Kim N, Kim JM, Huh CS, Ahn YT, Park SH, Shin CM, Park JH, Lee MK, Nam RH, Lee HS, Kim JS, Jung HV, Song IS (2012). Probiotic suppression of the H. pylori-induced responses by conjugated linoleic acids in a gastric epithelial cell line. Prostaglandins, Leukotrienes and Essential Fatty Acids 2012 86 225–231

[169] Weiss G, Christensen HR, Zeuthen LH, Vogensen FK, Jakobsen M, Frokiaer H. Lactobacilli and bifidobacteria induce differential interferon-beta profiles in dendritic cells. Cytokine 2011 56 520–530.

[170] Weiss G, Forster S, Irving A, Tate M, Ferrero RL, Hertzog P, Frøkiær H, Kaparakis-Liaskos M. *Helicobacter pylori* VacA suppresses *Lactobacillus acidophilus*-induced inter-

feron beta signaling in macrophages via alterations in the endocytic pathway. mBio 2013 4(3):e00609-12. doi:10.1128/mBio.00609-12.

[171] Yang YJ, Chuang CC, Yang HB, Lu CC and Sheu BS. Lactobacillus acidophilus ameliorates *H. pylori* induced gastric inflammation by inactivating the Smad7 and NF_B pathways. BMC Microbiology 2012 12:38

[172] Njume C, Afolayan AJ, Samie A, Ndip RN. Inhibitory and bactericidal potential of crude acetone extracts of Combretum molle (Combretaceae) on drug-resistant strains of *Helicobacter pylori*. Journal of Health Population and Nutrition 2011 29(5) 438-45.

[173] Okeleye BI, Bessong PO & Ndip RN. Preliminary phytochemical screening and in-vitro anti-*Helicobacter pylori* activity of extracts of the stem bark of *Bridelia micrantha* (Hochst., Baill., Euphorbiaceae). Molecules 2011 16(8) 6193-205.

[174] Nkomo LP, Green E, Ndip RN. Preliminary phytochemical screening and in vitro anti-*Helicobacter pylori* activity of extracts of the leaves of *Lippia javanica*. Health & Environmental Research Online 2011 5 (20) 2184-2192.

[175] Nethathe BB, Ndip RN. Bioactivity of *Hydonora africana* on selected bacterial pathogens: Preliminary phytochemical screening. African Journal of Microbiology Research 2011 5 2820–2826.

[176] Njume C, Jide AA, Ndip RN. Aqueous and Organic Solvent-Extracts of Selected South African Medicinal Plants Possess Antimicrobial Activity against Drug-Resistant Strains of *Helicobacter pylori*: Inhibitory and Bactericidal Potential. International Journal of Molecular Science 2011 12(9) 5652-65.

[177] Tan PV, Boda M, Etoa FX. In vitro and in vivo anti-*Helicobacter*/*Campylobacter* activity of the aqueous extract of *Enantia chlorantha*. Pharmaceutical Biology 2010 48(3) 349-56. doi: 10.3109/13880200903150377.

[178] Farag TH, Stoltzfus RJ, Khalfan SS, Tielsch JM. Unexpectedly low prevalence of *Helicobacter pylori* infection among pregnant women on Pemba Island, Zanzibar. Transactions of the Royal Society of Tropical Medicine and Hygiene 2007 101 915–922.

[179] Adeniyi CBA, Lawal TO and Mahady GB. *In vitro* susceptibility of *Helicobacter pylori* to extracts of *Eucalyptus camaldulensis* and *Eucalyptus torelliana.* Pharmaceutical Biology 2009 47(1) 99–102.

[180] Santos RC, Kushima H, Rodrigues CM, Sannomiya M, Rocha LR, Bauab TM, Tamashiro J, Vilegas W, Hiruma-Lima CA. Byrsonima intermedia A. Juss.: gastric and duodenal anti-ulcer, antimicrobial and antidiarrheal effects in experimental rodent models. *Journal of Ethnopharmacology* 2012 140(2) 203-12.

[181] Rozza AL, de Mello Moraes T, Kushima H, Nunes DS, Hiruma-Lima CA, Pellizzon CH. Involvement of glutathione, sulfhydryl compounds, nitric oxide, vasoactive intestinal peptide, and heat-shock protein-70 in the gastroprotective mechanism of *Cro-*

ton cajucara Benth. (Euphorbiaceae) essential oil. Journal of Medicinal Food. 2011 14(9) 1011-7.

[182] Quílez A, Berenguer B, Gilardoni G, Souccar C, de Mendonça S, Oliveira LF, Martín-Calero MJ, Vidari G. Anti-secretory, anti-inflammatory and anti-*Helicobacter pylori* activities of several fractions isolated from *Piper carpunya* Ruiz & Pav. Journal of Ethnopharmacology 2010 128(3) 583-9.

[183] Vega AE, Wendel GH, Maria AO, Pelzer L. Antimicrobial activity of *Artemisia douglasiana and dehydroleucodine* against *Helicobacter pylori*. Journal of Ethnopharmacology. 2009 124(3):653-5. doi: 10.1016/j.jep.2009.04.051

[184] Lima ZP, Calvo TR, Silva EF, Pellizzon CH, Vilegas W, Brito AR, Bauab TM, Hiruma-Lima CA. Brazilian medicinal plant acts on prostaglandin level and *Helicobacter pylori*. Journal of Medicinal Food 2008 11(4) 701-8. doi: 10.1089/jmf.2007.0676.

[185] Moraes Tde M, Rodrigues CM, Kushima H, Bauab TM, Villegas W, Pellizzon CH, Brito AR, Hiruma-Lima CA. *Hancornia speciosa*: indications of gastroprotective, healing and anti-*Helicobacter pylori* actions. Journal of Ethnopharmacology 2008 120(2) 161-8.

[186] Castillo-Juarez I, Rivero-Cruz F, Celis H, Romero I. Anti-Helicobacter pylori activity of anacardic acids from *Amphipterygium adstringens*. Journal Ethnopharmacology 2007 114 72-77.

[187] Mazzolin LP, Nasser AL, Moraes TM, Santos RC, Nishijima CM, Santos FV, Varanda EA, Bauab TM, da Rocha LR, Di Stasi LC, Vilegas W, Hiruma-Lima CA. *Qualea parviflora* Mart.: an integrative study to validate the gastroprotective, antidiarrheal, antihemorragic and mutagenic action. Journal of Ethnopharmacology 2010 127(2) 508-14.

[188] Heinrich M, Heneka B, Ankli A, Rimpler H, Sticher O, Kostiza T. Spasmolytic and antidiarrhoeal properties of the Yucatec Mayan medicinal plant *Casimiroa tetrameria*. Journal of Pharmacy and Pharmacology 2005 57(9) 1081-5.

[189] Sekiguchi H, Takabayashi F, Deguchi Y, Masuda H, Toyoizumi T, Masuda S, Kinae N. Leaf extract of Wasabia japonica relieved oxidative stress induced by Helicobacter pylori infection and stress loading in Mongolian gerbils. Bioscience Biotechnology and Biochemistry 2010 74(6) 1194-9.

[190] Wang YH, Wu JJ, and Lei HY. The Autophagic induction in *Helicobacter pylori*-infected macrophage. Experimental Biology and Medicine 2009 34171-180.

[191] Randhir R, Shetty K. Improved alpha-amylase and Helicobacter pylori inhibition by fenugreek extracts derived via solid-state bioconversion using *Rhizopus oligosporus*. Asia Pacific Journal of Clinical Nutrition 2007 16(3) 382-92.

[192] Wang G, Conover RC, Olczak AA, Alamuri P, Johnson MK, Maier RJ. Oxidative stress defense mechanisms to counter iron-promoted DNA damage in *Helicobacter pylori*. Free Radical Research 2005 39(11):1183-91.

[193] Nariman F, Eftekhar F, Habibi Z, Falsafi T. Anti-*Helicobacter pylori* activities of six Iranian plants. Helicobacter 2004 9(2) 146-51.

[194] Goel RK, Sairam K, Babu MD, Tavares IA, Raman A. In vitro evaluation of *Bacopa monniera* on anti-*Helicobacter pylori* activity and accumulation of prostaglandins. Phytomedicine 200310(6-7) 523-7.

[195] Moghaddam FM, Farimiani MM, Salahvarzi S, Amin G. Chemical constituents of dichloromethane extract of cultivated *Satureja khuzistanica*. Evidence-Based Complementary and Alternative Medicine 2007 4 95–98.

[196] Nariman F, Eftekhar F, Habibi Z, Massarrat S, Malekzadeh R. Antibacterial Activity of Twenty Iranian Plant Extracts Against Clinical Isolates of *Helicobacter pylori*. Iranian Journal of Basic Medical Sciences 2009 12(2) 105-111.

[197] Amin M, Anwar F, Naz F, Mehmood T, Saari N. Anti-*Helicobacter pylori* and urease inhibition activities of some traditional medicinal plants. Molecules 2013 18(2) 2135-49.

[198] Sharifi MS, Ebrahimi D, Hibbert DB, Hook J, Hazell SL. Bio-activity of natural polymers from the genus Pistacia: a validated model for their antimicrobial action. Global Journal of Health Science 2011 4(1):149-61

[199] Nakajima S, Fujita K, Inoue Y, Nishio M, Seto Y. Effect of the folk remedy, Bainiku-ekisu, a concentrate of *Prunus mume* juice, on *Helicobacter pylori* infection in humans. *Helicobacter* 2006 11(6) 589-91.

Chapter 10

Helicobacter pylori — Current Therapy and Future Therapeutic Strategies

Rajinikanth Siddalingam and
Kumarappan Chidambaram

Additional information is available at the end of the chapter

http://dx.doi.org/10.5772/58338

1. Introduction

Helicobacter pylori (H pylori) is a spiral-shaped bacterium that is attached to or just above the gastric mucosa. The organism can persist in the stomach indefinitely and may not cause clinical illness for many years after infection [1]. Indeed, a large number of infected patients never develop any symptoms [2, 3]. However, literature has also associated *H pylori* infection with gastritis and gastric malignancies (gastric adenocarcinoma and MALT-lymphoma) [4]. Chronic *H pylori* infection has also been associated with several extra intestinal diseases, such as autoimmune thrombocytopenia, sideropenic anemia and chronic urticaria but the pathogenesis is still not known [5]. *H pylori* gastric infection is one of the most prevalent infectious diseases worldwide with an estimate of 40%-50% of the world population [3]. Remarkable differences are due to geographical, socio-economic and demographic factors [6]. *H pylori* transmission is still not completely understood. In addition, among infected patients, the reasons why only some develop symptoms is still a matter of speculations. Studies suggested that *H.pylori* is also transmitted from domestic animals like cat and sheep, but humans are the primary reservoir of *H pylori* infection [7, 8]. Several tests are available to detect *H pylori* in patients with ulcer or dyspepsia. The more commonly used tests are the evaluation of biopsy specimens during upper gastrointestinal tract (GI)I endoscopy, the detection of serum anti *H pylori* antibodies and breath tests with 13C-labeled urea (9-11) The discovery that most upper gastrointestinal diseases are the consequence of *H pylori* infection that can be treated with antibacterials, is an important medical advance [12]. Although, in the last few decades, *H pylori* eradication has been standardized, occurrence of resistance to therapeutic regimens is a growing problem [3, 14]. The purpose of this paper is to provide an appraisal of the most effective, current treatments available for *H pylori*, and to speculate on the potential for newer approaches in treatment and prophylaxis in future.

2. Epidemiology and prevalence

Humans are the only host for *H.pylori*, which is found in stomach, duodenum, esophagus and rectum on areas of metaplastic gastric epithelium [15]. Other *H.pylori* species have been isolated from the animals [16]. Animal models of *Helicobacter* infection have been developed due to shared characteristics of other *H.pylori* like *H.mustelae* and *H. felis* with *H.pylori*. *H.pylori* exists the world over and its prevalence in the population increases with age [17, 18] In developed countries, prevalence increases with rate of 1% per year of age, where as it is rare in children, and reaches 70% in the seventh decade [19]. In developing countries, more than 50% children acquire the infection by the age of 10 years, and more than 80% of the population gets infected by the age of 20 years [20-22]. In asymptomatic individuals prevalence of *H.pylori* infection varies from 31%-84% [22]. *H.pylori* infection is chronic and once acquired remains life long, unless eradicated by antibiotics given for some other conditions [22]. Humoral and tissue immune response by the host is usually not sufficient to clear the infection. Though the mode of transmission is not yet well established, most probably it occurs by oral-oral or faeco-oral route and important risk factors are socioeconomic status and age [7, 8]. Overcrowding, poor socio-economic status and poor hygiene are associated with high infection rate. Re-infection rate after eradication is quite high in developing countries due to above mentioned risk factors [23].

Colonization of *H.Pylori* occurs by producing urease and gastric acid inhibitory protein. It can colonize only in gastric type epithelium and cannot stay anywhere else in the GI in the absence of gastric mucosa [24]. Metaplasia, which is present in more than 90% of patients of duodenal ulcer, occurs by replacing the columnar cells, normally covering the duodenal villi, by gastric type epithelium. Adhesion of *H.pylori* to the gastric epithelium occurs by tissue specific proteins. Colonization of the duodenal bulb by *H.pylori* leads to mucosal inflammation which makes it vulnerable to attack by acid or pepsin or bile resulting into ulceration, however, factors leading to gastric metaplasia in the duodenal bulb are not known. Stimulation of the immune system of *H.pylori* contributes to host damage and it evades the immunological clearance [25-2]).

3. Diseases associated with *H.pylori*

H.pylori infection is found to be associated with gastritis, non-ulcer dyspepsia (NUD), duodenal ulcer, gastric ulcer, gastric cancer, gastric lymphoma of mucosa associated lymphoid tissue (MALT) and even coronary heart disease [28, 29]. It has now been well established that *H.pylori* is the cause of almost all duodenal ulcers (DU) and chronic benign gastric ulcers (GU) which are not associated with nonsteroidal anti-inflammatory drugs (NSAID) [30]. More than 95%

of DU and 90% of GU are associated with *H.pylori* infection and there is a dramatic decrease in their relapse rate after the *H.pylori* eradication. Right now there is no convincing evidence that NUD symptoms are due to *H.pylori* infection. Prevalence of *H.pylori* infection is comparable between healthy individuals and patients with the symptoms of NUD. Recurrent abdominal pain in children suggestive of NUD subsides after the eradication of *H.pylori* which indirectly associates *H.pylori* infection with NUD. However, further studies are necessary to eradicate *H.pylori* completely in NUD. [31]

4. Current therapy of *H.pylori* infection

The objective of *H. pylori* treatment is the complete elimination of the organism from the GI of patients and once this has been achieved then the rate of reinfection is low. Development of a successful treatment for *H. pylori* infection has been fraught with difficulty. The survival capabilities of the *H.pylori* organism over a wide pH spectrum within the stomach make the task of eradication difficult [32]. The organism must be eradicated from each of these potential niches and this is a daunting task for any single antibiotic. Initial attempts to cure the infection showed that the presence of antibiotic susceptibility in vitro did not necessarily correlate with successful treatment. It was rapidly recognized that the therapy with a single antibiotic led to a poor cure rate and various antimicrobial mixtures were tried resulting in several effective combinations of antibiotics, bismuth and antisecretory drugs [33, 34].

It is vital that the infection be treated optimally with clinically relevant *H.pylori*– eradication regimens that has an acceptably high eradication rate and without major side effects and with minimal induction of bacterial resistance. The reasonable eradication targets would be ≥90% cure rate on per-protocol analysis, and ≥80% cure rate on intent-to-treat analysis [35]. Such goals have not been achieved with antibiotics alone. Because of luminal acidity influences the effectiveness of some antimicrobial agents that are active against *H. pylori.* In order to achieve the desirable eradication rate, the antibiotics are combined with proton-pump inhibitors or ranitidine bismuth citrate. So-called triple therapies, combinations of one anti secretory agent with two antimicrobial agents for 7 to 14 days, have been extensively evaluated, and several regimens have been approved by the Food and Drug Administration (FDA). Combination drug regimens are essential to maximize the chance of eradicating the infection and to minimize the risk of promoting antimicrobial (to metronidazole and clarithromycin) resistance [35].

The most widely used antimicrobials in these regimens are amoxicillin, clarithromycin, metronidazole, tetracycline, and bismuth. Resistance of *H pylori* to the limited range of antibiotics that have efficacy in its treatment can severely affect attempts to eradicate the bacteria. Resistance to tetracycline or amoxicillin is extremely rare [36, 37]. The issue of resistance primarily concerns the nitroimidazoles (metronidazole or tinidazole) and macrolides (clarithromycin) [38, 39]. Prevalence of *H pylori* resistance to metronidazole is approximately 25% in developing countries, because of the frequent use of nitroimidazoles to treat other diseases% [40, 41]. Increasing the dosage of metronidazole administered (e.g., from 1.0

to 1.5 g/day) generally improves the results of therapy when treating metronidazole-resistant *H.pylori* strains. Resistance to clarithromycin is becoming more prevalent in some European countries, where the prevalence may be as high as 17% [40, 41]. The clinical effect of clarithromycin resistance is essentially complete loss of any clarithromycin anti-*H pylori* effect; outcome of therapy can generally be predicted on the basis of what could be expected if only the other antimicrobials in the regimen are used [39].

4.1. First-line therapy of *H.pylori* infection

First-line *H. pylori* therapy should ideally be short, easy to administer, well tolerated and relatively cheap [42]. However, over and above these considerations, the prime objective of any treatment is to eradicate the infection in the maximum number of patients [43]. Some of the best validated first-line treatments for *H pylori* include amoxicillin or clarithromycin-based triple therapies, which consists of a proton pump inhibitor PPI (standard dose twice daily) combined with clarithromycin (500 mg twice daily) and either amoxicillin (1 g twice daily) or metronidazole (500 mg twice daily) for a minimum of 7 days. Bismuth-based quadruple therapies consisting of a histamine receptor antagonist or PPI combined with bismuth, tetracycline, and metronidazole [42, 43]. Another alternative approach is to include ranitidine bismuth citrate (RBC) in place of a PPI in clarithromycin triple therapy. These regimens have the propensity to eradicate 70 to 85% of the infection. However, the regimen, which employs a PPI with clarithromycin and amoxicillin is the most widely endorsed first-line regimen for *H pylori* [42, 43]. Any of the currently available PPIs may be used with equivalent treatment efficacy [44, 45] with the exception of esomeprazole as it is prescribed once daily because it is imperative that the standard dose of a PPI be prescribed twice daily in order to maximize treatment efficacy [46]. RBC is sometimes used in place of a PPI in countries outside the United States with at least equal and perhaps greater efficacy [47]. Metronidazole can be used as an alternative to amoxicillin, particularly in the setting of penicillin allergy or intolerance [42, 43].

Bismuth-based quadruple therapy is another option in penicillin allergic patients which yields similar eradication rates to clarithromycin triple therapies [48, 49]. A recent meta-analysis including five randomized trials reported intention-to-treat (ITT) and per protocol (PP) eradication rates of 79% and 85% for clarithromycin triple therapy and 80% and 87% for bismuth quadruple therapy, respectively [50]. Recently, simplified twice-daily dosing regimens for bismuth quadruple therapy have been successfully used in clinical trials [51].It is worth noting that the dosing of metronidazole used in the various bismuth quadruple therapies has not been consistent across studies. As higher doses of metronidazole (500 mg) may provide better cure rates than lower doses (250 mg), caution must be exercised when interpreting the data from comparative studies and pooled analyses involving quadruple therapies. Although there is no universal standard, there has been a desire to decrease the duration of therapy, particularly in countries outside the United States where treatment durations of at least 7 days have been recommended [42]. Until very recently, the recommended treatment duration in the United States has been 10–14 days due to lower eradication rates with 7-day regimens [52]. However, a large randomized US trial, rabeprazole-based triple therapy for 7 days was found to be as effective as 10 days of therapy (ITT eradication rates of

77% [71%–83%] vs. 78% [72%–84%], respectively) [53]. Based upon these results, 7-day rabeprazole-based triple therapy has been approved by the Food and Drug Administration for use in the United States. However there is some minor disagreement on the duration of treatment; the US guidelines recommend a 14-day course, whereas in Europe, a 7-day course is considered to be sufficient and Canadian and Asia–Pacific guidelines correspond largely to the Maastricht 2–2000 guidelines [54].

4.2. Second-line therapy of *H.pylori* infection

The choice of second-line treatment depends on which treatment approach was used initially, because retreatment with the same regimen is not recommended. If a clarithromycin-based regimen was used initially, a metronidazole-based regimen should be used as follow-up (in combination with a PPI, tetracycline, and bismuth), and vice versa. Prolonging the treatment period to 14 days is probably necessary. Because bacterial resistance to metronidazole or clarithromycin results primarily from previous treatment failures, first-choice treatment should never combine clarithromycin and metronidazole in the same regimen [55]. Second-line therapy has been extensively reviewed by several authors [55-57]. The assessment of *H pylori* sensitivity to antibiotics may be useful only after failure of the second-line therapy [58]

The most widely recommended second-line treatment for persistent *H pylori* infection is quadruple therapy with a PPI (standard dose twice daily), bismuth salt (subsalicylate or subcitrate 120 mg 4 times daily), metronidazole (500 mg thrice daily) and tetracycline (500 mg 4 times daily) for minimum of 7 days. Further failures should be managed by specialists. The Table 1 summarizes the suggested therapeutic regimens for eradication of *H pylori* infection. No other second-line treatment strategies have been widely endorsed; however, -line therapy should be [59] rifabutin-based triple therapy and furazolidone-based triple therapy [59, 60] have been investigated and suggested as alternatives to bismuth quadruple therapy (Table 1). As second-line therapy, the Maastricht 2-2000 Consensus Report suggests a quadruple therapy based on bismuth (120 mg, q.i.d.), tetracycline (500 mg, q.i.d.), metronidazole (500 mg, t.i.d.) and antisecretive agent (PPI, b.i.d.) for a minimum of 7 days [34]. Further trials have shown that replacing the proton pump inhibitor and the bismuth compound of the quadruple therapy by RBC also achieves good results, with an eradication rate ranging between 57%-95% [61, 62]. The failure of second line quadruple therapy is associated with its discontinuation because of high incidence of side effects (6%-68%) [63]. A triple therapy with the combination of levofloxacin, rabeprazole and tinidazole or amoxicillin has been proposed as an alternative to Maastricht. This protocol shows an eradication rate higher than 90% compared to quadruple therapies given for 7 days (63%) with a lower incidence of side effects [64]. Rifabutin has been shown to have a good eradication rate (87%), if administered at a high dose (300 mg) in combination with amoxicillin and PPI, as compared to quadruple therapy. Wong et al [65] showed that a combination of levofloxacin, rifabutin and rabeprazole has a high efficacy with an eradication rate >90%. Furazolidone is also used to replace metronidazole in quadruple therapy [66]. Different *in vivo* studies have confirmed the efficacy of regimens containing a high-dose furazolidone [200 mg, b.i.d.] as the second-line therapy in patients with metronidazole-resistance [66]. Many other combinations have been used with various rates of success.

Bacterial eradication may fail in up to 40% of cases after the suggested second-line regimens. As a consequence, to treat patients who have already undergone the first- and second-line therapies is a common challenge [67]. A recent rifabutin based triple therapy shown eradication rates of 100 and 87.5 % (Per Protocol and Intention-to-Treat analysis) in primary resistance to clarithromycin and tinidazole and 82.2 and 78.5% in secondary resistance [68].

4.3. Third-line rescue therapy for persistent *H.pylori* infection

Patients who fail both first- and second-line therapy are a clinical challenge. New modified eradication regimes involve the substitution of antibiotics used with other drugs, such as rifabutin, levofloxacin, and furazolidone [58-65] These antibiotics should be considered for third-line treatment. Currently, no widely endorsed treatment regimens are available, for persons with persistent *H.pylori* infection despite two or more previous courses of antibiotics (third-line therapy). A number of third-line regimens such as bismuth quadruple therapy, rifabutin-based triple therapy, levofloxacin-based triple therapy furazolidone-based triple therapy and Doxycycline-based therapy have been investigated and shown in Table 2.

The new fluoroquinolone, levofloxacin, has shown an excellent activity against a variety of Gram-positive and Gram-negative organisms which are resistant to the established agents Matsuzaki et al [69] studied several strains and reported that levofloxacin had an excellent and wide spectrum antibacterial activity compared with other fluoroquinolones and antibiotics tested [69]. A previous study has shown efficacy and safety of levofloxacin based triple therapy in *H.pylori* infection first-line therapy [70]. Recently, Gatta et.al [71] have proposed a third-line treatment after two eradication failed courses without fluoroquinolones, with standard dose of PPIs (b.i.d.), levofloxacin (250 mg, b.i.d.) and amoxicillin (1 g, b.i.d.) for 10 days. The eradications rates of 76.2% and 84.6% according to ITT and PP anlysis, respectively, have been achieved. The levofloxacin-based treatment could eradicate most of the strains (92.3%) which are resistant *in vitro* to both clarithromycin and metronidazole, but susceptible to levofloxacin. Furthermore, this drug combination, successfully employed as rescue therapy, is well tolerated and has no major side-effects [72].

Rifabutin, a spiropiperidyl derivative of rifamycin, has been shown to exhibit high in vitro activity against *H.pylori* [73, 74]. Furthermore, clinical trials have suggested that rifabutin may be a possible candidate for second or third line eradication combination therapy [75]. Furthermore, rifabutin is chemically stable at a wide pH range [74]. Recently, rifabutin-based rescue therapies (twice-daily standard-dose PPI plus amoxicillin 1 g twice daily or levofloxacin 500 mg once daily plus rifabutin 300 mg daily, for 7 days) have been shown to represent an encouraging strategy for eradication failures because they are effective against *H pylori* strains resistant to clarithromycin or metronidazole [75, 76]. However, rifabutin is very costly, and concerns still remain about the widespread use of this drug because of the possibility for accelerating development of drug resistance. Results of a recent study [59] suggest that a 10-day rescue therapy regimen based on the use of rabeprazole (20 mg twice daily) plus amoxicillin (1 g twice daily) plus levofloxacin (500 mg once daily) is more effective than standard quadruple regimen as a second-line option for *H.pylori* eradication. Additionally, a 7-day quadruple-therapy regimen containing amoxicillin and tetracycline has recently been proven

http://dx.doi.org/10.5772/58338

more effective than standard quadruple therapy with metronidazole and tetracycline to rescue failed triple therapy, by overcoming the antimicrobial resistance of *H.pylori* [77-81].

Doxycycline is a widely used tetracycline antibiotic for eradicating several infections. With respect to tetracycline, Doxycycline requires the administration of only two tablets per day, leading to a better compliance in patients undergoing eradication therapies. Furthermore, Heep et.al [82] have found no secondary resistance to doxycycline in *H.pylori* patients who failed one or more eradication therapies. Quadruple regimens represent the most widely used rescue therapy. Induction of metronidazole resistance has suggested a new protocol, namely replacing tetracycline with doxycycline (because it requires the administration of only two tablets per day) and metronidazole with amoxicillin (because its resistance is less 1%), one week quadruple therapy with doxycycline (100 mg, b.i.d.), amoxicillin (1 g, b.i.d.), omeprazole (20 mg, b.i.d.) and bismuth salts (120 mg, two tablets b.i.d). This treatment has proved to be a highly effective third-line 'rescue' therapy, achieving 91% eradication rate in patients harbouring metronidazole and clarithromycin resistant H pylori strains (by ITT analysis) [83]. This regimen shows excellent compliance (99%) with mild side-effects.

1.	Bismuth subsalicylate (120 mg q.i.d) + metronidazole (500 mg t.i.d) + tetracycline (.500 mg q.i.d) + proton pump inhibitor (standard dose b.i.d) for a minimum of 7 days
2.	Levofloxacin (250 mg b.i.d) + amoxicillin (1g mg b.i.d) + proton pump inhibitor (standard dose b.i.d) for 10 days

o.d = once daily; b.i.d = twice daily; t.i.d = three times daily; q.i.d = four times daily

Table 1. Second line therapy regimens of *H.pylori* infection.

1	Rifabutin (300 mg o.d) + amoxicillin (1g b.i.d)+ proton pump inhibitor (standard dose b.i.d) for 10 days
2	Furazolidone 200 mg bid + amoxicillin (1g b.i.d) + proton pump inhibitor (standard dose b.i.d) for 14 days
3	Furazolidone 200 mg bid + tetracycline (1g b.i.d) + proton pump inhibitor (standard dose b.i.d)+ bismuth (140 mg b.i.d) for 7 days
4	Doxycycline (100 mg, b.i.d.) + amoxicillin (1g b..id) + omeprazole (20 mg, b.i.d)+ bismuth salts (120 mg, b.i.d) for 7 days.

o.d = once daily; b.i.d = twice daily; t.i.d = three times daily; q.i.d = four times daily

Table 2. Third line rescue therapy regimens of *H.pylori* infection.

4.4. Failure of therapy

The reasons behind failure of these antibacterial treatments are not very clear, but are likely multifactorial [85-87]. Failure of therapy is most frequently associated with drug resistance and non-compliance, due to complexity of rgimens and associated side effects, e.g., nausea, diarrhea, taste disturbances, mucositis, and pseudo membranous colitis. The continuing emergence of resistance to the conventional antibacterials used to treat *H. pylori* infections is of major concern [85]. Resistance to nitroimidazoles (e.g. metronidazole) is extremely high in the developing world and rates of resistance(>50%) have been described in Western countries [39-41]. Strains of *H. pylori* which are resistant to clarithromycin are also now widespread e.g., 10–17% in most part of Europe [39].

5. Future therapeutic strategies

Resistance in *H. pylori* is anticipated to increase because the currently effective drugs are used to treat many other infections where also develops the drug resistance in body. So there is an urgent need for improvement over current regimens due high resistance over no of antibiotics using in current therapy and moreover current triple and quadruple therapies are may not be desirable for widespread eradication of *H. pylori* infection in future. The next generation of *H.pylori* therapeutic regimens should be simpler, novel and specific. There are some novel approaches available to achieve this goal, such as development of therapeutic vaccine, geonome bsed drug discovery, pathogen –host tissue adhesion inhibitor, and novel site specific drug delivery at specific site of *H.pylori* infection.

5.1. Vaccine development

The success of eradication of *H.pylori* by antibiotic therapy is being hampered by the increasing occurrence of antibiotic resistance *H.pylori* strains and patience compliance. Consequently investigative attention has been focused on development of an effective therapeutic vaccine. From mathematical [88] and animal models [89] of *H. pylori* colonization, the host response has been suggested to play an important role in bacterial growth regulation. Immunization against *H. pylori* may thus be considered as a strategy to deviate the immune response programmed by infection, i.e., the re-direction of a host response from natural infection leading to persistence of infection and gastric disease, to another state in the host response capable of attenuating or eliminating *H. pylori* and its associated gastric inflammatory sequelae. Evidence from both animal models and humans implicate *H. pylori* in the activation of B cell and T cell functions leading to heterogeneous systemic and local antibody responses, lymphoid follicle hyperplasia, and significant recruitment of CD4+and CD8+ T cells [90, 91].

Vaccination against H. pylori has been performed in several animal models. Although several studies showed the benefit of prophylactic as well as therapeutic vaccination in animals, bacterial eradication was not observed in humans [92]. Knockout studies in mice revealed that the Th2 response can be absent but immunization is still possible when using urease as an antigen [93, 94].

A number of novel approaches to delivery of *H. pylori* vaccine have been reported recently. Smythies et.al [95] reported on *H.pylori* vaccination based on a modified polio virus vector where the capsid genes are replaced with *H.pylori* urease B. Poliovirus UreB replicons were co-administered with a recombinant vaccinia virus engineered to express polio virus capsid proteins, resulting in a vaccine which can only undergo one round of infection. Mice which are transgenic for the human poliovirus receptor (C57BL/ 6/DAB) are susceptible to infection with poliovirus via the systemic route. Replicon vaccination resulted in clearance of an established *H.pylori* infection in 73% of mice compared to 31% of vector-immunized controls. Furthermore, immunization prevented an infection from becoming established in 80% of immunized mice. Bacterial ghosts (Gram-negative bacterial cell envelopes, devoid of cytoplasmic envelopes) have also been shown to have good adjuvant properties [96]. *H. pylori* ghosts induced protection in a mouse model without the use of an additional adjuvant, although batch-to-batch variations were observed and improvements are therefore required before this approach could have practical applications [97]. Sodium alginate microbeads have also been tested for controlled release of a model *H. pylori* vaccine [98]. Alginate beads are widely used for encapsulation of drugs, and the mild formulation conditions, and their reported muco-adhesive properties should make them ideal carriers for vaccine antigens. Recombinant urease encapsulated in alginate beads was administered to mice via the subcutaneous, nasal and oral routes. Unexpectedly, only subcutaneous delivery induced a significant antibody response and led to reductions in *H. pylori* colonization (as determined by urease test) indicating that this approach also needs further improvement [98].

DNA vaccines are a potentially attractive approach to vaccination, and a genomic library approach has shown encouraging preliminary results in mice [99]. Two recent studies have investigated the adjuvant properties of CpG motifs in the context of DNA immunization. Interestingly, a prototype immunization construct encoding the UreB subunit which included CpG motifs [100] induced significant increases in the expression of IL-10 and beta-defensins in the gastric mucosa. In an approach that aimed to induce and modulate the immune response by triggering a specific Toll-like receptor (TLR), Sommer et.al [101] immunized C57BL/6 mice with *H. pylori* lysate mixed with a synthetic CpG oligonucleotide targeted at TLR-9 (CpG oligonucleotide 1688). Immunization induced a Th1-biased immune response as expected, and immunized mice had 10-fold reduced levels of *H.pylori* in the gastric mucosa after challenge. Synthetic CpGs have recently been approved for human use as a therapy for genital warts [102], and so given the encouraging results from mice, this approach might also be applicable for a human *H.pylori* vaccine. However, DNA vaccination studies in human volunteers have reported only suboptimal immune responses [103] and it appears that the barriers to DNA uptake may be more difficult to overcome in humans [104]. To return to our original question regarding what we have learned from the mouse model, the data from animal models of *H. pylori* infection support the feasibility of both therapeutic and prophylactic vaccination, for neonates and adults. Furthermore, a variety of routes of application and adjuvants are effective. It is, however, clear that only a better understanding of the underlying immune mechanisms will make it possible to improve efficacy and to address the issue of post immunization gastritis.

5.2. Genome-based drug discovery

The recent availability of the genome sequences of two different isolates of *H.pylori* [105, 106] has provided much stimulus to research aimed at discovering and developing novel therapeutics to eradicate *H. pylori*. *H pylori* is a relatively simple organism with a small genome of *circa* 1.7 × 10^6 nucleotides, varying slightly according to the strain of the organism, and encoding around 1600 genes [107]. Of these, depending on the stringency of the comparison, roughly 55% have homologs of putative known identity in other organisms, while another 10% have database homologs of unknown identity. The remaining 35% are unique to *H pylori* at this time. This complement of 1600-1700 gene contain a relatively small number which encode proteins whose functions are essential to the viability of the bacterium. A genome-based strategy facilitates the expeditious advanced selection of novel lethal targets not used by current antimicrobials, thus providing the opportunity to identify novel classes of antibacterials. In the case of vaccine discovery and development, comparison of two genomes has allowed the identification of a "common set" of *H.pylori* genes, among which genes encode antigens [108].

The principle underlying genome based drug development is to identify those essential proteins which are specific to *H.pylori,* and then to isolate, identify and synthesize a small molecule chemical which inhibits the essential activity of such proteins [105]. This approach is designed both to identify a drug that will work as a monotherapy, which would be specific for *H pylori* and would not interfere with other organisms. In case of *H. pylori* drug discovery, the task is to identify those essential proteins which are specific for and conserved in *H. pylori.* Identification of essentiality involves a process whereby attempts are made to mutate a gene performed using an allelic recombination method via homologous recombination and so" knock-out" its function [106]. If a particular mutant can be generated, the disrupted gene does not code for a biological process that is required for viability in vitro. "Knock-out" mutagenesis experiments with selected members of the "common set" of *H. pylori* genes have allowed the identification of targets for drug discovery in a variety of *H. pylori* physiological functions [107, 108]. These targets include proteins involved in cell envelope synthesis/ integrity, cell division, protein synthesis, nucleic acid biosynthesis, gene expression and regulation, cell metabolism and energetics, as well as proteins encoded by *H. pylori* genes of unknown function [109]. Because many essential proteins are enzymes, it is possible to establish in vitro assays to detect the ability of compounds to interfere with their enzymatic activity. The selected essential protein target is overproduced in *E.coli,* purified, and employed to identify inhibitory compounds by High Throughput Screening [110, 111]. This involves the automated micro assay screening of the ability of large numbers of compounds (>200, 000) to inhibit the enzymatic activity of the target protein. Conformed "hits" are then tested for their ability to selectively kill *H.pylori* in vitro, and to eradicate *H.pylori* infection in an animal model. Lead compounds are subjected to chemical structure-activity relationship studies to improve antibacterial potency and selectivity, as well as solubility, oral bioavailability, duration of action and pharmacokinetic properties [101]. Understanding the mechanism of action of a particular target enzyme or molecular modeling based on three-dimensional crystal structure of the protein, with or without bound inhibitor(s), can be used to facilitate medicinal chemistry studies [112, 113]. As lead compounds are identified, the classical medicinal chemistry and combinatorial chemistry approaches are applied to improve the potency and the desired microbiological properties, with the ultimate goal of producing compounds suitable for human trials.

5.3. Novel drug delivery approaches

One of the reasons for incomplete eradication of *H.pylori* is probably due to the short residence time of antimicrobial agents in stomach so that effective antimicrobial concentration cannot be achieved in the gastric mucus layer or epithelial cell surfaces where *H.pylori* resides [114-116]. Conventional tablets and capsules are, in general used for eradication therapy but these do not remain in stomach for prolonged time therefore it is difficult to reach minimum inhibitory concentration in gastric mucus where *H.pylori* colonize. To overcome the problem, a new concept is proposed based on gstroretentive concept (Floating drug delivery systems and Mucoadhesive drug delivery systems) with site specific drug delivery [117]. It is expected that the topical delivery of narrow spectrum antibiotic through floating and bioadhesive drug delivery system may result in complete removal of organism from stomach.

5.4. Floating drug delivery systems (FDDS)

Floating drug delivery systems have a bulk density less than gastric fluids and so remain buoyant in the stomach without affecting the gastric emptying rate for a prolonged period of time. The FDDS can be divided into effervescent and non-effervescent systems. Effervescent floating dosage forms are matrix type systems prepared with the help of swellable polymers such as methylcellulose and chitosan and various effervescent compounds, such as sodium bicarbonate, tartaric acid, and citric acid. They are formulated in such a way that when comes in contact with the acidic gastric contents, $CO2$ is liberated and gets entrapped in swollen hydrocolloids, which provides buoyancy to the dosage forms. Non-effervescent floating dosage forms use a gel forming or swellable cellulose type of hydrocolloids, polysaccharides, and matrix-forming polymers like polycarbonate, polyacrylate, polymethacrylate, and polystyrene [118]. The formulation method includes a simple approach of thoroughly mixing the drug and the gel-forming hydrocolloid. After oral administration this dosage form swells in contact with gastric fluids and attains a bulk density of < 1. The air entrapped within the swollen matrix imparts buoyancy to the dosage form. The so formed swollen gel-like structure acts as a reservoir and allows sustained release of drug through the gelatinous mass. While the system floats on the gastric contents, the drug is released slowly at the desired rate from the system. After release of drug, the residual system is emptied from the stomach. The FDDS greatly improve the pharmacotherapy of the stomach through local drug release, leading to high drug concentrations at the gastric mucosa for eradicating *H.pylori* from the submucosal tissue of the stomach, making it possible to treat stomach and duodenal ulcers, and gastritis [119-121].

In our previous study [114] we have developed the floating in situ gelling system of amoxicillin and evaluated in vivo efficiency in Mongolian gerbil model, the result indicated that the floating in situ gel has promising potential for eradicating *H.pylori* infection. In this study the gelled solution floated in stomach for >20 h, and *the in vivo H.pylori* clearance efficiency was 10 time more than that of amoxicillin solution in gerbils model.

Yang et al [119] developed a swellable asymmetric triple-layer tablet with floating ability to prolong the gastric residence time of triple drug regimen (tetracycline, metronidazole, and clarithromycin) in *H.pylori*–associated peptic ulcers using hydroxy propyl methyl cellulose

(HPMC) and poly ethylene oxide (PEO) as the rate-controlling polymeric matrix. The design of the delivery system was based on the swellable asymmetric triple-layer tablet approach. Tetracycline and metronidazole were incorporated into the core layer of the triple-layer matrix for controlled delivery, while bismuth salt was included in one of the outer layers for instant release. According to the authors, the aim of such a device was to obtain a simple regimen for a standard triple therapy. Indeed, they obtained *in vitro* a duration of buoyancy and sustained release of metronidazole and tetracycline over prolong time of period. The rapid effect of the device would be due to the rapidly dissolving layer containing the bismuth salt, which disintegrated within 10–15 min in vitro. However, no in vivo data are available concerning the floating characteristics of the drug delivery system or its effect against *H.pylori.*

Umamaheshwari et al (120) developed several drug delivery systems especially designed to improve efficiency against *H.pylori*. In all of them, they used an antiurease drug, acetohydroxamic acid (AHA), as an active agent against the bacterium. *H. pylori* urease hydrolyses urea present in the gastric juice and extracellular fluid to generate ammonia and bicarbonate, which effectively neutralize an acidic pH in its environment [121, 122]. Thus, urease inhibitors hinder the bacterium to protect itself against low pH and avoid thus the problem of treatment of antibiotic-resistant strains [123].

The same authors developed polycarbonate microballoons by an emulsion (o/w) solvent evaporation technique. In vitro (i.e. in simulated gastric fluid) 74% to 85% of microballoons stayed buoyant up to 12 h and exhibited a sustained drug release profile. In vitro and in vivo growth inhibition studies were performed using cultures of *H. pylori* and *H. pylori*-infected Mongolian gerbils, respectively. Microballoons showed 10 times higher anti-*H. pylori* activity compared with AHA solution [124].

Umamaheshwari et al. [125] developed cellulose acetate butyrate coated floating microspheres of cholestyamine for targeting to *H.pylori* infection In vitro (drug release, buoyancy) and in vivo studies (gastric mucoadhesion in the rat stomach) led the authors to conclude that this drug delivery system possessed both floating and bioadhesive properties, and may be successful in the treatment of *H.pylori*. Katayama et al [126] deveolped a susrtained release liquid preparation of ampicillin using sodium alginate for the treatment of *H.pylori* infection. The gastroretentive property of the device was provided by the ability of sodium alginate to form a firm gel when an acid or di-or trivalent metal ions (Ca^{2+}, Ba^{2+}, Sr^{2+}) were added. The authors expected the solution to be able to spread out, adhere to the gastric mucosa, and release the antibiotic continuously (ampicillin). The alginate formulation gelled in stomach and delivered ampicillin locally in stomach and showed significant anti *H.pylori* effect in rat model.

5.5. Mucoadhesive drug delivery systems (MDDS)

Bioadhesive drug delivery systems are used to localize a delivery device within the lumen to enhance the drug absorption in a site-specific manner. Mucoadhesive drug carrier may prolong the residence time of drug in stomach because they adhere to mucus surface, resulting in an effective localizing drug concentration. Mucoadhesion is a very complex process and several theories have been put forward to explain the mechanism, including electrical, adsorption, and wetting and diffusion theories [127]. Because the mucosal surface is negatively charged, a positive charge on polymer might facilitate the mucoadhesion process. Some of the most promising charged excipients used commonly in these systems include polycarbophil, carbopol, lecithins, chitosan, carboxy methyl cellulose and gliadin, etc. Some investigators have tried a synergistic approach between floating and bioadhesion systems [120, 124, 128]. Among the mucoadhesive formulation, mucioadhesive microspheres have gained considerable attention due to their ability to adhere to mucus layer as well as release drugs locally at the infected cell line.

Nagahara et al [128] formulated mucoadhesive microspheres containing amoxicillin. They dispersed the drug and bioadhesive polymers (carboxyvinyl polymer and curdlan [polysaccharide]) in melted hydrogenated castor oil. They compared these microspheres with an amoxicillin suspension in infected Mongolian gerbils under feeding conditions. The microspheres with an amoxicillin dose of 1.0 mg/kg provided the same clearance rate (20%) as the amoxicillin suspension with a dose of 10 mg/kg. This means that the amoxicillin-microspheres provided 10 times greater anti-*H.pylori* activity than the amoxicillin suspension. Moreover, adhesion of microspheres on the stomach wall was observed (°47% and °20% remained in the stomach after 2 and 4 h, respectively). The authors concluded that these mucoadhesive microspheres containing an appropriate antimicrobial agent should be useful for the eradication of *H. pylori*.

Wang et al. [129] studied positively charged gelatin microspheres as gastric mucoadhesive drug delivery system for eradication of *H.pylori*. Umamaheshwari et.al [130] developed nonoparticles bearing amoxicillin using gliadin polymer rand evaluated in-vivo the anti *H.pylori* efficiency of nanoparicles in gerbil model, results were found to be promising molecule to eradicate of *H.pylori* infection. Radiet et.al [131] developed tetracycline-loaded crosslinked chitosan microspheres to increase the local concentration of the antibiotic in the stomach and, thus eradicate *H.pylori* infection. The microspheres were examined for gastric residence time and local tetracycline concentrations in fasted gerbils. The microspheres were found to reside in the stomach even after 10 h of administration.

Recently, Zhepeng et.al [132] also published a study on mucoadhesive microspheres containing amoxicillin by an emulsification/evaporation method, using ethylcellulose as matrix and carbopol 934P as a mucoadhesive polymer. This work showed that free amoxicillin was rapidly degraded in acidic medium; however, amoxicillin entrapped in the microspheres microspheres kept stable. Furthermore, studies on the *in vivo* clearance of *H.pylori* revealed that, in a single-dosage administration, the mucoadhesive microspheres had a better effectiveness than that of amoxicillin powder.Finally this study showed a complete eradication *of H.pylori* with microspheres in five of six rat stomachs, whereas amoxicillin powder showed four times less effectiveness. The authors found a tendency for an effective anti-*H.pylori* activity induced by mucoadhesive microspheres, but concluded that larger groups of animal are required to confirm these results.

Among all the drug delivery approaches (Dosage forms) described herein, some provide interesting solutions, although many of them present drawbacks. In the particular case of *H.pylori* eradication, the ideal dosage form should, to be really effective, not only stay in the stomach, but also target the bacterium. However, knowledge about this pathogen discovered twenty years ago is still poor. More data are necessary, for example, to identify an "ubiquitous" receptor (i.e. for all *H.pylori* strains) at the surface of the bacterium, which could provide a strong interaction with a ligand [133-135]. Thus, the development of an efficient gastroretentive dosage form against *H. pylori* is closely linked to a better understanding of its pathogenicity mechanisms.

6. Conclusion

Considerable advances have been made in understanding the evolution of the organism and pathogenesis of disease. Although combination therapies have high rates of eradication, the preferred therapy would be one which use a low dose of a single drug with a short duration treatment and without any adverse effect. The sequencing of two strains of *H.pylori* has provided a wealth of data that will be useful in understanding the pathogenesis of disease, microbial evolution and highlight potential therapeutic targets and potential vaccine candidates. In future, it is likely to advance understanding of disease progression and aid in the development of novel therapies. First aspect of research is that genomic studies are arousing considerable interest, and will certainly be followed up in future research for development of new therapies. A second area of research that is becoming increasingly important is the development of novel targeted drug delivery systems for *H.pylori* infection. The floating and mucoadhesive formulation of antibacterial drugs have shown good *H. pylori* clarence effect in both *in-vitro* and in-vivo animal model studies. However, extensive clinical studies are required in human to establish a correlation.

Author details

Rajinikanth Siddalingam and Kumarappan Chidambaram

Department of Pharmaceutical Technology, School of Pharmacy, Taylor's University, Subang Jaya, Kuala Lumpur, Malaysia

References

[1] Warren JR, Marshall B. Unidentified curved bacilli on gastric epithelium in active chronic gastritis. Lancet 1983; 11273-1275.

[2] McColl KEL, Murray L, El-Omar E, Dickson A, El-Nujumi A, Wirz A, Kelman A, Penny C, Knill-Jones R, Hilditch T. Symptomatic benefit from eradicating Helicobacter pylori infection in nonulcer dyspepsia. N Engl J Med 1998; 339 1869-1874.

[3] McNamara D, Buckley M, Gilvarry J, O'Morain C. Does Helicobacter pylori eradication affect symptoms in nonulcer dyspepsia: a five-year follow-up study. Helicobacter 2002 ;7, 317-321.

[4] Suerbaum S, Michetti P. *Helicobacter pylori* infections, New Engl J Med 347: 1175–1186, 2002.

[5] Gasbarrini A, Franceschi F, Armuzzi A, Ojetti V, Candelli M, Torre ES, De Lorenzo A, Anti M, Pretolani S, Gasbarrini G. Extradigestive manifestations of *Helicobacter pylori* gastric infection. Gut 1999; 45, 109-I12.

[6] Malaty HM, Graham DY. Importance of childhood socioeconomic status on the current prevalence of *Helicobacter pylori* infection. Gut, 35:742-745, 1994.

[7] Mitchell H, Megraud F, Epidemiology and diagnosis of *Helicobacter pylori* infection, Helicobacter 2002;7, 1-8–16..

[8] Brown, LM, Thomas, TL, Chang, YS.You, WC, Liu, WD,. Zhang, L, Pee, D, Gail, MH. *Helicobacter pylori* infection in rural China: demographic, lifestyle and environmental factors, Int. J. Epidemiol 2002, 31: 638–645.

[9] Howden CW, Hunt RH. Guidelines for the management of *Helicobacter pylori* infection, Am J Gastroenterol 1998;93:2330-2338.

[10] Drumm B, Koletzko S, Oderda G. *Helicobacter pylori* infection in children: a consensus statement. J Pediatr Gastroenterol Nutr 2000; 30, 207-213.

[11] Graham DY, Qureshi WA. Markers of infection. In: Mobley HLT, Mendz GL, Hazell SL, eds, *Helicobacter pylori:* physiology and genetics. Washington, D.C.: ASM Press, 2001 :499-510.

[12] Schmitz A, Josenhans C, Suerbaum S. Cloning and characterisation of the *Helicobacter pylori* flbA gene which codes for a membrane protein involved in coordinated expression of flagellar genes. J Bacteriol 1997; 179, 987-997.

[13] Nilius M, Malfertheiner P. *Helicobacter pylori* enzymes. Aliment Pharmacol Ther 1996; 10(Suppl 1):65-71.

[14] Graham DY, Klein PD, What you should know about the methods, problems, in terpretations and uses of urea breath tests. Am J Gastroenterol 1991; 86, 1118-1122.

[15] Megraud F. Epidemiology of *Helicobacter pylori* infection: where are we in 1995? Eur J Gastroenterol Hepatol 1995 ; 7, 292-295.

[16] Mendal MA, Goggin PM, Molineaus N, Childhood living conditions and *Helicobacter pylori* seropositivity in adult life. Lancet, 1995 ;332: 896-897.

[17] Noach LA, Rolf TM, Bosma NB. Gastric metaplasia and *Helicobacter pylori* infection. Gut 1993; 34, 1510-1514.

[18] Rahman MM, Mahalanabis D, Sarker SA, Bardhan PK, Alvarez JO, Hildebrand P, Beglinger C, Gyr K. *Helicobacter pylori* colonization in infants and young children is not necessarily associated with diarrhea. J Trop. Pediatr 1998; 44, 283–287.

[19] Robert WF, John C, Helicobacter in the developing world. Microbes and Infection 2003; 5, 705–713.

[20] Dunn BE, Cohen H, Blaser MJ. *Helicobacter pylori*, Clin. Microbiol. Rev, 1997; 10, 720–741.

[21] Go MF. Review article: natural history and epidemiology of *Helicobacter pylori* infection. Aliment Pharmacol. Therapeutics, 2002; 16 (1) 3–15.

[22] Bardhan PK. Epidemiological features of *Helicobacter pylori* infection in developing countries. Clin. Infect. Dis 1997; 25, 973–978.

[23] Lindkvist P, Enquselassie F, Asrat D, Muhe L, Nilsson I, Giesecke J. Risk factors for infection with *Helicobacter pylori*—a study of children in rural Ethiopia. Scand J Infect Dis 1998;30, 371–376.

[24] Mobley HLT. *Helicobacter pylori* urease. In: Achtman M, Suerbaum S, eds, *Helicobacter pylori:* molecular and cellular biology. Wymondham, United Kingdom: Horizon Scientific Press 2001; 155-1570.

[25] Weeks DL, Eskandari S, Scott DR, Sachs G. A H+-gated urea channel: the link between *Helicobacter pylori* urease and gastric colonization. Science 2000;28, 482-485.

[26] Josenhans C, Suerbaum S, *Helicobacter* motility and chemotaxis. In: Achtman M, Suerbaum S, eds. *Helicobacter pylori:* molecular and cellular biology. Wymondham, United Kingdom: Horizon Scientific Press, 2001; 171-184.

[27] Ilver D, Arnqvist A, Ogren J. *Helicobacter pylori* adhesin binding fucosylated histo-blood group antigens revealed by retagging. Science 1998; 279, 373-377.

[28] Rogha M, Nikvarz M, Poumoghaddas Z, Shirneshan K, Dadkhah D, Pourmoghaddas M. Is helicobacter pylori infection a risk factor for coronary heart disease?. ARYA Atheroscler 2012; 8(1): 5-8.

[29] Rogha M, Dadkhah D, Poumoghaddas Z, Shirneshan K, Poumoghaddas M. Association of Helicobacter pylori infection with severity of coronary heart disease et al. ARYA Atheroscler 2012; 7(4): 138-41.

[30] Saad R, Chey WD. A clinician's guide to managing Helicobacter pylori infection. Cleve Clin J Med 2005;72(1) 109-118.

[31] McCarthy C, Patchett S, Collins RM. Long-term prospective study of *Helicobacter pylori* in non-ulcer dyspepsia. Dig Dis Sci 1995', 40, 114-119.

[32] Miehlke S, Bayerdorffer E, Graham DY. Treatment of *Helicobacter pylori* infection. Semin Gastrointest Dis 2001; (1), 167–179.

[33] Ricci V, Zarrilli R, Romano M. Voyage of *Helicobacter pylori* in human stomach: odyssey of a bacterium. Dig Liver Dis 2002; 34 (1)2–8.

[34] Graham DY. Therapy of *Helicobacter pylori*: current status and issues. Gastroenterology 2000; 118, S2–8.

[35] Mégraud F, O'Morain C, Malfertheiner P. on behalf of the Working Party of the European *Helicobacter pylori* Study Group. Guidelines for clinical trials in *Helicobacter*

pylori infection. Statistical annex: statistical aspects of clinical trials in *Helicobacter pylori* infection. Gut 1997; 41, S19–23.

[36] Gerrits MM, Schuijffel D, van Zwet AA, Kuipers EJ, Vandenbroucke-Grauls CM, Kusters JG. Alterations in penicillin-binding protein 1A confer resistance to beta-lactam antibiotics in Helicobacter pylori. *Antimicrob Agents Chemother2002;* 46, 2229–2233.

[37] Kwon DH, Kim JJ, Lee M, et al. Isolation and characterization of tetracycline-resistant clinical isolates of Helicobacter pylori. *Antimicrob Agents Chemother 2000;* 44, 203–3205.

[38] Megraud F. Epidemiology and mechanism of antibiotic resistance in Helicobacter pylori. *Gastroenterology 1998;* 115:1272–1278.

[39] Huang J, Hunt RH. The importance of clarithromycin dose in the management of Helicobacter pylori infection: a meta-analysis of triple therapies with a proton pump inhibitor, clarithromycicn and amoxicillin or metronidazole. *Aliment Pharmacol Ther 1999;* 13:719–729.

[40] Iovene MR, Romano M, Pilloni AO, et al. Prevalence of antimicrobial resistance in eighty clinical isolates of Helicobacter pylori. *Chemotherapy 1999;* 45, 8–14.

[41] Debets-Ossenkopp YJ, Herscheid AJ, Pot RG, Kuipers EJ, Kusters JG, Vanderbroucke-Grauls CM. Prevalence of Helicobacter pylori resistance to metronidazole, clarithromycin, amoxicillin, tetracycline and trovafloxacin in The Netherlands. *J Antimicrob Chemother 1999;* 43:415–511.

[42] Malfertheiner P, Megraud F, O'Morain C, Hungin AP, Jones R, Axon A, Graham DY, Tytgat G. Current concepts in the management of Helicobacter pylori infection, the Maastricht 2-2000 Consensus Report. Aliment Pharmacol Ther 2002;, 16:167-180.

[43] Coelho LG, Leon-Barua R, Quigley EM. Latin-American Consensus Conference on Helicobacter pylori infection. Latin-American National Gastroenterological Societies affiliated with the Inter-American Association of Gastroenterology (AIGE). Am J Gastroenterol 2000; 95, 2688-2691, 2000.

[44] Ulmer HJ, Beckerling A, Gatz G. Recent use of proton pump inhibitor-based triple therapies for the eradication of H pylori: a broad data review. Helicobacter 2003; 8, 95-104.

[45] Vergara M, Vallve M, Gisbert JP, Calvet X. Meta-analysis: comparative efficacy of different proton-pump inhibitors in triple therapy for Helicobacter pylori eradication.Aliment Pharmacol Ther 2003;18:647-654.

[46] Vallve M, Vergara M, Gisbert JP, Calvet X. Single vs. double dose of a proton pump inhibitor in triple therapy for Helicobacter pylori eradication: a meta-analysis. Aliment Pharmacol Ther 2002; 16:1149-1156.

[47] Buzas GM, Jozan J. Eradication of Helicobacter pylori infection in Europe: a meta-analysis based on congress abstracts, 1997-2002. Orv Hetil 2002; 145:2035-2041.

[48] Fischbach LA, van Zanten S, Dickason J. Meta-analysis: the efficacy, adverse events, and adherence related to first-line anti-Helicobacter pylori quadruple therapies. Aliment Pharmacol Ther 2004 ; 20, 1071-1082.

[49] Gene E, Calvet X, Azagra R, Gisbert JP. Triple vs. quadruple therapy for treating Helicobacter pylori infection: a meta-analysis. Aliment.Pharmacol.Ther 2003; 17:1137-1143.

[50] Gene E, Calvet X, Azagra R, Gisbert JP. Triple vs quadruple therapy for treating Helicobacter pylori infection: an updated meta-analysis. Aliment. Pharmacol.Ther 2003;18, 543-544.

[51] Graham DY, Belson G, Abudayyeh S, Osato MS, Dore MP, El-Zimaity HM. Twice daily (mid-day and evening) quadruple therapy for *H. pylori* infection in the United States. Dig Liver Dis 2004 ;36:384-387.

[52] Howden CW, Hunt RH. Guidelines for the management of Helicobacter pylori infection. Ad Hoc Committee on Practice Parameters of the American College of Gastroenterology. Am J Gastroenterol 1998;93:2330-2338.

[53] Vakil N, Lanza F, Schwartz H, Barth J. Seven-day therapy for Helicobacter pylori in the United States. Aliment Pharmacol Ther, 2004;20, 99-107.

[54] Suerbaum S, Michetti P. *Helicobacter pylori* infection. N Engl J Med 2002; 347(15) 1175-1186.

[55] Peitz U, Sulliga M, Wolle K, et al. High rate of post-therapeutic resistance after failure of macrolide-nitroimidazole triple therapy to cure Helicobacter pylori infection: impact of two second-line therapies in a randomised study. *Aliment Pharmacol Ther 2002;*16:315–324.

[56] McLoughlin RM, O'Morain CA, O'Connor HJ. Eradication of *Helicobacter pylori*: recent advances in treatment. Fundam Clin Pharmacol 2005; 19: 421-427.

[57] Gisbert JP, Pajares JM. Review article: *Helicobacter pylori* 'rescue' regimen when proton pump inhibitor-based triple therapies fail. Aliment Pharmacol Ther 2003;16:1047-1057.

[58] Bilardi C, Dulbecco P, Zentilin P, Reglioni S, Iiritano E, Parodi A, Accornero L, Savarino E, Mansi C, Mamone M, Vigneri S, Savarino V. A 10-day levofloxacinbased therapy in patients with resistant Helicobacter pylori infection: a controlled trial. Clin Gastroenterol Hepatol 2004;2:997-1002.

[59] Nista EC, Candelli M, Cremonini F, Cazzato IA, Di Caro S, Gabrielli M, Santarelli L, Zocco MA, Ojetti V, Carloni E, Cammarota G, Gasbarrini G, Gasbarrini A. Levofloxacin-based triple therapy vs. quadruple therapy in second-line Helicobacter pylori treatment: a randomized trial. Aliment Pharmacol Ther2003;, 18:627-633.

[60] Perri F, Festa V, Clemente R, Villani MR, Quitadamo M, Caruso N, Bergoli ML, Andriulli A. Randomized study of two "rescue" therapies for Helicobacter

pyloriinfected patients after failure of standard triple therapies. Am J Gastroenterol 2001; 96:58-62.

[61] Zullo A, Hassan C, Campo SM, Lorenzetti R, Febbraro I, De Matthaeis M, Porto D, Morini S. A triple therapy regimen after failed *Helicobacter pylori* treatments. Aliment Pharmacol Ther 2001; 15: 1193-1197.

[62] Michopoulos S, Tsibouris P, Bouzakis H, Balta A, Vougadiotis J, Broutet N, Kralios N. Randomized study comparing omeprazole with ranitidine as anti-secretory agents combined in quadruple second-line *Helicobacter pylori* eradication regimens. Aliment Pharmacol Ther 2000; 14: 737-744.

[63] Gomollon F, Ducons JA, Ferrero M, Garcia Cabezudo J, Guirao R, Simon MA, Montoro M. Quadruple therapy is effective for eradicating *Helicobacter pylori* after failure of triple proton-pump inhibitor-based therapy: a detailed, prospective analysis of 21 consecutive cases. *Helicobacter* 1999; 4: 222-225.

[64] Watanabe Y, Aoyama N, Shirasaka D, Maekawa S, Kuroda K, Miki I, Kachi M, Fukuda M, Wambura C, Tamura T, Kasuga M.Levofl oxacin based triple therapy as a second-line treatment after failure of *helicobacter pylori* eradication with standard triple therapy. Dig Liver Dis 2003; 35: 711-715.

[65] Wong WM, Gu Q, Lam SK, Fung FM, Lai KC, Hu WH, Yee YK, Chan CK, Xia HH, Yuen MF, Wong BC. Randomized controlled study of rabeprazole, levofl oxacin and rifabutin triple therapy vs. quadruple therapy as second-line treatment for *Helicobacter pylori* infection. Aliment Pharmacol Ther 2003; 17:553-560.

[66] Ebrahimi-Dariani N, Mirmomen S, Mansour-Ghanaei F, Noormohammadpoor P, Sotodehmanesh R, Haghpanah B, Bahrami H. The efficacy of furazolidone-based quadruple therapy for eradication of *Helicobacter pylori* infection in Iranian patients resistant to metronidazole-based quadruple therapy. Med Sci Monit 2003: 9: PI105-PI108.

[67] Isakov V, Domareva I, Koudryavtseva L, Maev I, Ganskaya Z. Furazolidone-based *pylori* resistant to metronidazole. Aliment Pharmacol Ther 2002; 16:1277-1282.

[68] Toracchioa S, Capodicasab S, Sorajac DB, Cellinic L, Marziob L. Rifabutin based triple therapy for eradication of *H. pylori* primary and secondary resistant to tinidazole and clarithromycin. Digestive Liver Disease 2005;37: 33–38.

[69] Matsuzaki K, Koyama H, Chiba A, Omika K, Harada S, Sato Y, et.al. In vitro activities of levofloxacin and other antibiotics against fresh clinical isolates. Jpn J Antibiot 1999;52:571–84.

[70] Cammarota G, Cianci R, Cannizzaro O, Cuoco L, Pirozzi Gasbarrini A, et al. Efficacy of two one-week rabeprazole /levofloxacin-based triple therapies for *Helicobacter pylori* infection. Aliment Pharmacol Ther 2000; 14:1339–43.

[71] Gatta L, Zullo A, Perna F, Ricci C, De Francesco V, Tampieri A, Bernabucci V, Cavina M, Hassan C, Ierardi E, Morini S, Vaira D. A 10-day levofl oxacin-based triple therapy

in patients who have failed two eradication courses. Aliment Pharmacol Ther 2005; 22: 45-49.

[72] Zullo A, Hassan C, De Francesco V, Lorenzetti R, Marignani M, Angeletti S, Ierardi E, Morini S. A third-line levofloxacinbased rescue therapy for *Helicobacter pylori* eradication. Dig Liver Dis 2003; 35: 232-236.

[73] Kunin CM. Antimicrobial activity of rifabutin. Clin Infect Dis 1996;22 :1:S3–13.

[74] Heep M, Beck D, Bayerdorffer E, Lehn N. Rifampin and rifabutin resistance mechanism in *Helicobacter pylori*. Antimicrob Agents Chemother 1999;43:1497–1499.

[75] Perri F, Festa R, Clemente R, Quitadamo M, Andriulli A. Rifabutin-based "rescue therapy" for *Helicobacter pylori* infected patients after failure of standard regimens. Aliment Pharmacol Ther 2000;14:311–316.

[76] Wong WM, Gu Q, Lam SK, et al. Randomized controlled study of rabeprazole, levofloxacin and rifabutin triple therapy vs quadruple therapy as second-line treatment for Helicobacter pylori infection. *Aliment Pharmacol Ther 2003;*17:553–560.

[77] Chi CH, Lin C-Y, Sheu B-S, Yang H-B, Huang A-H, Wu J-J. Quadruple therapy containing amoxicillin and tetracycline is an effective regimen to rescue failed triple therapy by overcoming the antimicrobial resistance of Helicobacter pylori. *Aliment Pharmacol Ther 2003;* 18:347–353.

[78] Gisbert JP, Calvet X, Bujanda L, Marcos S, Gisbert JL, Pajares JM. "Rescue" therapy with rifabutin after multiple *Helicobacter pylori* treatment failures. *Helicobacter,* 2003;8: 90-94.

[79] Canducci F, Ojetti V, Pola P, Gasbarrini G, Gasbarrini A. Rifabutin-based *Helicobacter pylori* eradication 'rescue therapy'.Aliment Pharmacol Ther 2001; 15: 143-149.

[80] Borody TJ, Pang G, Wettstein AR, Clancy R, Herdman K, Surace R, Llorente R, Ng C. Efficacy and safety of rifabutincontaining 'rescue therapy' for resistant *Helicobacter pylori* infection. Aliment Pharmacol Ther 2006; 23: 481-488.

[81] Kwon DH, Lee M, Kim JJ, Kim JG, El-Zaatari FA, Osato MS, Graham DY. Furazolidone- and nitrofurantoin-resistant *Helicobacter pylori*: prevalence and role of genes involved in metronidazole resistance. Antimicrob Agents Chemother 2001; 45:306-308.

[82] Heep M, Kist M, Strobel S, Beck D, Lehn N. Secondary resistance among 554 isolates of *Helicobacter pylori* after failure of therapy. Eur J Clin Microbiol Infect Dis 2000; 19: 538-541.

[83] Xiao SD, Liu WZ, Hu PJ, Ouyang Q, Wang JL, Zhou LY, Cheng NN. A multicentre study on eradication of *Helicobacter pylori* using four 1-week triple therapies in China. Aliment Pharmacol Ther 2001;15: 81-86.

[84] Qasim A, Sebastian S, Thornton O, Dobson M, McLoughlin R, Buckley M, O'Connor H, O'Morain C. Rifabutin- and furazolidone- based *Helicobacter pylori* eradication therapies after failure of standard first- and second-line eradication attempts in dyspepsia patients. Aliment Pharmacol Ther 2005; 21: 91-96.

[85] Cammarota G, Martino A, Pirozzi G, Cianci R, Branca G, Nista EC, Cazzato A, Cannizzaro O, Miele L, Grieco A, Gasbarrini A, Gasbarrini G. High effi cacy of 1-week doxycycline- and amoxicillin- based quadruple regimen in a culture-guided, third-line treatment approach for *Helicobacter pylori* infection. AlimentPharmacol Ther 2004; 19: 789-795.

[86] Pipkin, GA, Dixon JS, Williamson R, Wood JR.Clarithromycin dual therapy regimens for eradication of *Helicobacter pylori*. Helicobacter, 1997; 159-171.

[87] Megraud F. Resistance of *Helicobacter pylori* to antibiotics: the main limitation of current proton-pump inhibitor triple therapy. Eur J Gastroenterol Hepatol 1999; 11 (2) S35–37.

[88] Vaira D, Ali A, Gatta L, O'Morain C. Treatment of *Helicobacter pylori*. Curr Opin Gastroent 1999;14 (1) S71–78.

[89] Lind T, Megraud F, Unge P,. The MACH2 Study: role of omeprazole in eradication of *Helicobacter pylori* with 1-week triple therapies. Gastroenterology 1999;116: 248–253.

[90] Wang J, Tauchi Y, Deguchi Y, Morimotov K, Tabata Y, Ikada Y. Positively charged gelatin microspheres as gastric mucoadhesive drug delivery system for eradication of *H. pylori*,. Drug Delivery 2003 ; 7(4) : 237– 243.

[91] Blaser MJ, Kirschner D. Dynamics of *Helicobacter pylori* colonization in relation to the host response. Proc Natl Acad Sci USA 1999; 96: 8359–8364.

[92] Dubois A, Berg DE, Incecik ET, Fiala N,. Host specificity of *Helicobacter pylori* strains and host responses in experimentally challenged nonhuman primates. Gastroenterology 1999; 116: 90–96.

[93] Fox JG, Perkins S, Yan L,. Local immune response in *Helicobacter pylori* infected cats and identi. cation of *H. pylori* in saliva, gastric fluid and faeces. Immunology 1996;88: 400–406.

[94] Wotherspoon AC, Doglioni C, Diss TC. Regression of primary low grade B cell gastric lymphoma of mucosa-associated lymphoid tissue after eradication of *Helicobacter pylori*. Lancet 1993; 342: 575–577.

[95] Smythies, LE., Novak, MJ., Waites, KB., Lindsey, JR., Morrow, CD., Smith, PD. Poliovirus replicons encoding the B subunit of *Helicobacter pylori* urease protect mice against *H. pylori* infection. Vaccine 2005; 23: 901–909.

[96] Hoffelner, H., Haas, R. Recombinant bacterial ghosts: versatile targeting vehicles and promising vaccine candidates. Int J Med Microbiol 2004; 294:303–311.

[97] Panthel, K, Jechlinger, W, Matis, A, Rohde, M, Szostak, M, Lubitz, W, Haas, R Generation of Helicobacter pylori ghosts by PhiX protein E-mediated inactivation and their evaluation as vaccine candidates. Infect Immun 2003b; 71: 109–116.

[98] Leonard, M, De Boisseson, MR, Hubert, P, Dalencon, F, Dellacherie, E Hydrophobically modified alginate hydrogels as protein carriers with specific controlled release properties. J Control Release, 2004; 98: 395–405.

[99] Dzwonek, A, Mikula, M, Woszczynski, M, Hennig, E, Ostrowski, J. Protective effect of vaccination with DNA of the *H. pylori* genomic library in experimentally infected mice. Cell Mol Biol Lett 2004; 9: 483–495.

[100] Hatzifoti, C, Bajaj-Elliott, M, Dorrell, N, Anyim, M, Prentice, MB, Nye, KE, Wren, B, Morrow, WJ. A plasmid immunization construct encoding urease B of *Helicobacter pylori* induces an antigen-specific antibody response and upregulates the expression of betadefensins and IL-10 in the stomachs of mmunized mice. Vaccine 2004; 22: 2651–2659.

[101] Sommer, F., Wilken, H., Faller, G., Lohoff, M. Systemic Th1 immunization of mice against Helicobacter pylori infection with CpG oligodeoxynucleotides as adjuvants does not protect from infection but enhances gastritis. Infect Immun 2004;72: 1029–1035.

[102] Garland, SM. Imiquimod. Curr Opin Infect Dis 2003; 16: 85–89.

[103] Wang R, Epstein, J, Charoenvit Y, Baraceros FM, Rahardjo N, Hoffman SL. Induction in humans of CD8+ and CD4+ Tcell and antibody responses by sequential immunization with malaria DNA and recombinant protein. J Immunol 2004;172: 5561–5569.

[104] Manoj S, Griebel PJ, Babiuk LA, van Drunen Littel-van den Hurk S. Modulation of immune responses to bovine herpesvirus-1 in cattle by immunization with a DNA vaccine encoding glycoprotein D as a fusion protein with bovine CD154. Immunology 2004;112: 328–338.

[105] Alm RA, Ling L-SL, Moir DT, ae.al. Genomic –sequence comparision of two unrelated isolates of human gastric pathogen Helicobacter pylori. Nature 1999; 397: 176-180.

[106] McClain MS, Shaffer CL, Israel DA, Peek RM Jr, Cover TL. Genome sequence analysis of Helicobacter pylori strains associated with gastric ulceration and gastric cancer BMC Genomics. 2009; 5;10-3

[107] Tomb JF, White O, Kerlavage AR. The complete genome sequence of the gastric pathogen Helicobacter pylori. Nature 1997;, 388:539-547.

[108] Axon, A T R. Treatment of Helicobacter pylori: future therapeutic and prophylactic perspectives. *Gut* 1998;43;70-73.

[109] Tatusov RL., Koonin EV, Lipman.D.J. A genomic perspective on protein families. Science 1997;278:631–637.

[110] Beier, D, Frank R. Molecular characterization of two-component systems of *Helicobacter pylori*. J Bacteriol 2000;182:2068–2076.

[111] Bereswill S, Lichte F, Greiner S, Waidner B, Fassbinder F, Kist N. The ferric uptake regulator (Fur) homologue of *Helicobacter pylori*: functional analysis of the coding gene and controlled production of the recombinant protein in *Escherichia coli*. Med Microbiol Immunol 1999;188:31–40.

[112] Dorrell N, Wren, BW. Helicobacter pylori research from genes to genome biology: a new era in. *Gut 1998;* 42;451-453.

[113] Donald T. Moir 1, Karen J, Roberta S, Gerald F. Vovis1 Genomics and Antimicrobial Drug Discovery. Antimicrob. Agents Chemother 1999;43:3:439–446.

[114] Rajinikanth PS and Mishra B. Floating in situ gelling system for stomach site-specific delivery of clarithromycin to eradicate *H. pylori*. J. Contr. Rel 2008; 4(1), 33-41.

[115] P.S.Rajinikanth, and B.Mishra, Development and in vitro evaluation of floating in situ gelling system of acethydroxamic acid for clearance of *H.pylori*. Drug. Dev. Ind. Pharm 2008;34, 577-584.

[116] Shah S, Qaqish R, Patel V, Amiji M. Evaluation of the factors influencing stomach-specific delivery of antibacterial agents for *Helicobacter pylori* infection. J. Pharm Pharmacol 1999; 51: 667–672.

[117] Yokel RA, Dickey KM, Goldberg AH. Selective adherence of a sucralfate-tetracycline complex to gastric ulcers: implications for the treatment of *Helicobacter pylori*. Biopharm Drug Dispos 1995; 16: 475–479.

[118] Myung-Kwan C, Hongkee S, Hoo-Kyun C. Preparation of mucoadheive microspheres containing antimicrobial agents for eradication of *H.pylori*. Int J Pharm 2005; 297 : 172-179.

[119] Yang L, Eshrafh J, Fassihi R. A new intragastric delivery system for the treatment *of Helicobacter pylori* associated gastric ulcer: in vitro evaluation. J Contr Rel 1999; 57: 215-225.

[120] Umamaheshwari RB, Jain S, Bhadra D, Jain NK. Floating microspheres bearing acetohydroxamic acid for the treatment of Helicobacter pylori. J Pharm. Pharmacol 2003;55 :12: 1607– 1613.

[121] P.S.Rajinikanth, and B.Mishra, Development and evaluation of floating–mucoadhesive microspheres of clarithromycin for eradication of *H.pylori*. Chem. Pharm. Bull 2008;52(12), 45-53.

[122] P.S.Rajinikanth, J.Balasubramaniam and B.Mishra Development and evaluation of a novel floating in situ gelling system of amoxicillin for eradication of *H.pylori.* International Journal of Pharmaceutics 2007; 335, 114-122.

[123] P.S.Rajinikanth and B.Mishra, Preparation and In Vitro Characterization of Gellan based Floating Beads of Acetohydroxamic Acid for Eradication of *H.pylori.*, Acta Pharmaceutica 2007; 57 (1), 413–427.

[124] Umamaheshwari RB Jain S, Tripathi PK, Agrawal GP, Jain NK. Floating-bioadhesive microspheres containing acetohydroxamic acid for clearance of Helicobacter pylori, Drug Deliv 9 :4 :223– 231, 2002.

[125] Umamaheshwari RB, Jain S, Jain JK. Anew approach in gastroretentive drug delivery system using cholestyramine. Drug delivery 2003;1(10):151-160.

[126] Kattayama H, Nishimura T, Ochi S, Tsuruta Y,. Sustained release liquid preparation using sodium alginate for eradication of *Helicobacter pylori*.. Bio Pharm Bull 1999; 55-60.

[127] Park H, Rabinson JR. Mechanism of bioadhesion of poly(acrylic acid) hydrogels. Pharm Res 1987; 4 : 457-464.

[128] Nagahara N, Akiyama Y, Nakao M, Tada M, Kitano M, Ogawa Y. Mucoadhesive microspheres containing amoxicillin for clearance of *Helicobacter pylori*. Antimicrob Agents Chemother 1998;42 : 2492–2494.

[129] Wang J, TabataY, Bi D, Morimoto K. Evaluation of gastric mucoadhesive properties of aminated gelatin microspheres. J Contr Rel 2002; 73 : 223–231.

[130] Umamaheshwar RB, Ramteke S, Jain JK. Anti–*Helicobacter Pylori* Effect of mucoadhesive nanoparticles bearing amoxicillin in experimental gerbils model., AAPS PharmSci Tech 2004;, 5 (2) Article 32.

[131] Radi H, Mansoor A. Stomach anti *H.pylori* therapy I: Preparation and characterization of tetracycline – loaded chitosan microspheres. Int J Pharm 2002; 235 : 87-94.

[132] Zhepeng L, Weiyue L, Quian L, Xuhui Z, Pengyun Z. In vitro and in vivo studies on mucoadgesive microspheres of amoxicillin. J Contr Rel 2002;102 :135-144.

[133] Osaki T, Yamaguchi H, Taguchi H, Fukada M, Kawakami H, Hirano H, Kamiya S. Interleukin-8 induction and adhesion of the coccoid form of *Helicobacter pylori*. J Med Microbiol 2002;51 :4: 295– 299.

[134] Sisto F, Brenciaglia MI, Scaltrito MM, Dubini F. *Helicobacter pylori*: ureA, cagA and vacA expression during conversion to the coccoid form. Int J Antimicrob Agents 2000;15 (4)277–282.

[135] Khin, MM, Hua JS, Ng HC, Wadstrom T, Bow H. Agglutination of Helicobacter pylori coccoids by lectins. World J Gastroenterol 2000;6(2)202– 209.

Chapter 11

Floating Drug Delivery Systems for Eradication of *Helicobacter pylori* in Treatment of Peptic Ulcer Disease

Yousef Javadzadeh and Sanaz Hamedeyazdan

Additional information is available at the end of the chapter

http://dx.doi.org/10.5772/57353

1. Introduction

Peptic ulcer (gastric or duodenal ulcer) is one of the most common disorders affecting the gastrointestinal system. The lifetime cumulative incidence of peptic ulcer disease is more than 10% of adult population in western countries (Ofman et al., 2000). The pathophysiology of peptic ulcer disease is an imbalance between mucosal defense factors (bicarbonate, mucin, prostaglandin, nitric oxide and other peptides and growth factors) and injurious factors (acid and pepsin). The management and prevention of these acid-related disorder are possible either by decreasing the level of gastric acidity or by enhancing mucosal protection (Brunton et al., 2008). Various factors, including genetic, diet, pharmacologic and psychologic might contribute to peptic ulcers (Wyatt, 1989). *Helicobacter pylori* (*H. pylori*) is a prominent etiologic factor influencing peptic ulcer disease (Hauser et al., 2005). Regarding the fact that *H. pylori* play a dominant role in the majority of peptic ulcers, prevention of relapse is focused on eradication of this organism from the stomach.

Nowadays it is believed that, *H. pylori* and non-steroidal anti-inflammatory drugs (NSAID) are the two major contributing factors causing peptic ulcer disease (Graham, 1996). *H. pylori* is found in approximately 100% of chronic active antral gastritis cases; 90% to 95% of duodenal ulcer patients and 50% to 80% of gastric ulcer patients (Kluwer, 2004). Owing to the fact that chronic infection with *H. pylori* weakens the natural defenses of the lining of the stomach against the ulcerating action of acid, medications that neutralize stomach acid, antacids, and medications that decrease the secretion of acid in the stomach such as H_2-blockers and proton pump inhibitors (PPIs) have been used effectively for many years to treat ulcers. Obviously, antacids, H_2-blockers and PPIs not only would have no effect on *H. pylori* eradication from the stomach, but also the ulcers are frequently returned promptly after these medications are discontinued. Accordingly, eradication of *H. pylori* also is important in the treatment of the pylori-related ulcers which could be achieved through the commonly used antibiotics.

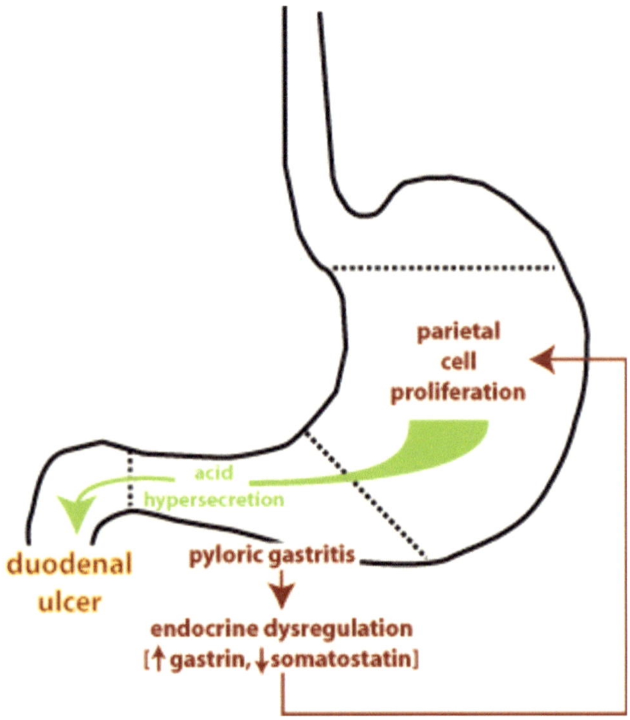

Figure 1. *H. pylori* in peptic ulcers.

Not surprisingly, the wide range of effective medicinal agents available today is one of the greatest scientific achievements. Regardless of the effectiveness and safety of the medicines embedded in dosage forms, the pharmaceutical concept of the latter is growing to be ever more eminent in the management of different diseases. The oral dosage forms of the medications available for *H. pylori* eradication, typically, possess several physiological restrictions such as non-uniform drug absorption profiles, incomplete drug release and shorter residence time of the dosage form in the stomach (MotlekarYouan, 2006; Adibkia et al., 2011; GisbertCalvet, 2011). Rate of the transition for a dosage form through the gastrointestinal (GI) tract is highly affected by the physiological properties of the GI tract as well as the formulation properties (Bardonnet et al., 2006a; Khobragade et al., 2009). Hence, suitable pharmaceutical dosage forms in *H. pylori* eradication is also an important basic principle of the drug delivery system dominating these constraints and offering a proper delivery strategy that would function independent of the digestive state, clinical condition, or GI motility of the individual. Since the bioavailability of drugs often depends on the GI transit rate of the dosage form, it appears necessary to establish an appropriate sustained release system for drug delivery (Hu et al., 2010; JavadzadehHamedeyazdan, 2012).

http://dx.doi.org/10.5772/57353

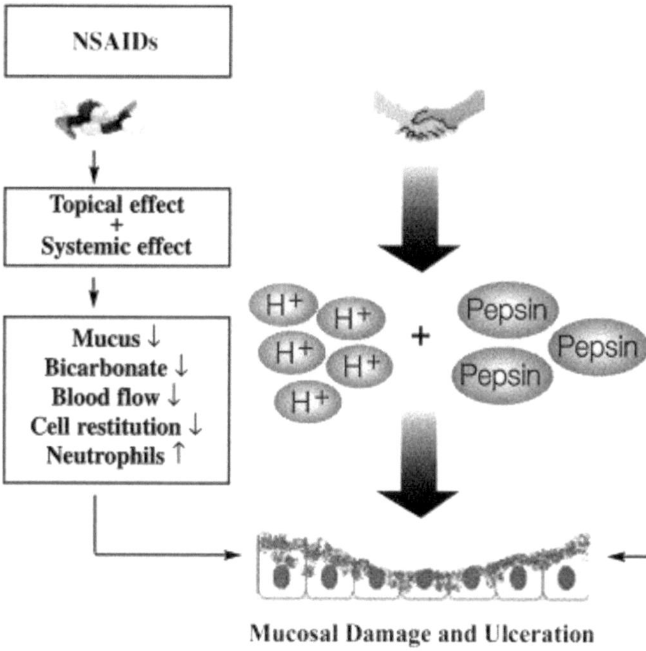

Figure 2. Major factors causing mucosal damage and ulceration (Peura, 2004).

2. Prolongation of GI retention

Scientific and technological advancements have been made in the research and development of different types of drug delivery systems. Keeping up with the rapid development in designing novel drug delivery systems, it is advisable to explore the existing delivery concept and new intra gastric delivery systems which would be expected to overcome the current medication limitations of the treatment of *H. pylori* associated peptic ulcer. It is obvious that formulating dosage forms that retained in the stomach for a prolonged and predictable period of time seem to be advantageous in *H. pylori* eradication.

The most feasible method for achieving a prolonged and predictable drug delivery in the GI tract is to control the gastric residence time by gastro retentive and sustained release dosage forms that have some beneficial in safety and efficacy over normal release systems. This method of application is especially helpful in delivery of sparingly soluble and insoluble drugs used in *H. pylori* eradication. It is acknowledged that, as the solubility of a drug decreases, the time available for drug dissolution becomes less adequate and so the transit time becomes an important factor affecting drug absorption in drugs with lower solubility. Other drug candidates suitable for gastroretentive drug delivery systems include those drugs that are locally active in the stomach, drugs with narrow absorption window in GI tract, drugs that are unstable in the intestinal or colonic environment, drugs that act locally in the proximal part of GI tract or disturb normal colonic microbes like antibiotics and also drugs that exhibit low solubility at high pH values. Concerning the pharmacotherapy of the stomach through local drug release of gastroretentive dosage forms, bringing about high levels of drug concentrations at the gastric mucosa (eradication of *H. pylori* from the submucosal tissue of the stomach), and treating stomach and duodenal ulcers, gastritis and oesophagitis, the risk of gastric carcinoma would be drastically reduced. In contrast, there are drugs that do not fit in gastroretentive drug delivery systems; Drugs that have very limited acid solubility, drugs that suffer instability in the gastric environment, and drugs intended for selective release in the colon should follow other techniques of drug delivery to reach for their intended site of action. Hence, gastroretentive dosage forms despite providing rather constant drug concentrations in the bloodstream for longer periods of time do not fulfill this benefit with several groups of drugs (Javadzadeh-Hamedeyazdan, 2012; Pahwa et al., 2012b).

One of the advantages of the sustained release dosage forms is that medication is administered less often than other dosage forms reducing fluctuations of drug concentration in the bloodstream. As a result, the patient is not repeatedly subjected to different levels of drug which are less or more than adequate. Nor does the blood chemistry undergo frequent chemical imbalances, which might be risky to the patient's health. Additionally, through gastroretentive dosage forms not only the bioavailability and therapeutic efficacy of drugs are improved but also it may allow for a possible reduction in the dose because of the steady therapeutic levels of drugs. Drugs that have poor solubility in higher pH, absorption windows in stomach, requiring local delivery in stomach could be delivered ideally to the site of action by the gastroretentive formulations. On the other hand, drugs that cause irritation to gastric mucosa and the ones meet first-pass metabolism or have stability problems in gastric fluids are not appropriate for these kinds of drug delivery systems (JavadzadehHamedeyazdan, 2012; Pahwa et al., 2012a; Pawar et al., 2012).

In brief, gastric retention is a means to enable a delivery strategy that will function irrespective of the digestive state, clinical condition, or GI motility of the individuals with longer drug residence time in the stomach being advantageous in superior drug bioavailabilities and also in certifying local action of some drugs in the upper part of the GI tract, that are used in *H. pylori* eradication (Bardonnet et al., 2006b; Nama et al., 2008; Badhan et al., 2009; Shah et al., 2009; AdebisiConway, 2013).

3. *H. pylori* associated peptic ulcer

3.1. Acidic condition of stomach

The human stomach can produce and secrete about 2.2 to 3 L of gastric acid per day with basal secretion levels being typically highest in the evening. Normally no bacteria or viruses can survive in this medium that is composed of digestive enzymes and concentrated hydrochloric acid. Consequently, stomach has been regarded as a sterile ingestion organ for its hostile and acidic environment that could be considered as a barrier for invasion of various microorganisms. However, this notion has been totally changed since *H. pylori* as a major cause of peptic ulcer disease and gastritis in human was firstly isolated by Marshall and Warren in 1983 (Yang et al., 1999). *H. pylori*, a spiral-shaped gram-negative rod, is classified as *Campylobacter pyloridis* due to its similar histological and growth properties to the *Campylobacter* species. Based on the unique morphological and biochemical characteristics, *Campylobacter pyloridis* was regrouped into a new genus *Helicobacter* (Brooks et al., 2004).

3.2. Pathogenesis of *H. pylori*

H. pylori is associated with antral gastritis, peptic ulcer disease (gastric and duodenal ulcer disease) and gastric carcinoma, however, it initially induces chronic gastritis to develop peptic ulcer rather than directly causing the ulcer disease (Wyatt, 1989). Ever since, *H. pylori* grows optimally at a pH of 6-7, it would not grow at the pH of the gastric lumen. Gastric mucus is relatively impermeable to acid and has a strong buffering capacity so deep mucus layer near the epithelial surface where the pH is about physiologic of 7.4 is an appropriate place for *H. pylori* growth. The bacterium produces a protease modifying the gastric mucus to reduce the ability of acid to diffuse through the mucus. In addition, *H. pylori* also has potent urease activity, which yields production of ammonia and further buffering of acid, which may directly damage the cells, too (Brooks, Butel et al., 2004; Abe et al., 2011). Although, the mechanisms by which *H. pylori* causes mucosal inflammation and damage, are not well known but they may involve both bacterial and host factors. Compared to other infectious diseases, the *H. pylori* associated morbidity is relatively high, which is about 10% for peptic ulcer disease and 0.5% for gastric adenocarcinoma (Kusters, 2001). Once *H. pylori* eradication has been achieved, re-infection rates are less than 0.5% per year, and ulcer recurrence rates are dramatically reduced (Kluwer, 2004). Since, there is not any clear hypothesis about spread of *H. pylori*, prevention is rather difficult issue. Then in treatment of peptic ulcer disease, clinicians are logically focusing on the eradication of *H. pylori* (Ables et al., 2007; Yamaoka, 2010).

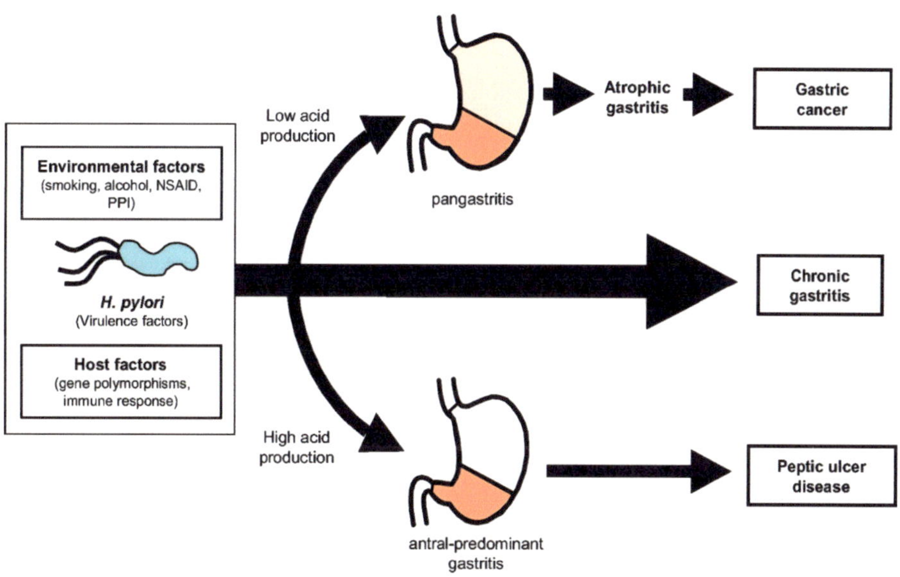

Figure 3. Pathogenesis of *H. pylori* (Kusters et al., 2006).

3.3. Treatments for *H. pylori* associated peptic ulcer disease

Basically, the goals for peptic ulcer treatments have been defined as: alleviation of symptoms, healing of the ulceration, prevention of recurrence of ulcer. Primarily, before the bacterium was found, it was believed that stomach ulcers occur when excess acid damaged the gastric mucosa so the treatment was based on reduction or neutralization of that acid (Gisbert et al., 2010; GisbertPajares, 2010). Patients were treated with long-term suppressive therapy by giving acid-blocking medications, for instance, H_2-blockers and, more recently, proton pump inhibitors (BreuerGraham, 1999). This kind of treatment could certainly relieve ulcer-related symptoms, heal gastric mucosal inflammation and even heal the ulcer. Unfortunately, it has a high recurrence rate just owing to the lack of basic treatment of the infection and eradication of the bacterium, *H. pylori* (Brunton, Parker et al., 2008). The identification of *H. pylori*, and understanding of *H. pylori* associated peptic ulcer disease have greatly changed therapeutic regiments covering peptic ulcer disease. Eradication of *H. pylori* is now recognized to be the correct approach in the treatment of the disease (Yang, Eshraghi et al., 1999; Chuah et al., 2011). The treatment of peptic ulcer with antibiotics is recognized as the choice treatment for patients (Beales, 2001). Savings of costs and time are the major benefits of this protocol to therapy with acid reducing medications. The same drug and dosage regimens could be applied to the treatment for both gastric and duodenal ulcer as there are no important differences between these two ulcer diseases (DzieniszewskiJarosz, 2006). Antibiotics and agents used to eradicate *H. pylori*, attack three main areas, i.e. the bacterium cell wall, the ribosome and nuclear DNA. For instance, metronidazole, a nitroimidazole antiprotozoal drug that also has potent antibacterial activity against anaerobes, including bacteroides and clostridium species, can disrupt the bacterial DNA helix preventing replication and interrupting gene expression, bismuth salt may disrupt bacterial cell wall or membrane (Malfertheiner, 1996).

3.3.1. Combination therapy

Although *H. pylori* is sensitive to many antibiotics *in vitro*, this sensitivity is not correlated with eradication of the organism *in vivo* (Drumm, 1990). Recurrence of the infection is common after treatment of *H. pylori* by bismuth alone or monotherapy antibiotic (Rauws et al., 1988; Oderda et al., 1989; Chang et al., 2009). It has been postulated that the failure of antibiotic monotherapy to clear *H. pylori in vivo* may be due to the lack of efficacy of the antibiotics in the acid environment of the stomach (Drumm, 1990). Other possible reason of failure could be the area that *H. pylori* colonized and resistance to bacteria. As a result of failure of single antibiotic therapies, combination regiments are suggested to increase the rate of *H. pylori* eradication. Nonetheless, many regimens for *H. pylori* eradication have been proposed, the ideal regimen in this setting should achieve a cure rate of >80% (Brunton, Parker et al., 2008).

3.3.2. Triple combination therapy

Triple combination therapy, using two antibacterial antibiotics and a proton pump inhibitor, had achieved a high eradication rate and seems to be the most effective regimens for *H. pylori* eradication (AxonMoayyedi, 1996; Ishizone et al., 2007). Proton pump inhibitors promote eradication of *H. pylori* through several mechanisms: direct antimicrobial properties (minor);

raising intra-gastric pH and lowering the minimal inhibitory concentrations of antibiotics against *H. pylori.* One of the principal treatment regimens consists of a 10–14 day regimen of "triple therapy": a proton pump inhibitor (standard dose, b.i.d.), clarithromycin, (500 mg, b.i.d.) and amoxicillin (1 g, b.i.d.). For patients who have allergy to penicillin, metronidazole, 500 mg twice daily, should be substituted for amoxicillin. Moreover, after completion of triple therapy, the proton pump inhibitor has been recommended to be continued once daily for a total of 4–6 weeks to ensure complete ulcer healing (Katzung, 2006). Other triple therapies that are being mentioned in other reference includes combinations of bismuth salts and various antibiotics (Rauws, Langenberg et al., 1988).

3.3.3. Quadruple combination therapy

In the case of *H. pylori* eradication quadruple therapy has been offered for 14 days: Proton pump inhibitor twice a day, metronidazole 500 mg three times daily, bismuth subsalicylate 525 mg, tetracycline 500 mg four times daily or H_2-receptor antagonist twice a day, bismuth subsalicylate 525 mg, metronidazole 250 mg, tetracycline 500 mg four times daily (Brunton, Parker et al., 2008). Antibiotics from systemic circulation have to traverse the epithelial layer (Malfertheiner, 1996; Hsu et al., 2011). Seeing as, in systemic administration of drugs the gastric emptying makes the effective local concentrations of drugs difficult to maintain, the effects of drug is not local and is through its systemic absorption, the frequent doses of oral antibiotics are required leading to higher drug dosages, lower patient compliance, and adverse drug effects.

3.4. Drug delivery systems for *H. pylori* eradication

3.4.1. Importance of drug delivery systems in treatment of diseases

It is judicious to be reminiscent of the GI tract being a primary site for the absorption of drugs with a variety of limitations making the *in vivo* performance of drug delivery systems uncertain. Despite tremendous advancement in drug delivery, the oral rout still remains the preferred route for the administration of therapeutic agents in consequence of the low cost of therapy, and ease of administration, as well as patient compliance. However, oral dosage forms hold several physiological restrictions like non-uniform absorption profiles, incomplete drug release and shorter residence time of the dosage form in the stomach (Adibkia, Hamedeyazdan et al., 2011). Undoubtedly, rate of drug transition through the gastrointestinal (GI) tract is highly controlled by the physiological properties of the GI tract as well as the formulation properties. Since, bioavailability of drugs in this route of administration often depends on the GI transit rate of the dosage form it is of value to distinguish between an appropriate drug delivery system for an especial objective in treatment of diseases. Acquiring a clear notion of why certain medications are prone to problems in reaching the desired efficiency and bioavailability, to dominate the relative constraints offering successful medication therapy recalling some fundamental characteristics of the stomach would be of note.

3.4.2. Stomach and drug delivery systems

As far as we know, the stomach is a muscular, hollow, dilated part of the alimentary canal which functions as an important organ of the human body located between the esophagus and the small intestine. Surface epithelium of stomach retains its integrity throughout the course of its lifetime, even though it is constantly exposed to a high concentration of hydrochloric acid and powerful enzymes. This self protection mechanism is due to the fact that the specialized goblet cells located in the stomach and continuously secrete a large amount of mucus that remains closely applied to the surface epithelium (Chein, 1992). In general, stomach is an important site of enzyme production with small surface area, offering an imperfect site of absorption (Chein, 1992). The main function of stomach is to store food temporarily, grind it, and then release it slowly in to the duodenum. The process of gastric emptying occurs both during fasting and fed states; however, the pattern of motility differs markedly in the two states. Fasted state is characterized by an inter-digestive series of electrical events which cycle both through the stomach and small intestine every 2–3 h which is called the inter-digestive myoelectric cycle or migrating myoelectric complex (Fell, 1996). In the fed state, the gastric emptying rate is slowed since the feeding results in a lag time prior to the onset of gastric emptying, depending upon the physiological state of the subject and the design of pharmaceutical formulation, the emptying process can last from a few minutes to 12 h. Alterations in gastric emptying occurs due to factors such as age, race, sex, and disease states, as they may seriously affect the release of a drug from the drug delivery system (SinghKim, 2000).

The complex and highly variable nature of gastric emptying process making the *in vivo* performance of conventional drug delivery systems uncertain draw researchers' attention to find a clue and dominate these constraints and present suitable drug delivery strategies that would serve independent of the digestive state, clinical condition, or GI motility of the individual. Conventional oral dosage forms provide a specific drug concentration in the systemic circulation without offering any control over the rate of drug delivery, whilst controlled-release drug delivery systems provide drug release at a predetermined, predictable, and controlled rate of drug release (Hwang et al., 1998). Nevertheless, in some cases the insufficient residency of drugs in the vicinity of absorption site for the life time of drug delivery restricts the use of controlled-release drug delivery systems. The inadequate drug residence in the vicinity of absorption site might arise from differences in GI transit time of drugs in individuals, and physical properties of the object ingested as well as the physiological conditions of the alimentary canal. Correspondingly, medications with sustained drug release forms have some benefits over normal release systems in safety and efficacy in reducing the frequency of drug dosage, together with the diminished incidence of adverse drug reactions. Hence, if medications used in *H. pylori* eradication therapy are used in terms of sustained release dosage forms some advantages are fulfilled seeing as the medications are administered less often than other dosage forms, fluctuations of drug concentration in the blood would be reduced, and the patient is not repeatedly subjected to amounts of the drug which are less or more than adequate, nor the blood chemistry experience frequent chemical imbalances, which might be detrimental to the patient's health (Klausner et al., 2003; Javadzadeh et al., 2007; Tang et al., 2007; Javadzadeh et al., 2009; Javadzadeh et al., 2012). Several methods have been developed for extension of GI transit time via enhancing the residence time of drug delivery systems in the stomach.

3.4.3. *Floating drug delivery systems*

One of the approaches followed to extend the residency of medications in the stomach is floating dosage forms with lower density than the gastric fluids to be capable of floating on the gastric juice in the stomach (SinghKim, 2000; Adibkia, Hamedeyazdan et al., 2011). According to the mechanism of buoyancy, two evidently different technologies are applied in development of floating dosage forms, effervescent and non-effervescent systems. In general, the principle rule is indelible in all approaches and that is to float on gastric juice with a specific density of less than 1.004 g/cm of the gastric juice in the stomach.

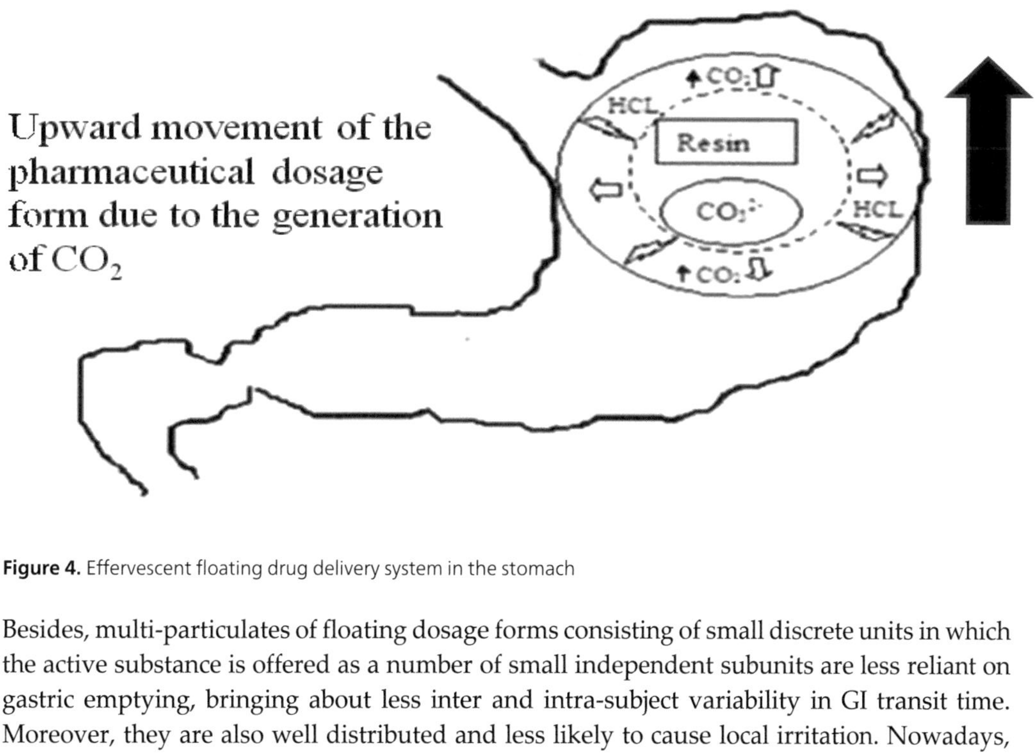

Figure 4. Effervescent floating drug delivery system in the stomach

Besides, multi-particulates of floating dosage forms consisting of small discrete units in which the active substance is offered as a number of small independent subunits are less reliant on gastric emptying, bringing about less inter and intra-subject variability in GI transit time. Moreover, they are also well distributed and less likely to cause local irritation. Nowadays, much emphasis is being laid on the development of multi particulate dosage forms rather than single unit systems due to potential benefits of them such as increased bioavailability, reduced risk of systemic toxicity, reduced risk of local irritation as well as predictable gastric emptying (MohamadDashevsky, 2007; GuptaPathak, 2008).

A number of factors that affect gastric emptying of a dosage form, such as density, size, and shape of dosage form, concomitant intake of food and drugs such as anticholinergic agents (e.g., atropine, propantheline), opiates (e.g., codeine), prokinetic agents (e.g., metoclopramide, cisapride), and biological factors like gender, posture, age, body mass index, and disease states (e.g., diabetes, Crohn's disease) could be controlled by these floating dosage forms providing a more convenient medication therapy (SinghKim, 2000).

These systems are also appropriate for drugs which are locally active to the gastric mucosa in the stomach, such as administration of metronidazole (MZ) as an antibiotic for *H. pylori* eradication in the treatment of peptic ulcer disease (Murata et al., 2000; Rajinikanth et al., 2007; RajinikanthMishra, 2007; RajinikanthMishra, 2008). Treatment of *H. pylori* infection by topical administration of antimicrobial agents has been reported. In order to avoid the side effects of standard triple therapy, Satoh used a technique of instilling a combination of bismuth subnitrate, amoxicillin and metronidazole into the stomach via a naso-gastric tube for 1 hour. He found that topical therapy was highly successful with high eradication rate of *H. pylori* and none-ulcer dyspepsia as well. Although this local administration successfully avoids some of the side effects of standard triple therapy, it is inconvenient and still complicated to patient when compared to oral dosage delivery system (Satoh, 1996). Elsewhere, the hydrodynamically balanced delivery system of Clarithromycin was developed which, after oral administration had the ability of prolonged gastric residence time with the desired *in vitro* release profile for the localized action in the stomach, in the treatment of *H. pylori* mediated peptic ulcer. In this study, wet granulation technique was applied for preparing of floating tablets of Clarithromycin. The proportion of sodium bicarbonate was varied to get the least possible lag time, also the polymer part varied to get the desired release. The formulation that developed using 66.2% Clarithromycin, 12% HPMC K4M polymer, 8% sodium bicarbonate gave floating lag time less than 3 min with a floating time of 12 h, and an *in vitro* release profile very near to the desired release. *In vivo* radiographic studies also suggested that the tablet had increased gastric residence time for the effective localized action of the antibiotic (Clarithromycin) in the treatment of *H. pylori* mediated peptic ulcer. The mechanism of release of Clarithromycin from the floating tablets was anomalous diffusion transport and followed by zero order kinetics (Nama, Gonugunta et al., 2008). In another study by Pornsak Sriamornsak, oil-entrapped calcium pectinate gel floating beads were prepared using selected oils that were floated immediately and remained floating for 24 hours. They concluded that this lasting intra-gastric buoyancy of a controlled release dosage form may also provide a suitable manner to deliver drugs that are locally active to the gastric mucosa in the stomach and, hence, achieve a site-specific therapeutic action (e.g., antibiotic administration for *H. pylori* eradication in the treatment of peptic ulcer disease (Sriamornsak et al., 2004). Then again, in another study Sriamornsak et al. evaluated the effects of some variables on release behavior of metronidazole from floating emulsion gel beads of calcium pectinate. They detected a notable prolongation drug release profile by coating the beads with Eudragit or by hardening with glutaraldehyde, whereas no clear effect on drug release was obtained using PEG10000, glyceryl monostearate and Eudragit as additives in the formulations (Sriamornsak, Thirawong et al., 2004; Sriamornsak et al., 2005).

Considering the fact that prolongation of the local availability of the antibacterial agents show positive effects of increasing in the effectiveness of *H. pylori* treatment ensuring a high drug concentration in the gastric mucosa, we had tried to formulate metronidazole in floating pharmaceutical dosage forms to encounter higher concentrations of the antibacterial agent in the gastric mucosa and clarify the mechanism of the release obtaining a general kinetic model for drug release profiles. In our previously published papers, we had reported the use of two different mechanisms in preparation of metronidazole floating matrix tablets including: A low density producing agent (gas generating agent/porous agent) and hydrocolloid-forming polymer(s) (Asnaashari et al., 2011). Carbonate acted as the gas generating agent when it came into contact with an acidic environment of the stomach under fed condition which got entrapped inside the system, producing bubbles, decreasing the density of the formulation. Preparing a low-density system using calcium silicate a characteristically porous structure with many pores and a large pore volume which forms a porous buoyant system (Jain et al., 2005). The hydrocolloids such as HPMC, carbopol, psyllium in the metronidazole formulations were hydrated and formed a colloid gel barrier that controled the rate of drug release, around its surface with thickness growing by time and increasing of volume due to hydration that in a bulk density less than 1 g/cm3 remaining buoyant on the gastric fluid. The established suitable release metronidazole floating matrix tablets could ensure a more localized drug concentration which might be useful for *H. pylori* eradication. In other survey, we had prepared alginate beads of metronidazole employing gas generating and porous agents followed by physicochemical evaluations for the prepared formulations (Javadzadeh et al., 2010). Alginates due to their high biocompatibility and nontoxic nature in oral administration that also demonstrate protective effect on the mucous membranes of the upper GI tract are a remarkable natural polymers found in brown algae that have been studied for a variety of biomedical applications. Sodium-Alginate beads (Na-Alg) have been developed in recent years as a unique vehicle for drug delivery. Alginates, which are naturally substances, are found in brown algae and can be considered as block polymers, which mainly consist of mannuronic acid (M), guluronic acid (G) and mannuronic-guluronic (MG) blocks. Alginate is known to be nontoxic when taken orally and also have protective effect on the mucous membranes of the upper gastrointestinal tract. The alginate beads with the structure of spherical gels are taken shape through dropwise addition of aqueous alginate solution to the aqueous solution containing calcium ions and/or other di and polyvalent cations (10). The pH dependent reswelling property of dried alginate beads let them to be administrated as controlled release system in gastrointestinal tract. The drug release from pharmaceutical dosage forms is a major determinant in their biological effect, thus evaluation of drug release kinetic is of paramount importance in the field. The findings of our study revealed high compatibility of the alginate beads in achieving a suitable floating pharmaceutical dosage forms which could control metronidazole release from the beads with a definite kinetic of drug release. Identifying drug release kinetics of a drug which is an important variable in obtaining one or two physically meaningful parameters in relating the drug release parameter with important parameters such as *in vivo* drug bioavailability is of substantial value in pharmaceutical manufacturing.

Hence, developing an efficient floating dosage form is reliant to a better understanding of the relation among the physiological properties of the GI tract, formulation variables and the performance of these floating systems *in vivo* and clinical stages, leading to a superior floating drug delivery system in special cases like *H. pylori* eradication.

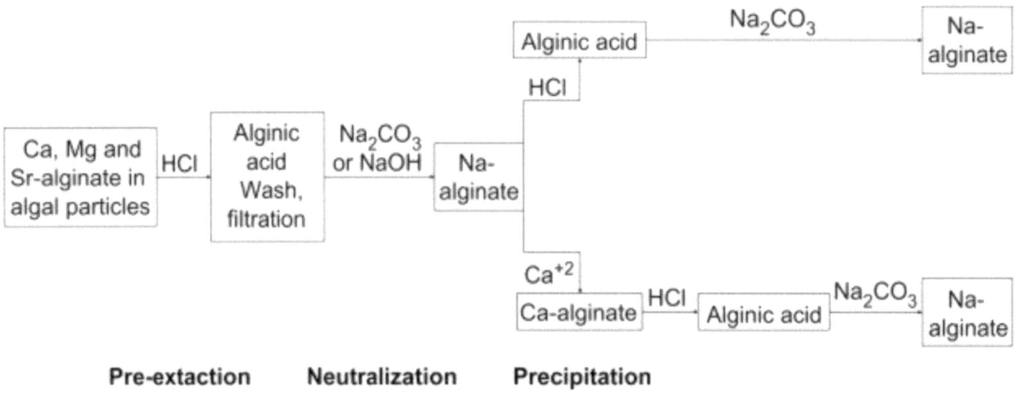

Figure 5. Alginates in floating drug delivery systems

4. Conclusion

Overall, developing an efficient floating dosage form for *H. pylori* eradication could be established by the combination of two buoyancy mechanisms, gas generating systems with swellable polymers, being advantages in view point of obtaining an appropriate floating lag time and duration of buoyancy which guarantees the optimum efficiency of the pharmaceutical dosage form. Nonetheless, further investigations may focus on the compatibility of the mentioned concepts in the interplay of the pharmacokinetic and pharmacodynamic parameters *in vivo* and also in clinical aspect to provide the effectiveness of the floating drug delivery systems in *H. pylori* eradication therapies.

Author details

Yousef Javadzadeh and Sanaz Hamedeyazdan

Biotechnology Research center, Tabriz University of Medical Sciences, Iran

References

[1] Abe, T., Kodama, M., Murakami, K., Matsunari, O., Mizukami, K., Inoue, K., Uchida, M., Okimoto, T., Fujioka, T., Uchida, T., Moriyama, M. & Yamaoka, Y. (2011). Impact of Helicobacter pylori CagA diversity on gastric mucosal damage: an immunohistochemical study of East-Asian-type CagA. *J. Gastroenterol. Hepatol.*, Vol.26, No.4, pp. 688-693.

[2] Ables, A.Z., Simon, I. & Melton, E.R. (2007). Update on Helicobacter pylori treatment. *Am. Fam. Physician.*, Vol.75, No.3, pp. 351-358.

[3] Adebisi, A.O. & Conway, B.R. (2013). Preparation and characterisation of gastroretentive alginate beads for targeting H. pylori. *J Microencapsul*, pp.

[4] Adibkia, K., Hamedeyazdan, S. & Javadzadeh, Y. (2011). Drug release kinetics and physicochemical characteristics of floating drug delivery systems. *Expert Opin. Drug Deliv.*, Vol.8, No.7, pp. 891-903.

[5] Asnaashari, S., Khoei, N.S., Zarrintan, M.H., Adibkia, K. & Javadzadeh, Y. (2011). Preparation and evaluation of novel metronidazole sustained release and floating matrix tablets. *Pharm. Dev. Technol.*, Vol.16, No.4, pp. 400-407.

[6] Axon, A.T. & Moayyedi, P. (1996). Eradication of Helicobacter pylori: omeprazole in combination with antibiotics. *Scand. J. Gastroenterol. Suppl.*, Vol.215, pp. 82-89.

[7] Badhan, A.C., Mashru, R.C., Shah, P.P., Thakkar, A.R. & Dobaria, N.B. (2009). Development and evaluation of sustained release gastroretentive minimatrices for effective treatment of H. pylori infection. *AAPS PharmSciTech*, Vol.10, No.2, pp. 459-467.

[8] Bardonnet, P.L., Faivre, V., Pugh, W.J., Piffaretti, J.C. & Falson, F. (2006a). Gastroretentive dosage forms: overview and special case of Helicobacter pylori. *J. Control. Release*, Vol.111, No.1-2, pp. 1-18.

[9] Bardonnet, P.L., Faivre, V., Pugh, W.J., Piffaretti, J.C. & Falson, F. (2006b). Gastroretentive dosage forms: overview and special case of Helicobacter pylori. *J Control Release*, Vol.111, No.1-2, pp. 1-18.

[10] Beales, I.L. (2001). Efficacy of Helicobacter pylori eradication therapies: a single centre observational study. *BMC Gastroenterol.*, Vol.1, pp. 7.

[11] Breuer, T. & Graham, D.Y. (1999). Costs of diagnosis and treatment of Helicobacter pylori infection: when does choosing the treatment regimen based on susceptibility testing become cost effective? *Am. J. Gastroenterol.*, Vol.94, No.3, pp. 725-729.

[12] Brooks, G., Butel, J., Morse, S., Melnick, J., Jawetz, E. & Adelberg, E. (2004). *Jawetz, Melnick, & Adelberg's Medical Microbiology*. United States of America, McGraw-Hill Professional.

[13] Brunton, L., Parker, K., Blumenthal, D. & Buxton, L. (2008). *Goodman & Gilman's Manual of Pharmacology and Therapeutics*. United States of America, McGraw-Hill Companies.

[14] Chang, W.L., Sheu, B.S., Cheng, H.C., Yang, Y.J., Yang, H.B. & Wu, J.J. (2009). Resistance to metronidazole, clarithromycin and levofloxacin of Helicobacter pylori before and after clarithromycin-based therapy in Taiwan. *J. Gastroenterol. Hepatol.*, Vol.24, No.7, pp. 1230-1235.

[15] Chein, Y.W. (1992). *Novel Drug Delivery System*. New York, Marcel Dekker, Inc.

[16] Chuah, S.K., Tsay, F.W., Hsu, P.I. & Wu, D.C. (2011). A new look at anti-Helicobacter pylori therapy. *World J. Gastroentero.*, Vol.17, No.35, pp. 3971-3975.

[17] Drumm, B. (1990). Helicobacter pylori. *Arch. Dis. Child.*, Vol.65, No.11, pp. 1278-1282.

[18] Dzieniszewski, J. & Jarosz, M. (2006). Guidelines in the medical treatment of Helicobacter pylori infection. *J. Physiol. Pharmacol.*, Vol.57 Suppl 3, pp. 143-154.

[19] Fell, J.T. (1996). Targeting of drugs and delivery systems to specific sites in the gastrointestinal tract. *J. Anat.*, Vol.189 (Pt 3), pp. 517-519.

[20] Gisbert, J.P. & Calvet, X. (2011). Review article: the effectiveness of standard triple therapy for Helicobacter pylori has not changed over the last decade, but it is not good enough. *Aliment. Pharm. Ther.*, Vol.34, No.11-12, pp. 1255-1268.

[21] Gisbert, J.P., Calvet, X., O'Connor, A., Megraud, F. & O'Morain, C.A. (2010). Sequential therapy for Helicobacter pylori eradication: a critical review. *J. Clin. Gastroenterol.*, Vol.44, No.5, pp. 313-325.

[22] Gisbert, J.P. & Pajares, J.M. (2010). Treatment of Helicobacter pylori infection: the past and the future. *Eur. J. Intern. Med.*, Vol.21, No.5, pp. 357-359.

[23] Graham, D.Y. (1996). Nonsteroidal anti-inflammatory drugs, Helicobacter pylori, and ulcers: where we stand. *Am. J. Gastroenterol.*, Vol.91, No.10, pp. 2080-2086.

[24] Gupta, R. & Pathak, K. (2008). Optimization studies on floating multiparticulate gastroretentive drug delivery system of famotidine. *Drug Dev. Ind. Pharm.*, Vol.34, No. 11, pp. 1201-1208.

[25] Hauser, K., Longo, B. & Jameson, F. (2005). *Harrison's Principles of Internal Medicine*. United States of America, McGraw-Hill companies.

[26] Hsu, P.I., Wu, D.C., Wu, J.Y. & Graham, D.Y. (2011). Modified sequential Helicobacter pylori therapy: proton pump inhibitor and amoxicillin for 14 days with clarithromycin and metronidazole added as a quadruple (hybrid) therapy for the final 7 days. *Helicobacter*, Vol.16, No.2, pp. 139-145.

[27] Hu, L.D., Xing, Q.B., Shang, C., Liu, W., Liu, C., Luo, Z.L. & Xu, H.X. (2010). Preparation of rosiglitazone maleate sustained-release floating microspheres for improved bioavailability. *Pharmazie*, Vol.65, No.7, pp. 477-480.

[28] Hwang, S.J., Park, H. & Park, K. (1998). Gastric retentive drug-delivery systems. *Crit Rev Ther Drug Carrier Syst*, Vol.15, No.3, pp. 243-284.

[29] Ishizone, S., Maruta, F., Suzuki, K., Miyagawa, S., Takeuchi, M., Kanaya, K., Oana, K., Hayama, M., Kawakami, Y. & Ota, H. (2007). *In vivo* bactericidal activities of Japanese rice-fluid against H. pylori in a Mongolian gerbil model. *Int. J. Med. Sci.*, Vol.4, No.4, pp. 203-208.

[30] Jain, S.K., Awasthi, A.M., Jain, N.K. & Agrawal, G.P. (2005). Calcium silicate based microspheres of repaglinide for gastroretentive floating drug delivery: preparation and *in vitro* characterization. *J. Control. Release*, Vol.107, No.2, pp. 300-309.

[31] Javadzadeh, Y., Asnaashari, S. & Hamedeyazdan, S. (2012). Recrystallization of Drugs: Significance on Pharmaceutical Processing Recrystallization. K. Sztwiertnia. Croatia, InTech.

[32] Javadzadeh, Y. & Hamedeyazdan, S. (2012). Novel Drug Delivery Systems for Modulation of Gastrointestinal Transit Time Recent Advances in Novel Drug Carrier Systems. A. D. Sezer. Croatia, InTech: 393-418.

[33] Javadzadeh, Y., Hamedeyazdan, S., Adibkia, K., Kiafar, F., Zarrintan, M.H. & Barzegar-Jalali, M. (2010). Evaluation of drug release kinetics and physico-chemical characteristics of metronidazole floating beads based on calcium silicate and gas-forming agents. *Pharm. Dev. Technol.*, Vol.15, No.4, pp. 329-338.

[34] Javadzadeh, Y., Jafari-Navimipour, B. & Nokhodchi, A. (2007). Liquisolid technique for dissolution rate enhancement of a high dose water-insoluble drug (carbamazepine). *Int J Pharm*, Vol.341, No.1-2, pp. 26-34.

[35] Javadzadeh, Y., Mohammadi, A., Khoei, N.S. & Nokhodchi, A. (2009). Improvement of physicomechanical properties of carbamazepine by recrystallization at different pH values. *Acta Pharm*, Vol.59, No.2, pp. 187-197.

[36] Katzung, B. (2006). *Basic and Clinical Pharmacology*. San Francisco, mc graw hill pressed.

[37] Khobragade, D.S., Parshuramkar, P.R., Ujjainkar, A.P., Mahendra, A.M., Phapal, S.M. & Patil, A.T. (2009). Conception and evaluation of sustained release polymeric matrix beads for enhanced gastric retention. *Curr. Drug. Deliv.*, Vol.6, No.3, pp. 249-254.

[38] Klausner, E.A., Lavy, E., Friedman, M. & Hoffman, A. (2003). Expandable gastroretentive dosage forms. *J. Control. Release*, Vol.90, No.2, pp. 143-162.

[39] Kluwer, W. (2004). *Drug Facts and Comparisons*. St. Louis, USA., Facts and Comparisons.

[40] Kusters, J.G. (2001). Recent developments in Helicobacter pylori vaccination. *Scand. J. Gastroenterol. Suppl.*, No.234, pp. 15-21.

[41] Kusters, J.G., van Vliet, A.H. & Kuipers, E.J. (2006). Pathogenesis of Helicobacter pylori infection. *Clin Microbiol Rev*, Vol.19, No.3, pp. 449-490.

[42] Malfertheiner, P. (1996). Management of Helicobacter pylori-positive peptic ulcer disease. *Scand. J. Gastroenterol. Suppl.*, Vol.215, pp. 69.

[43] Mohamad, A. & Dashevsky, A. (2007). *In vitro* and *in vivo* performance of a multiparticulate pulsatile drug delivery system. *Drug Dev. Ind. Pharm.*, Vol.33, No.2, pp. 113-119.

[44] Motlekar, N.A. & Youan, B.B. (2006). The quest for non-invasive delivery of bioactive macromolecules: a focus on heparins. *J. Control. Release*, Vol.113, No.2, pp. 91-101.

[45] Murata, Y., Sasaki, N., Miyamoto, E. & Kawashima, S. (2000). Use of floating alginate gel beads for stomach-specific drug delivery. *Eur. J. Pharm. Biopharm.*, Vol.50, No.2, pp. 221-226.

[46] Nama, M., Gonugunta, C.S. & Reddy Veerareddy, P. (2008). Formulation and evaluation of gastroretentive dosage forms of Clarithromycin. *AAPS PharmSciTech*, Vol.9, No.1, pp. 231-237.

[47] Oderda, G., Dell'Olio, D., Morra, I. & Ansaldi, N. (1989). Campylobacter pylori gastritis: long term results of treatment with amoxycillin. *Arch. Dis. Child.*, Vol.64, No.3, pp. 326-329.

[48] Ofman, J.J., Etchason, J., Alexander, W., Stevens, B.R., Herrin, J., Cangialose, C., Ballard, D.J., Bratzler, D., Elward, K.S., FitzGerald, D., Culpepper-Morgan, J. & Marshall, B. (2000). The quality of care for Medicare patients with peptic ulcer disease. *Am. J. Gastroenterol.*, Vol.95, No.1, pp. 106-113.

[49] Pahwa, R., Saini, N., Kumar, V. & Kohli, K. (2012a). Chitosan-based gastroretentive floating drug delivery technology: an updated review. *Expert Opin Drug Deliv*, Vol.9, No.5, pp. 525-539.

[50] Pahwa, R., Singh, M., Kumar, V. & Kohli, K. (2012b). Recent advances and patent perspectives in gastroretentive technology. *Recent Pat Drug Deliv Formul*, Vol.6, No.3, pp. 278-290.

[51] Pawar, V.K., Kansal, S., Asthana, S. & Chourasia, M.K. (2012). Industrial perspective of gastroretentive drug delivery systems: physicochemical, biopharmaceutical, technological and regulatory consideration. *Expert Opin Drug Deliv*, Vol.9, No.5, pp. 551-565.

[52] Peura, D.A. (2004). Prevention of nonsteroidal anti-inflammatory drug-associated gastrointestinal symptoms and ulcer complications. *Am J Med*, Vol.117 Suppl 5A, pp. 63S-71S.

[53] Rajinikanth, P.S., Balasubramaniam, J. & Mishra, B. (2007). Development and evaluation of a novel floating in situ gelling system of amoxicillin for eradication of Helicobacter pylori. *Int. J. Pharm.*, Vol.335, No.1-2, pp. 114-122.

[54] Rajinikanth, P.S. & Mishra, B. (2007). Preparation and in vitro characterization of gellan based floating beads of acetohydroxamic acid for eradication of H. pylori. *Acta Pharm.*, Vol.57, No.4, pp. 413-427.

[55] Rajinikanth, P.S. & Mishra, B. (2008). Floating in situ gelling system for stomach site-specific delivery of clarithromycin to eradicate H. pylori. *J. Control. Release*, Vol.125, No.1, pp. 33-41.

[56] Rauws, E.A., Langenberg, W., Houthoff, H.J., Zanen, H.C. & Tytgat, G.N. (1988). Campylobacter pyloridis-associated chronic active antral gastritis. A prospective study of its prevalence and the effects of antibacterial and antiulcer treatment. *Gastroenterology*, Vol.94, No.1, pp. 33-40.

[57] Satoh, K. (1996). Treatment of Helicobacter pylori infection by topical administration of antimicrobial agents. *Scand. J. Gastroenterol. Suppl.*, Vol.214, pp. 56; discussion 57-60.

[58] Shah, S.H., Patel, J.K. & Patel, N.V. (2009). Gastroretentive floating drug delivery systems with potential herbal drugs for Helicobacter pylori eradication: a review. *Zhong Xi Yi Jie He Xue Bao*, Vol.7, No.10, pp. 976-982.

[59] Singh, B.N. & Kim, K.H. (2000). Floating drug delivery systems: an approach to oral controlled drug delivery via gastric retention. *J. Control. Release*, Vol.63, No.3, pp. 235-259.

[60] Sriamornsak, P., Thirawong, N. & Puttipipatkhachorn, S. (2004). Morphology and buoyancy of oil-entrapped calcium pectinate gel beads. *AAPS J.*, Vol.6, No.3, pp. e24 (21-27).

[61] Sriamornsak, P., Thirawong, N. & Puttipipatkhachorn, S. (2005). Emulsion gel beads of calcium pectinate capable of floating on the gastric fluid: effect of some additives, hardening agent or coating on release behavior of metronidazole. *Eur. J. Pharm. Sci.*, Vol.24, No.4, pp. 363-373.

[62] Tang, Y.D., Venkatraman, S.S., Boey, F.Y. & Wang, L.W. (2007). Sustained release of hydrophobic and hydrophilic drugs from a floating dosage form. *Int. J. Pharm.*, Vol. 336, No.1, pp. 159-165.

[63] Wyatt, J.I. (1989). The role of Campylobacter pylori in the pathogenesis of peptic ulcer disease. *Scand. J. Gastroenterol. Suppl.*, Vol.157, pp. 7-11; discussion 21-12.

[64] Yamaoka, Y. (2010). Mechanisms of disease: Helicobacter pylori virulence factors. *Nat. Rev. Gastroenterol. Hepatol.*, Vol.7, No.11, pp. 629-641.

[65] Yang, L., Eshraghi, J. & Fassihi, R. (1999). A new intragastric delivery system for the treatment of Helicobacter pylori associated gastric ulcer: *in vitro* evaluation. *J. Control. Release*, Vol.57, No.3, pp. 215-222.

Chapter 12

Empirical Versus Targeted Treatment of *Helicobacter pylori* Infections in Southern Poland According to the Results of Local Antimicrobial Resistance Monitoring

Elżbieta Karczewska, Karolina Klesiewicz,
Paweł Nowak, Edward Sito, Iwona Skiba,
Małgorzata Zwolińska–Wcisło, Tomasz Mach and
Alicja Budak

Additional information is available at the end of the chapter

http://dx.doi.org/10.5772/57387

1. Introduction

1.1. General information

Helicobacter pylori (*H. pylori*) is a spiral-shaped, Gram-negative, microaerophilic bacterium inhabiting human gastric mucosa and playing an essential role in dyspepsia, gastritis, gastric ulcer disease and duodenal ulcer disease [1-6]. Moreover, in 1994 the International Agency for Research on Cancer of the World Health Organization (IARC/WHO) concluded that *H. pylori* is a class I carcinogen, involved in gastric cancer and mucosa-associated lymphoid tissue (MALT) lymphoma [2, 7-11]. Furthermore, increasing number of studies showed the association between *H. pylori* infections and pathogenesis of extragastric diseases. The most convincing data appeared in case of iron-deficiency anemia (IDA) of unknown origin and idiopathic thrombocytopenia purpura (ITP) [12]. Eradication of *H. pylori* in IDA patients resulted in normalization of hemoglobin level while in ITP patients lead to a favorable platelet response [13]. Moreover, the findings and ongoing research concerning *H. pylori* infections suggest its association with other diseases such as: heart or vascular diseases (ischemic heart disease, coronary artery disease, cardiac syndrome x), neurological diseases (stroke, Alzheimer's or Parkinson's diseases) as well as obesity, diabetes mellitus, asthma or diseases of oral mucosa [1, 14-18].

H. pylori infection is one of the most common bacterial infections, with the estimated prevalence reaching 50% of the human population worldwide. Nevertheless, the occurrence of *H. pylori* infections correlate with the socioeconomic status and are often reflected in their geographical distribution. The frequency of this infection is markedly higher in the developing countries (80-90%) rather than in the developed countries (<40%) [4]. In Europe the incidence of *H. pylori* varies and can be associated with geographical location and the percentage of compatriots of non-European origin [19]. Current studies show the declining trend in the prevalence of *H. pylori* infections in developed countries such as Denmark or Czech Republic [20, 21], while the frequency of this infection in Asia–Pacific region ranges from 15.5% in Australia, 71.7% in Shanghai China, to 94.3% in Eastern Siberia [6].

The Polish multi-center study performed between 2000 and 2003 revealed that the incidence of *H. pylori* infections was 84% in adult patients [22], whereas our research, conducted in southern Poland between 2009 and 2011, showed that the rate of *H. pylori* infection among adults was 23% [23].

*H. pylor*i has evolved numerous strategies for survival in the gastric niche (especially due to the release of urease, an enzyme, which increases the pH value of the environment around the bacterial cells) [24]. Furthermore, the clinical course of *H. pylori* infection depends from both the bacterial virulence factors and the host susceptibility (e.g. diet, genetic predispositions, degree of the immune response to infection) [3, 7, 25].

It was concluded that untreated *H. pylori* infection led to acid-related disorders of the digestive system. Great majority of individuals colonized by *H. pylori* developed co-existing chronic gastritis, which in subsets of patients could evolve to duodenal or gastric ulcer as well as gastric cancer [7, 8, 26, 27]. Experiments performed in animal models (Mongolian gerbils) confirmed the progressive sequence of lesions from chronic gastritis to gastric cancer by gastric atrophy, intestinal metaplasia, and dysplasia [28]. Figure 1 illustrates the sequential steps of diseases resulting from *H. pylori* infection.

H. pylori infection significantly enhances the risk of development of peptic ulcer disease (up to 15 times) as well as gastric cancer (up to 6 times) [1, 7, 24]. Peptic ulcer disease (PUD) – gastric and/or duodenal ulcer – develops in about 15% of *H. pylori* infected patients, whereas the progression to neoplastic lesions may occur only in a small fraction of patients with *H. pylori* infection. Gastric cancer arises in about 1-5% of patients and MALT cancer in <1% of infected subjects [7, 8, 27, 29].

The information presented above highlights the importance of an effective treatment against *H. pylori*. Furthermore, the increasing resistance of *H. pylori* to antibiotics/chemotherapeutics currently used in empirical therapy justifies the need for continuous surveillance of antibiotic resistance as well as compliance to guidelines of the European Helicobacter Study Group (EHSG) [1].

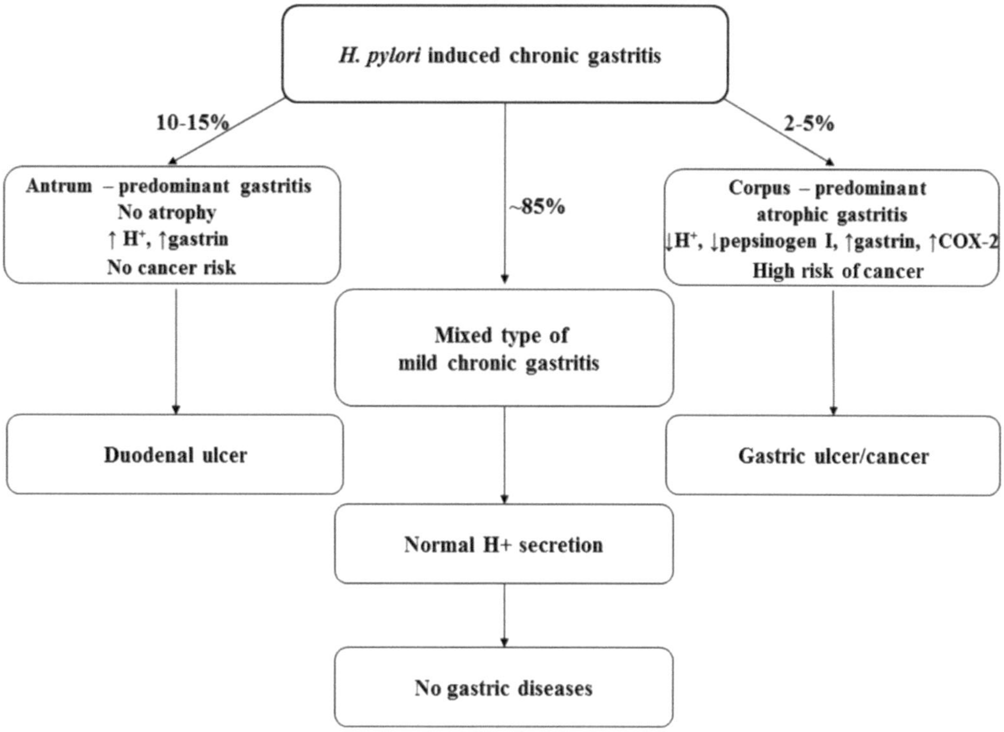

Figure 1. Sequential steps of diseases resulting from *H. pylori* infection *(based on fig. 3 Konturek et. al J Physiol Pharmacol. 2009* [8]).

1.2. Virulence factors (VF)

The pathogenesis of *H. pylori* is determined by wide spectrum of virulence factors, which can be divided into two major groups:

1. VF secreted into the bacterial extracellular environment (e.g. immunogenic protein CagA, vacuolating cytotoxin VacA, secreted enzymes: urease, aliphatic amidase, catalase, oxidase, superoxide dismutase, phospholipases, glycosulfatase and proteolitic enzymes).

2. VF associated with the bacterial surface (e.g. outer membrane proteins, adhesins, flagella, LPS) [24, 25].

CagA. One of the most important *H. pylori* virulence factors is highly immunogenic protein CagA. It is encoded by cytotoxin associated gene (*cag*A gene), which is located on the *cag* pathogenicity island (*cag* PAI) and carried by 56-90% of *H. pylori* strains [8, 24, 29-32]. CagA protein (after translocation into the host cells by the type IV cag secretion system) stimulates epithelial cells to produce the following cytokines: interleukin IL-8 (strong chemotactic factor and activator of inflammatory process on the mucous membrane), IL-6, IL-1β, and tumor necrosis factor α (TNF-α; enhances the inflammatory process) [31, 33, 34] and is also responsible for changes in the host cells such as proliferation, motility, and polarity [25,

35]. Patients infected with *cag*A positive strains usually exhibit a higher inflammatory response and are at a higher risk of developing gastric ulcer disease, atrophic gastritis, or gastric cancer [3, 8, 24, 36, 37].

VacA. Another major *H. pylori* virulence determinant is vacuolating cytotoxin A (VacA). This protein is involved in various mechanisms of programmed cell death (including apoptosis and necrosis) in the target host cells [38]. While VacA encoding gene (*vac*A) occurs in almost all *H. pylori* strains, only approximately 50% of isolates express active protein. Moreover, variations in the *vac*A gene structure considering signal (s) as well as middle (m) region result in differences in vacuolating activity of this cytotoxin [7, 8, 24, 34, 39]. *H. pylori* strains carrying s1/m1 allelic form of *vac*A gene have higher vacuolating activity than isolates with s1/m2 or s2/m1 alleles. Furthermore, polymorphisms among the *vac*A signal region (s1, s1a, s1b, s2) and middle region (m1, m2) are also correlated with the intensity of inflammation process and the severity of gastric epithelial cell injury, respectively. While strains possessing *vac*A s1a genotype cause stronger inflammation process than isolates carrying *vac*A s1b or *vac*A s2 genotype, the strains harboring *vac*A m1 genotype cause more severe gastric epithelial cell injury than the *vac*A m2 strains [34, 40]. Moreover, the infection with *H. pylori* strains possessing *vac*A s1/m1 allele is strongly associated with peptic ulcer disease and gastric cancer [7, 40]. A third polymorphic determinant of vacuolating activity of *vac*A gene was described in mid region and termed the intermediate (i), but its role in the pathogenesis of *H. pylori* infection remains debatable [41].

H. pylori is described as one of the most important risk factors contributing to the development of gastric cancer in more than 50% of cases, while CagA and VacA as major virulence determinants play an important role in this process [2, 7, 8]. Due to the presence/absence of CagA and VacA, *H. pylori* strains were divided into two types: type I (possessing *cag*A gene and expressing vacuolating cytotoxin) and type II (lacking the *cag*A gene and with no expression of vacuolating cytotoxin). Strains belonging to the type I (CagA+, VacA+ phenotype) are more virulent, as their infections are associated with increased risk of peptic ulcer disease and gastric cancer. Strains of the type II (CagA-, VacA- phenotype) are less virulent. Furthermore, an intermediate type of *H. pylori* strain has been described. Isolates belonging to this group have independent expression of CagA and VacA cytotoxins and represent a moderate level of virulence [24, 34, 42].

Urease and aliphatic amidase. Remarkable capacity of *H. pylori* to colonize highly acidic environment of stomach is mostly attributed to the production of urease. This enzyme hydrolyzes urea (to ammonia and carbon dioxide), which results in an increase of pH value in the environment surrounding the bacterium. A similar effect is produced by aliphatic amidase, which also contributes to the pH value of the gastric environment [43]. Furthermore, ammonia which is the product of enzymatic hydrolysis of urea, shows toxicity against epithelial cells [24, 25, 32].

Other pathogenic enzymes.*H. pylori* produces many other groups of enzymes responsible for the pathogenesis. While catalase, oxidase, and superoxide dismutase play a role in protecting the bacterial cells from phagocytosis, phospholipase A2, phospholipases C, and glycosulfatase damage the cells of the mucous membrane [44-48]. Furthermore, *H. pylori* secretes numerous proteolytic enzymes responsible for the gastric mucus degradation [49].

Adhesins. Adherence of *H. pylori* to the host cell receptors triggers cellular changes, which include signal transduction cascades, leading to infiltration of inflammatory cells and to persistence of the organism. *H. pylori* adhesins are proteins, glycoconjugates, or lipids, which are involved in the initial stages of colonization by mediating the interactions between the bacterium and the host cell surface (AlpA, AlpB, BabA, Hsp60, Hsp70, LPS core, LPS O antigen (Lewis X), Nap) [8, 50, 51].

Outer membrane proteins. Outer inflammatory protein (OipA) is an outer membrane inflammatory-related protein significantly associated with the development of duodenal ulcers and gastric cancer. OipA plays an important role in induction of the mucosal cytokines and in gastric mucosal inflammation [7, 8, 36]. The outer membrane proteins contributing to the adherence of *H. pylori* are represented by: SabA, AlpAB [32, 36].

Flagella.*H. pylori* possess up to 6 unipolar flagella composed of two proteins: FlaA and FlaB [24, 52]. Due to the flagella, *H. pylori* is motile and can move within stomach niche between regions of low pH value to regions with higher pH value, which is more hospitable for these bacteria [8, 53]. The motility is also necessary for the successful colonization of the stomach mucosa [52].

LPS. Lipopolysaccharide of *H. pylori* is a unique and a potent immunogen. LPS of *H. pylori* contains O-antigen structures, which resemble human glycosphingolipids due to the presence of common host carbohydrate residues [54]. LPS contains structures like Lewis X and Lewis Y antigens, which are similar to antigens of human blood groups, which occur also in the human gastric epithelium. Due to molecular mimicry, bacteria are able to escape the host immune response. Moreover, the specific structure of *H. pylori* LPS is crucial for the adhesion to epithelial cells and colonization process of the human stomach by *H. pylori* [24, 54, 55].

While in the majority of people *H. pylori* colonization is asymptomatic, long-term carriage significantly increases the risk of development of site-specific diseases [7, 8, 34, 36]. It was also concluded that untreated *H. pylori* infection may lead to serious implications such as gastritis, gastric ulcer disease and gastric cancer, therefore it is crucial to provide effective treatment. Moreover, it was proved that introduction of early effective treatment of *H. pylori* infection in cases of peptic ulcer disease can prevent these patients from developing gastric cancer [1, 26].

1.3. Treatment guidelines

Several recommendations concerning diagnosis and treatment regimen were issued as the infection treatment is often unsuccessful. The first guidelines on diagnostic and therapeutic approaches for the *H. pylori* infection were issued in the United States of America. The second recommendations were introduced by Polish Society of Gastroenterology *Helicobacter pylori* Working Group (PSG-E/HPWG) in 1996. The next guidelines of the PSG-E/HPWG on diagnostic and therapeutic approaches for the *H. pylori* infection were issued in 2000, 2004 and 2008 [22, 56, 57]. The European Helicobacter Study Group (EHSG) took the initiative of introducing recommendations for the clinical management of *H pylori* infection in 1996 in Maastricht and since then four consensus reports have been issued (1997, 2000, 2005, 2012) [1, 5, 58, 59].

Recommendations for the management of *H. pylori* infection are constantly evolving along with the development of knowledge concerning this bacterium and its infections [1]. Current guidelines on the management of *H. pylori* infections were produced by EHSG in 2012 (Maastricht IV/Florence Consensus Report) and should be introduced in the management of this infection in European countries. Despite that fact, the recent Polish recommendations issued in 2008 still support the Third Maastricht Consensus Report (2005). Nevertheless, the new Polish guidelines are under development and will be issued in the near future.

The European Helicobacter Study Group and the Polish Society of Gastroenterology recommend therapeutic regimens, which include three types of drugs: 1) antisecretory (proton pump inhibitors (PPI)), 2) cytoprotectants (drugs containing bismuth salts), and 3) antibiotics/chemotherapeutics (clarithromycin, amoxicillin, metronidazole, tetracycline, levofloxacin, and rifabutin) [1, 22].

The treatment regimens of *H. pylori* infections according to the PSG-E guidelines (2008) [22] are presented in Table 1.

Treatment strategy	**Time of treatment**
The First-Line Treatment (one of the following):	
PPI, amoxicillin (1000 mg) and metronidazole (500 mg) twice a day	
PPI, clarithromycin (500 mg), and metronidazole (500 mg) twice a day	10–14 days
PPI, amoxicillin (500 mg), and clarithromycin (500 mg) twice a day	
The Second-Line Treatment (one of the following):	
PPI, amoxicillin (1000 mg), and metronidazole (500 mg) twice a day and tetracycline (250 mg) three times a day	10–14 days
PPI, amoxicillin (1000 mg), and metronidazole (500 mg) twice a day and bismuth salts (120 mg) four times a day	
The Third-Line Treatment:	
Evaluation of the susceptibility of the strains to the currently used antimicrobial agents: amoxicillin, metronidazole, clarithromycin, and tetracycline	14 days
Possible introduction of levofloxacin	*(prolonged if the previous treatments were shorter)*
Adding a probiotic	

Table 1. Proposed strategy of the first, second and third – line treatment of *H. pylori* infection *(table based on the guidelines of PSG-E Consensus Report, 2008 [22])*

According to the Maastricht IV/Florence Consensus Report guidelines, the treatment regimen should be selected according to the areas of low (<20%) and high (>20%) clarithromycin resistance, to provide the most effective therapy. Figure 2 presents the current EHSG guidelines.

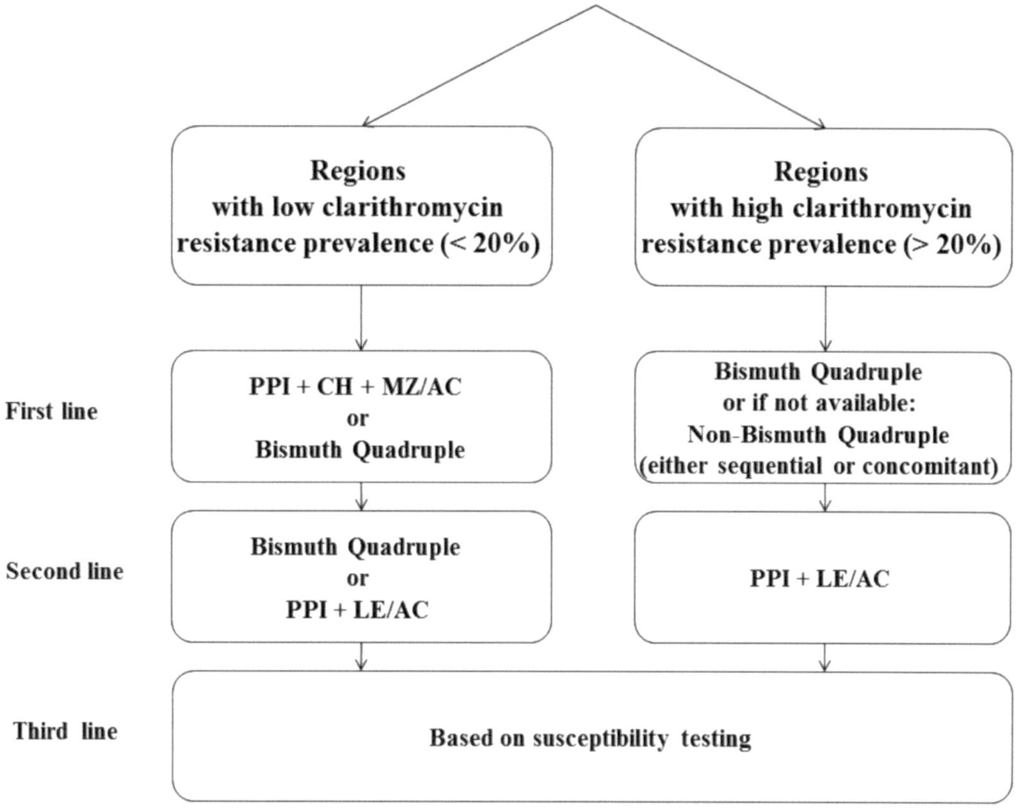

PPI – proton pump inhibitor, **CH** – clarithromycin, **MZ** – metronidazole, **AC** – amoxicillin, **LE** – levofloxacin
Bismuth quadruple therapy: PPI, bismuth, metronidazole, and tetracycline (10 days)
Non-bismuth quadruple sequential therapy: 5-day period with PPI, amoxicillin, followed by 5-day period with PPI, clarithromycin, and metronidazole (or tinidazole)
Non-bismuth quadruple concomitant therapy: clarithromycin, amoxicillin, and metronidazole + PPI (10-14 days)

Figure 2. Treatment schemes of *Helicobacter pylori* infection considering the regions of low and high prevalence of clarithromycin-resistant strains (based on the Maastrich/Florence IV Consensus Report) [1].

In regions with high prevalence of resistance to clarithromycin (>20%), it is recommended to abandon clarithromycin in the empirical treatment of *H. pylori* infections, if the antibiotic susceptibility cannot be tested. As the first line empirical treatment, the bismuth–containing quadruple therapy is recommended. If the bismuth salts are not available in certain countries (e.g. Poland), then non-bismuth quadruple therapies (sequential or concomitant) could be prescribed. Non-bismuth quadruple sequential therapy consists of 5-days of PPI plus amoxicillin, followed by 5-day period with PPI, clarithromycin, and metronidazole (or tinidazole), whereas non-bismuth quadruple concomitant therapy comprises simultaneous use of clarithromycin, amoxicillin, metronidazole, and PPI for 10-14 days. Although both non-bismuth quadruple therapies contain clarithromycin, these regimens could be applied only as targeted therapy based on testing of the bacterial susceptibility to clarithromycin. In regions, where bismuth salts are not available and high clarithromycin resistance occurs, targeted therapy with clarithromycin seems to be the best option.

After failure of the first line treatment, the second line treatment regimen with PPI, levofloxacin, and amoxicillin should be prescribed. It should be emphasized that levofloxacin cannot be used in patients with chronic bronchitis or pneumonia, who may have taken fluoroquinolones, hence it is recommended to perform susceptibility testing to levofloxacin. Moreover, increasing resistance rate to antimicrobial agents should be taken into account [1], for instance in Poland we noted an increasing resistance rate to levofloxacin [23]. Susceptibility testing conducted before treatment, can protect against increasing resistance rate.

If the second line regimen failed, a third line treatment based on antimicrobial susceptibility testing should be introduced. If susceptibility testing is not available, the empirical third line regimen should contain antimicrobials not used previously. Except for the drugs already mentioned, rifabutin is a therapeutic option (its use is limited to mycobacterial infections) [1].

Taking into account the EHSG recommendations, the rationale is to perform susceptibility testing whenever possible to prevent the increase of drug resistance, especially in regions where the resistance to clarithromycin is high.

1.4. Antimicrobial agents and bacterial resistance

Recent data show that combination of standard therapeutic strategies have lost some efficacy. This fact is attributed to increasing antimicrobial resistance of *H. pylori* strains.

Clarithromycin. Among antimicrobial agents used in the treatment of *H. pylori* infections, clarithromycin was considered to be one of the most effective drugs; nonetheless emergence of clarithromycin resistance became the major risk factor of the treatment failure. In susceptible strains, the eradication rates amounted to 87.7%, whereas in resistant strains the rates decreased to 18.3% [5]. One of the most significant factors contributing to clarithromycin resistance is the extensive use of macrolides, particularly in the treatment of upper and lower respiratory tract infections in children [60]. Furthermore, studies conducted between 2001 and 2008 in 18 European countries confirmed the correlation between antibiotic resistance of *H. pylori* strains and outpatient antibiotic consumption in adults. According to this multi-center study, *H. pylori* clarithromycin resistance rates in Europe amounted to 17.5% and were considerably higher in western/central and southern Europe (>20%) than in the northern European countries (<10%) [61]. In Poland, the prevalence of *H. pylori* resistance to clarithromycin was 28% (data published by PSG-E) [22]. Nevertheless, according to our recent study conducted in the years 2006-2008 and 2009-2011, resistance of *H. pylori* strains isolated in southern Poland was also high and amounted to 34% and 22%, respectively [23, 62].

The major mechanism responsible for *H. pylori* clarithromycin resistance is associated with the decrease in the binding of the antibiotic to the ribosome which is caused by the occurrence of the point mutations within the peptidyltransferase-encoding region of 23S rRNA. The most frequently reported point mutation is A-G transition at position 2143 (A2143G), which occurs in 69.8% of *H. pylori* strains resistant to clarithromycin, while the less common mutations are represented by A2142G and A2143C. Furthermore, other mutations, such as A2115G, G2141A,

C2147G, T2190C, C2195T, A2223G, and C2694A, might also be associated with clarithromycin resistance. Molecular assays have a significant impact on improving the availability and accuracy of the data concerning *H. pylori* clarithromycin resistance, resulting in faster and better selection of effective therapy [60, 63].

Metronidazole. Another antimicrobial agent, recommended in the therapy of *H. pylori* infection is metronidazole. Metronidazole has a higher resistance rate than clarithromycin, but it is of secondary importance and can be partly overcome. Treatment with this antimicrobial agent is effective, however, with the exception of the regions where metronidazole resistance reaches 40%. The resistance of *H. pylori* strains to metronidazole amounted to 34.9%, in Europe [5, 61]. In Poland, the resistance rate to metronidazole is higher (46%), according to PSG-E data (2008) [22], whereas in southern Poland, according to our recent study, it is 44% [62].

Common use of metronidazole in parasitic as well as gynecological diseases results in high resistance rates of *H. pylori* strains isolated from both tropical residents and female patients and contributes to overall resistance of the bacterium population [60].

Mechanism of metronidazole resistance in *H. pylori* is not completely understood and, according to some authors, it is related to mutations in *rdx*A (which encodes an oxygen-insensitive NADPH nitroreductase) and *frx*A genes (which encode NADPH flavin oxidoreductase) [60, 64].

Levofloxacin. Levofloxacin is another antimicrobial agent recommended in *H. pylori* treatment, however rapid acquisition of levofloxacin resistance may contribute to the reduction of its future efficiency. In Europe, the resistance rate of *H. pylori* to levofloxacin amounted to 14.4% between 2001 and 2008. Increasing rates of quinolone resistance are attributed to frequent use of these agents in the therapy of the respiratory and urinary tract infections. While in countries with lower quinolone consumption (e.g. Norway) the resistance rate of *H. pylori* strains remains lower, in countries with high use of quinolones (e.g. Italy) the resistance rate is higher [61]. According to data published by PSG-E, the population of *H. pylori* strains in Poland is susceptible to ciprofloxacin [22]. Nevertheless, we reported that levofloxacin resistance rate in southern Poland amounted to 16% in 2011 and in comparison with previous years, the figure had grown [23].

The resistance to fluoroquinolones in *H. pylori* strains is due to the point mutations occurring in *gyr*A gene at the 87 and 91 positions. Furthermore, some studies revealed a correlation between the resistance to levofloxacin and norfloxacin and the point mutation in the position 463 of *gyr*B gene [60, 65].

Amoxicillin and Tetracycline. According to current surveys, the resistance to amoxicillin as well as tetracycline is either very low or even absent, indicating their present clinical irrelevance. While amoxicillin resistance is most likely associated with mutational changes in the penicillin-binding encoding gene (*pbp*D), the tetracycline resistance is based on changes in three nucleotides in the 16S rRNA (AGA 926-928→TTC) [22, 60, 62].

Rifabutin. Rifabutin is one of the antimicrobial agents recommended as an alternative in the third line treatment, after two treatment failures. Prevalence of *H. pylori* resistance to this antibiotic is not well known but it is presumed to be very low, because its use is limited to mycobacterial infection [1]. Moreover, rifabutin is very expensive and causes adverse events like leukopenia, thrombocytopenia or clinically important impairment of liver functions [66, 67]. However, increase in rifabutin consumption may contribute to rapid emergence of resistance. The mechanism of resistance to this antibiotic is mediated by mutations in the *rpo*B gene [1, 60].

1.5. Resistance rate in Poland

Summing up the current and previous data concerning the prevalence of *H. pylori* resistance in Poland, we revealed some differences. The results presented in Polish multi-center study performed between 2000 and 2003 revealed that 28% of the analysed *H. pylori* strains were resistant to clarithromycin, 46% to metronidazole, while all strains were susceptible to amoxicillin and tetracycline [22].

Our studies conducted in the years 2006-2009 and 2010-2012 showed that the resistance rates of *H. pylori* to clarithromycin in southern Poland were 34% and 22%, respectively [23, 62]. Moreover, we reported that the percentage of *H. pylori* strains resistant to metronidazole and levofloxacin accounted for 44% and 6%, respectively. Furthermore, we confirmed the coexistence of resistance to more than one antimicrobial agent: a) resistance to metronidazole and clarithromycin in 23% of the strains, b) resistance to metronidazole, clarithromycin, and levofloxacin in 4% of the strains [62]. Additionally, in our recent studies we demonstrated that in southern Poland the number of *H. pylori* strains resistant to levofloxacin increased significantly; from 5% in the years 2006-2008 to 16% in 2009-2011 [23].

As it was previously emphasized, the Maastricht IV/Florence Consensus Report recommends that treatment regimen should be selected according to areas of low (<20%) and high (>20%) clarithromycin resistance [1]. Referring to available data concerning clarithromycin resistance rates in Poland, this country should be classified as a high clarithromycin resistance region [22, 23, 62].

Although the current Polish guidelines (PSG–E, 2008) on diagnostic and therapeutic approaches to the *H. pylori* infection recommend clarithromycin in the first line treatment, the rationale is to either abandon clarithromycin in an empirical treatment or apply clarithromycin in therapy, but only with prior susceptibility testing.

2. Problem statement

Dynamic growth of *H. pylori* resistance to antimicrobial agents used in empirical treatment becomes an increasingly important problem. While *H. pylori* resistance is often associated with the antibiotic consumption and may vary according to region, it is recommended to constantly monitor the resistance rates of this bacterium. Furthermore, in the areas of high clarithromycin resistance rates as well as increasing resistance to other antibiotics/chemotherapeutics (used in *H. pylori* treatment), it is worth consideration to replace empirical therapy with targeted therapy based on prior susceptibility testing. Moreover, early effective treatment of *H. pylori* infection in patients with peptic ulcer disease can prevent gastric cancer.

3. Aplication area

Data concerning *H. pylori* resistance rates enable to introduce the most effective schemes of infection treatment [5].

4. Research course

1. Monitoring of *H. pylori* resistance to antimicrobial agents used in empirical therapy (according to the Maastricht IV/ Florence Consensus Report) in southern Poland.
2. Selection of the appropriate treatment regimen in *H. pylori* infections in southern Poland, according to the current recommendations and local clarithromycin resistance rates (Maastricht IV/ Florence Consensus Report).
3. Introduction of treatment guided by antimicrobial susceptibility testing in *H. pylori* infections in southern Poland, taking into account: a) high level of clarithromycin resistance, b) increasing resistance rates to levofloxacin, c) persisting high metronidazole resistance rate.
4. Application of molecular method in detection of clarithromycin resistance.

5. Materials and methods

Clinical specimens. The study covered a group of 316 adult dyspeptic patients with therapeutic indications for gastroscopy, who applied to the Falck Medycyna Outpatient Clinic of Gastroenterology (Krakow, Poland) and the Chair of Gastroenterology, Hepatology and Infectious Diseases, Jagiellonian University Medical College (Krakow, Poland).

All patients enrolled to the study underwent gastroscopy in the years 2010-2013. Two biopsy specimens (one from antrum and the second from the body of the stomach) were taken from each patient during gastroscopy. The biopsy specimens were transferred into transport medium (Portagerm Pylori, bioMérieux, France) and transported to the laboratory (Department of Pharmaceutical Microbiology, Jagiellonian University Medical College, Krakow, Poland) for further investigations.

Analysis of endoscopy and histopathological examination enabled to qualify patients into two groups:

1. Subjects with peptic ulcer diseases (PUD) including individuals with peptic and/or duodenal ulcers.

2. Subjects with non-ulcerous dyspepsia (NUD) comprising patients without any pathological changes found in endoscopy and patients with erosive and non-erosive diseases including esophagitis, gastritis or duodenitis.

***H. pylori* microbiological culture and identification.** Gastric biopsy specimens were homogenized in glass sterile mortars and inoculated onto both non selective (Schaedler agar with 5% sheep blood, bioMérieux, France) and selective (Schaedler agar with 5% sheep blood and selective supplement Dent, Oxoid, UK) media. Simultaneously, direct Gram-stained slides and urease tests were performed from the biopsy specimens to confirm the presence of *H. pylori*.

The culture was carried out for 3 to 10 days under microaerophilic conditions at 37°C. The cultured strains were identified according to:

1. Macroscopic appearance of the colonies;
2. Gram–stained slides prepared from bacterial colonies;
3. Biochemical tests (urease, catalase, and oxidase).

The study was approved by the Bioethical Commission of the Jagiellonian University (Krakow, Poland). Before entering our study, each patient signed the informed consent document.

Susceptibility testing. Susceptibility of *H. pylori* strains to the recommended antimicrobial agents (clarithromycin, metronidazole, levofloxacin, tetracycline, and amoxicillin) was quantitatively assessed by the use of strips impregnated with antimicrobial agents gradient (E-test, bioMérieux, France), which enabled to determine the minimal inhibitory concentration (MIC). The colonies from pure *H. pylori* culture were suspended in 0.85% aqueous NaCl solution in order to obtain an equivalent of 3.0 McFarland units. The bacterial suspension was spread onto Schaedler agar medium with 5% sheep blood (bioMérieux, France) with sterile cotton swabs. Single E-test stripes were applied onto the separate, inoculated agar plates and incubated according to the manufacturer recommendations (E-test technical manual, bioMérieux, France).

Results of the susceptibility testing were interpreted according to EUCAST guidelines (breakpoint values were presented in Table 2) [68].

Quality control of the susceptibility testing was performed with *H. pylori* ATCC 43504 strain.

DNA extraction.*H. pylori* culture (incubated for 72 hours on solid medium) was suspended in 1 ml of 0.85% aqueous NaCl solution and centrifuged (12000 rpm/3 min.). Genomic DNA was extracted using the Sherlock AX isolation kit (A&A Biotechnology, Poland) according to the manufacturer's recommendations. DNA quantification was performed by spectrophotometry at 260 nm. The purity of DNA was evaluated by the ratio of the absorbance at 260 and 280 nm (A260/A280). The obtained DNA was stored at -20°C.

PCR identification of *H. pylori*. To confirm *H. pylori* microbiological identification, all analysed strains were subjected to 16S rRNA PCR assay using primers HP-1 and HP-2 described by Kargar et al. [69]. PCR reaction was performed in a final volume of 25 μl containing: 2 μl of genomic DNA, 2 μl of each primer, 5 μl of GoTaq® Flexi Buffer, 1.5 μl of

Antibiotic agent	MIC breakpoints (mg/L)	
	S ≤	R >
Amoxicillin	0.12	0.12
Clarithromycin	0.25	0.5
Levofloxacin	1	1
Metronidazole	8	8
Rifampicin	1	1
Tetracycline	1	1

Table 2. EUCAST clinical breakpoint for *H. pylori* [68].

$MgCl_2$ (25 mM), 0.5 µl of PCR Nucleotide Mix (10 mM each), 0.125 µl of GoTaq® DNA Polymerase (5u/µl) and Nuclease-Free Water (Promega, USA). The following amplification conditions were used: the initial denaturation at 95°C for 2 min., 35 cycles of 95°C for 60 s, 58°C for 60 s, 72°C for 60 s and the final elongation at 72°C for 5 min. The expected 109-base-pair PCR product was visualized after electrophoresis on an 2% agarose gel stained with ethidium bromide.

***cag*A and *vac*A genes detection.** The DNA from analysed *H. pylori* strains was subjected to PCR assay detecting the *cag*A gene with the use of primers D008 and R008 described previously by Chen et al. [70]. The PCR reaction was carried out as described above for the 16s rRNA PCR assay. PCR cycling conditions consisted of initial denaturation at 94°C for 5 min., 33 cycles: 94°C for 60 s, 60°C for 60 s, 62.5°C for 60 s, 72°C for 60 s and the final elongation at 72°C for 5 min. The expected product of 298-base-pairs was visualized after agarose gel electrophoresis. Furthermore, we performed the PCR assay to detect the *vac*A gene. A 229-base-pair fragment of *vac*A was amplified with the primer pair VAC3624F and VAC3853R described previously by Chisholm et al. [71]. The PCR reaction was carried out in the total volume of 25 µl as described above. The following amplification conditions were used: the initial denaturation at 95°C for 2 min., 35 cycles of 95°C for 30 s, 53°C for 30 s, 72°C for 30 s and the final elongation at 72°C for 5 min. The expected product was visualized after agarose gel electrophoresis.

Detection of clarithromycin resistance by RFLP-PCR analysis. The most prevalent point mutations responsible for clarithromycin resistance (A2143G and A2142G) were detected by PCR followed by RFLP analysis. A 425-base-pair fragment of the 23S rRNA was amplified with the primers K1 and K2 described by Agudo et al. [63]. PCR amplification of DNA was performed in a final volume of 25 µl as described above for the 16S rRNA PCR assay. The cycling program was: 1 cycle at 95°C for 2 min.; 35 cycles of 95°C for 30 s, 60°C for 30 s, 72°C for 30 s and a final elongation step at 72°C for 5 min. The amplicon was digested with Eco31I (BsaI) enzyme (Thermo Scientific, USA) for 30 min. at 37°C and 5 min. at 65°C to detect A2143G mutation [63] or with BbsI enzyme (New England Biolabs, USA) for 24 h at 37°C to detect A2142G mutation [72]. The restriction products were analysed by electrophoresis on an 2% agarose gel. Enzyme Eco31I digested the A2143G-positive *H. pylori* PCR amplicon into 304- and 101-base-pair fragments, while BbsI enzyme cut the A2142G-positive *H. pylori* PCR product into 332- and 93-base-pair fragments.

6. Results

Prevalence of *H. pylori* infection. Among 316 patients with dyspeptic symptoms admitted to the study between November 2010 and June 2013, the presence of *H. pylori* infection was confirmed in 73 cases (according to rapid urease test and bacterial culture). Therefore, the prevalence of *H. pylori* infection in patients with dyspeptic symptoms from southern Poland amounted to 23.1% (73/316). Taking into account the analysis of endoscopy and histopathological examination among 73 *H. pylori*-positive patients, 26% (19/73) were qualified into the I group (patients with PUD), whereas 74% (54/73) patients were qualified into the II group (patients with NUD).

Susceptibility testing. The susceptibility testing of 73 *H. pylori* strains to the recommended antimicrobial agents showed that 51.7% of isolates were resistant to one or more drugs, while 49.3% of strains were susceptible to all tested antibiotics/chemotherapeutics. The resistance rates of *H. pylori* strains to the assayed antimicrobial agents were presented in Table 3 (data include strains resistant to one, two or four antibiotics/chemotherapeutics).

The rate of resistance of *H. pylori* strains to clarithromycin amounted to 23.3% (17/73). According to the Maastricht/Florence IV Consensus Report, southern Poland should be qualified as an area of high clarithromycin resistance. Consequently, the use of clarithromycin in *H. pylori* infections in this region should be either abandoned (as an empirical treatment) or applied but only with prior susceptibility testing. Due to this fact, it seems reasonable to change the current Polish recommendation (PSG-E, 2008) concerning clarithromycin use in the treatment of *H. pylori* infections.

Furthermore, the resistance rates to metronidazole and levofloxacin were 39.7% (29/73) and 12.3% (9/73), respectively.

Antimicrobial agents	N (%) of resistant strains (n = 73)
Clarithromycin	17 (23.3)
Metronidazole	29 (39.7)
Levofloxacin	9 (12.3)
Amoxicillin	1 (1.4)
Tetracycline	0 (0)

Table 3. Resistance rates of *H. pylori* to clarithromycin, metronidazole, levofloxacin, amoxicillin, and tetracycline in southern Poland (the data include strains resistant to one, two or four antibiotics/chemotherapeutics).

We also reported the presence of one strain (1,4%; 1/73) resistant to amoxicillin. Resistance to amoxicillin is an uncommon phenomenon and it is the first report of an amoxicillin-resistant strain in southern Poland. All examined *H. pylori* strains were susceptible to tetracycline.

Moreover, we analysed the co-occurrence of resistance to more than one antimicrobial agent among *H. pylori* isolates (Table 4).

Our studies showed the presence of 35.6% (26/73) of single-resistant, 8% (13/73) of double-resistant and 1.4% (1) of quadruple-resistant strains (susceptibility testing for each tested isolate included: clarithromycin, metronidazole, levofloxacin, and amoxicillin).

Antimicrobial agents		**N (%) of resistant strainsn n=73**
	Clarithromycin	6 (8.2)
single-resistant strains	Metronidazole	16 (21.9)
	Levofloxacin	4 (5.4)
	Clarithromycin + Metronidazole	9 (12.3)
double-resistant strains	Metronidazole + Levofloxacin	3 (4.1)
	Clarithromycin + Levofloxacin	1 (1.4)
quadruple-resistant strains	Clarithromycin + Metronidazole + Levofloxacin + Amoxicillin	1 (1.4)

Table 4. Co-occurrence of resistance to various antibiotics/chemotherapeutics among H. pylori strains isolated in southern Poland.

The MICs obtained in our study ranged from 0.016 mg/L to 256 mg/L for clarithromycin [Figure 3], from 0.016 mg/L to 256 mg/L for metronidazole [Figure 4], from 0.002 mg/L to 12 mg/L for levofloxacin [Figure 5], and from 0.016 mg/L to 0.125 mg/L for both amoxicillin [Figure 6] and tetracycline [Figure 7].

The mean MIC values were as follows: 19.2 mg/L for clarithromycin, 75.2 mg/L for metronidazole, 0.61 mg/L for levofloxacin, 0.018 mg/L for amoxicillin, and 0.024 mg/L for tetracycline.

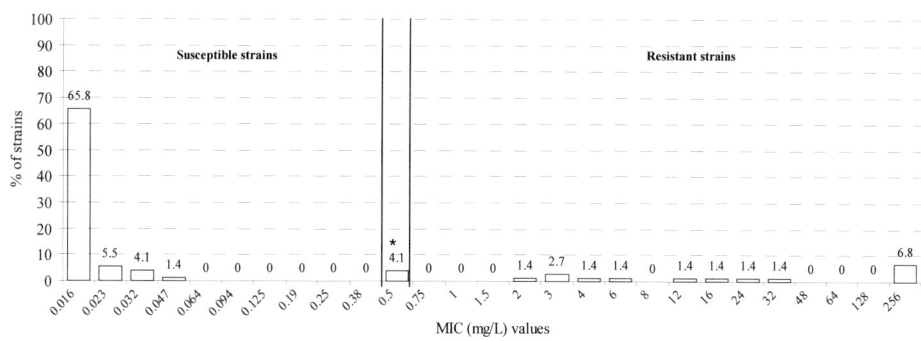

Figure 3. The distribution of clarithromycin MICs among *H. pylori* strains (Clinical breakpoints according to EUCAST: resistant MIC>0.5 mg/L; susceptible MIC≤0.25 mg/L); * strains with MIC value of 0.5 mg/L were considered as resistant to clarithromycin according to the results of PCR–RFLP analysis.

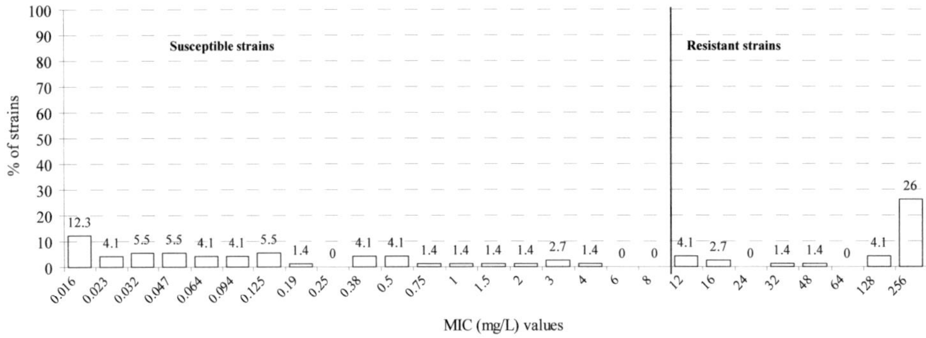

Figure 4. The distribution of MICs among *H. pylori* strains (Clinical breakpoints according to EUCAST: resistant MIC>8 mg/L; susceptible MIC≤8 mg/L).

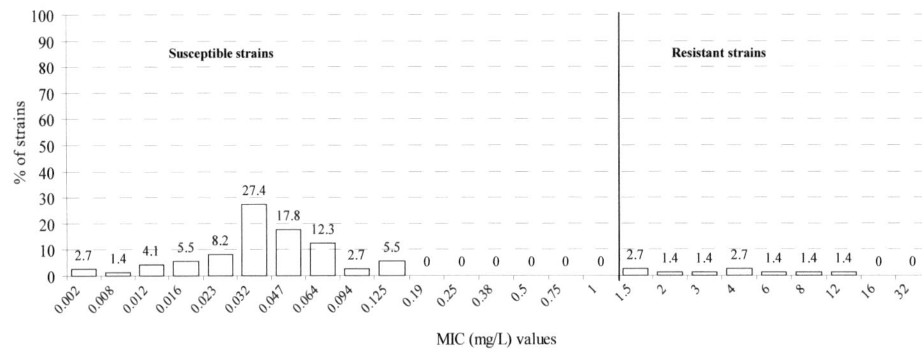

Figure 5. The distribution of levofloxacin MICs among *H. pylori* strains (Clinical breakpoints according to EUCAST: resistant MIC>1 mg/L; susceptible MIC≤1 mg/L).

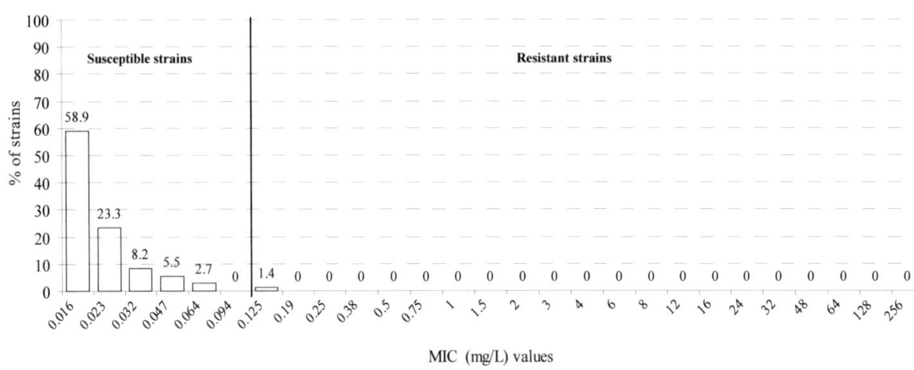

Figure 6. The distribution of amoxicillin MICs among *H. pylori* strains (Clinical breakpoints according to EUCAST: resistant MIC>0.12 mg/L; susceptible MIC≤0.12 mg/L).

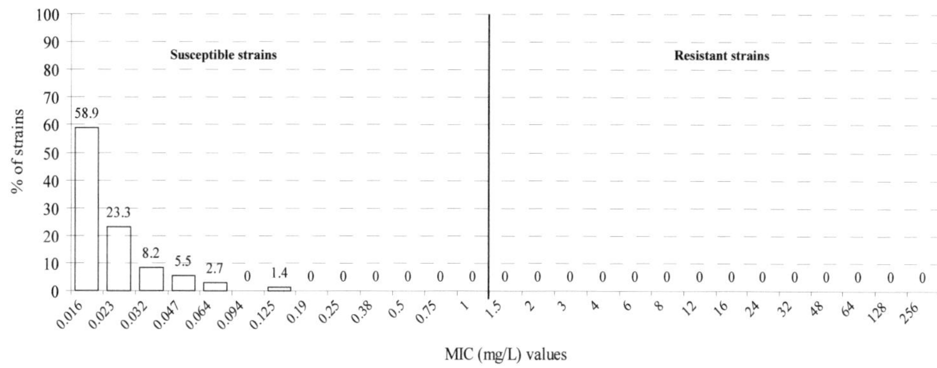

Figure 7. The distribution of tetracycline MICs among *H. pylori* strains (Clinical breakpoints according to EUCAST: resistant MIC>1 mg/L; susceptible MIC≤1 mg/L).

The quantitative E-test method allowed us to observe the dynamically increasing resistance of *H. pylori* to antimicrobials during the monitoring.

In Poland, *H. pylori* resistance rate to clarithromycin exceeded 20% [22, 23, 62]. Our recent study revealed that this rate remained at the same high level or even increased to 23.3%. Therefore the current Polish guidelines (PSG–E, 2008) should be changed according to EHSG (2012). EHSG recommended abandoning clarithromycin in empirical treatment or susceptibility testing prior to the administration of this drug in regions with high prevalence of resistant *H. pylori* strains (>20%).

Moreover, it is worth emphasizing that our study showed that 6.8% of analysed strains demonstrated high clarithromycin MIC values: 256 mg/L.

Furthermore, we revealed persistent, high-level resistance to metronidazole (39.7% of isolates). Twenty-six percent of *H. pylori* strains displayed the metronidazole MIC values as high as 256 mg/L. Additionally, the resistance rate to levofloxacin increased in comparison to our previous studies (5% in the years 2006-2008 [62] *vs.* 12.3% currently).

Although the amoxicillin MIC values are still low, emergence of a resistant *H. pylori* isolate was a new phenomenon. It was the first amoxicillin-resistant *H. pylori* strain isolated in southern Poland.

The reason as to why *H. pylori* resistance to antibiotics/chemotherapeutics has to be monitored, are the results of our study. Moreover, in order to obtain effective regimen for the cure of *H. pylori* infection, it seems reasonable to perform susceptibility testing prior to the treatment.

PCR identification of *H. pylori*. Microbiological identification of all 73 *H. pylori* isolates was confirmed by PCR targeting the 16S rRNA gene (representative samples are presented in Figure 8).

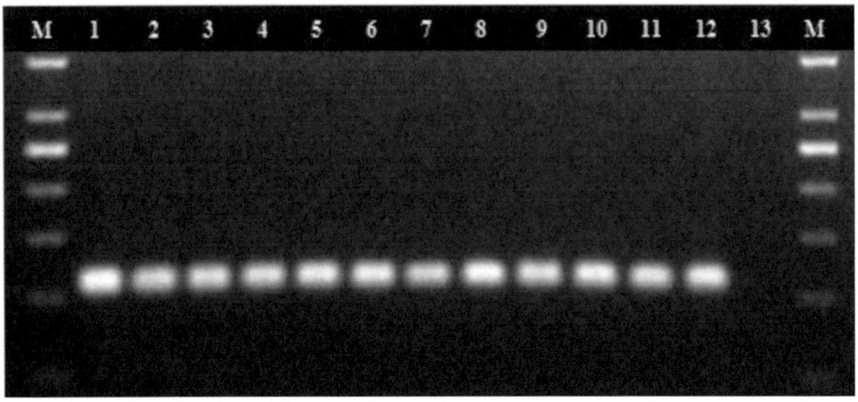

Figure 8. Representative samples of 16S rRNA PCR assay. Lines: 1-11 - selected *H. pylori* strains isolated from patients enrolled to the study, 12 - positive control (109 bp), 13 - negative control; M - molecular weight marker (O'GeneRuler 50 bp DNA Ladder, Thermo Scientific, USA).

cag*A *and vac*A genes distribution.cag*A and *vac*A genes have been identified as being virulence-associated and may have important clinical and epidemiological implications [73]. While *cag*A is carried by 56-90% of *H. pylori* strains [8, 24, 29-32], *vac*A is present in all identified *H. pylori* isolates [74]. The occurrence of *cag*A and *vac*A genes was tested in all 73 strains.

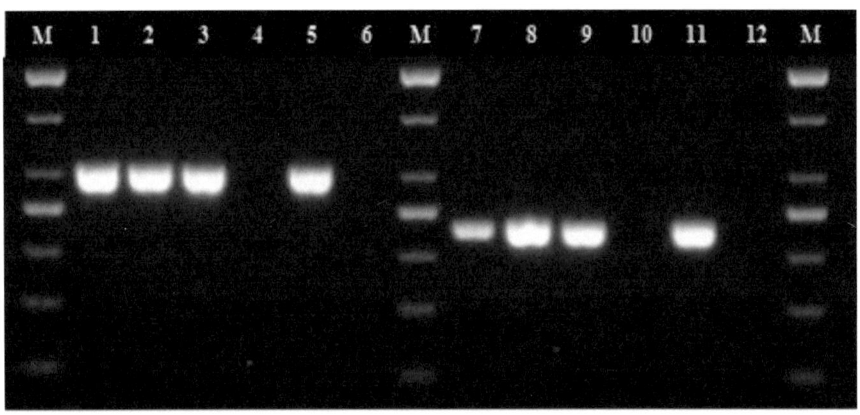

Figure 9. Representative samples of *cag*A and *vac*A genes detection. A) *cag*A detection: lines: 1-4 - selected *H. pylori* strains isolated from patients enrolled to the study, 5 - positive control (298 bp), 6 - negative control; B) *vac*A detection: lines: 7-10 - selected *H. pylori* strains isolated from patients enrolled to the study, 11 - positive control (229 bp), 12 - negative control; M - molecular weight marker (O'GeneRuler 50 bp DNA Ladder, Thermo Scientific, USA).

The cytotoxin associated gene - *cag*A - was detected in 80.8% of *H. pylori* strains (59/73), whereas *cag*A-negative strains accounted for 19.2% (14/73) (representative samples are shown in Figure 9). The occurrence of *vac*A gene was confirmed in 89% (65/73) of strains, while 11% (8/73) of strains were *vac*A-negative. The absence of *vac*A gene in 11% of assayed *H. pylori* strains was associated with limited sensitivity of the method used in this study [71].

Table 5 shows the relationship between the distribution of *cag*A and *vac*A genes and the clinical diagnosis.

Among 19 patients with peptic ulcer disease (PUD), 78.9% (15/19) were infected with *H. pylori cag*A-positive strains, while 21.1% (4/19) with strains *cag*A-negative. Moreover, 84.2% (16/19) of patients with PUD were infected with *H. pylori vac*A-positive strains and 15.8% (3/19) with strains *vac*A-negative. Double positive *H. pylori* strains (*cagA*-positive and *vacA*-positive) occurred in 63.2% (12/19) of patients with peptic ulcer disease.

Among the group of patients with NUD, 81.5% (49/54) of isolated *H. pylori* strains carried *cag*A gene, but only 18.5% (10/54) were *cag*A-negative. Although none of these patients developed ulceration during the study, it is probable that these infections, if untreated, may lead to serious consequences such as peptic ulcer disease or even gastric cancer, due to the fact that the *cag*A-positive *H. pylori* strains increase the likelihood of developing these diseases.

The *cag*A-positive, *vac*A-positive *H. pylori* genotype was the most common one in both: groups of patients: with PUD as well as with NUD, whereas the duble-negative genotype was not found.

Genotype	N (%) of strains	
	PUD n=19	NUD n=54
cagA +	15 (78.9)	44 (81.5)
cagA -	4 (21.1)	10 (18.5)
vacA +	16 (84.2)	49 (90.7)
vacA -	3 (15.8)	5 (9.3)
cagA + *vacA* +	12 (63.2)	39 (72.5)
cagA + *vacA* -	3 (15.8)	5 (9.3)
cagA - *vacA* +	4 (21.1)	10 (18.5)
cagA - *vacA* -	0 (0)	0 (0)

PUD – peptic ulcer disease

NUD – non-ulcer dyspepsia

Table 5. Relationship between distribution of *cag*A and *vac*A genes and the clinical diagnosis.

PCR-RFLP analysis of *H. pylori* resistance to clarithromycin. Molecular analysis of clarithromycin resistance mechanism was conducted on 73 *H. pylori* strains. The results of PCR-RFLP analysis are shown in Figure 10 and Table 6.

Among the 17 clarithromycin-resistant isolates, Eco31I (BsaI) digested PCR amplicons of 12 (70.6%) strains to 304-base-pair and 101-base-pair, indicating that the strains contained A2143G mutation in the 23S rRNA gene. Furthermore, BbsI enzyme cut products of 3 (17.6%) strains to 332-base-pair and 93-base-pair suggesting that the isolates had A2142G mutation.

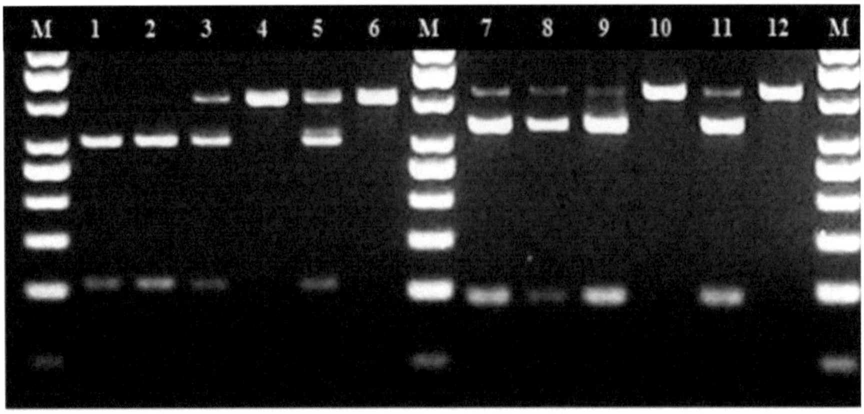

Figure 10. Restriction endonuclease analysis of 23S rRNA amplicons (425 bp) digested with Eco31I (BsaI) and BbsI enzymes. A) detection of A2143G mutation: lines: 1-4 - selected *H. pylori* strains isolated from patients enrolled to the study, 5 - positive control (digestion products of 304 and 101 bp), 6 - negative control; B) detection of A2142G mutation: lines: 7-10 - selected *H. pylori* strains isolated from patients enrolled to the study, 11 - positive control (digestion products of 332 and 93 bp), 12 - negative control; M – Molecular Weight Marker (50 bp O'Gene Ruler, Thermo Scientific, USA).

RFLP analysis of 11.8% (2/17) clarithromycin-resistant isolates gave negative results for both assayed mutations. Resistance to clarithromycin in these isolates (negative for both A2413G and A2142G) might be associated with other mutations in the 23S rRNA such as A2142C, T2245C, T2717C, A2115G, G2141A, T2182G, or T2182C as well as efflux pump [63].

Digestion of PCR products of 100% (56/56) strains not resistant to clarithromycin revealed the absence of the tested mutations. Moreover, our studies suggest that the presence of A2142G mutation is more related to the high clarithromycin MIC level than the A2143G mutation.

Type of mutation	N (%) of strains	
	Clarithromycin–resistant n=17	**Clarithromycin–susceptible n=56**
A2143G	12 (70.6)	0 (0)
A2142G	3 (17.6)	0 (0)
not detected	2 (11.8)	56 (100)

Table 6. Prevalence of A2143G and A2142G mutations in the group of 73 tested *H. pylori* strains.

7. Conclusions

Results of our studies concerning the resistance rates of *H. pylori* strains isolated from subjects in southern Poland suggest the need for constant monitoring of the resistance to a set of antimicrobial agents routinely used for empirical therapy. We observed high level of clarithromycin resistance rate (>20%), which resulted in the necessity of either to abandon clarithromycin in an empirical treatment or to perform susceptibility testing prior to application of clarithromycin-containing treatment.

We also noted the increase in *H. pylori* resistance to levofloxacin and persistent high level resistance to metronidazole, which resulted in the necessity of treatment guided by antimicrobial susceptibility testing.

To conclude, antimicrobial susceptibility testing can improve treatment outcomes and reduce the outpatient antibiotic consumption, while the introduction of molecular methods for clarithromycin resistance testing allows better and more efficient management of *H. pylori* infections.

8. Further research

Our further investigations will be concerned with the application of the PCR-RFLP method in detection of less frequent 23S rRNA gene mutations associated with clarithromycin resistance. Furthermore, we will focus on direct detection of *H. pylori* in biopsy specimens as well as characterization of the resistance determinants.

Acknowledgements

This work was supported by a research grant funded by the Polish Government in the years 2011-2013 (NN404547640)

Author details

Elżbieta Karczewska[1], Karolina Klesiewicz[1], Paweł Nowak[1], Edward Sito[2], Iwona Skiba[1], Małgorzata Zwolińska–Wcisło[3], Tomasz Mach[3] and Alicja Budak[1]

1 Department of Pharmaceutical Microbiology, Jagiellonian University Medical College, Krakow, Poland

2 Falck Medycyna Outpatient Clinic of Gastroenterology, Krakow, Poland

3 Chair of Gastroenterology, Hepatology and Infectious Diseases, Jagiellonian University Medical College, Krakow, Poland

References

[1] Malfertheiner P, Megraud F, O'Morain CA, Atherton J, Axon AT, Bazzoli F, et al. European Helicobacter Study Group. Management of Helicobacter pylori infection--the Maastricht IV/ Florence Consensus Report. Gut. 2012;61(5):646-664. doi: 10.1136/gutjnl-2012-302084. http://gut.bmj.com/content/61/5/646.long (accessed 10 July 2013).

[2] International Agency For Research on Cancer. IARC. Monograph on the Evaluation of Carcinogenic Risks to Humans, Schistosomes, Liver Flukes and Helicobacter pylori. Lyon, France: IARC, 1994;61:177-242.

[3] Ando T, Goto Y, Maeda O, Watanabe O, Ishiguro K, Goto H. Causal role of Helicobacter pylori infection in gastric cancer. World J Gastroenterol. 2006;12(2):181-186. http://www.wjgnet.com/1007-9327/full/v12/i2/181.htm (accessed 10 July 2013).

[4] Perez-Perez GI, Rothenbacher D, Brenner H. Epidemiology of Helicobacter pylori infection. Helicobacter. 2004;9(Suppl 1):1-6.

[5] Malfertheiner P, Megraud F, O'Morain C, Bazzoli F, El-Omar E, Graham D, et al. Current concepts in the management of Helicobacter pylori infection: the Maastricht III Consensus Report. Gut. 2007;56(6):772-81. doi:10.1136/gut.2006.101634 http://gut.bmj.com/content/56/6/772.long (accessed 10 July 2013).

[6] Goh KL, Chan WK, Shiota S, Yamaoka Y. Epidemiology of Helicobacter pylori infection and public health implications. Helicobacter. 2011;16(Suppl 1):1-9. doi: 10.1111/j.1523-5378.2011.00874.x. http://onlinelibrary.wiley.com/doi/10.1111/j.1523-5378.2011.00874.x/full (accessed 12 July 2013).

[7] Wroblewski LE, Peek Jr. RM, Wilson KT. Helicobacter pylori and Gastric Cancer: Factors That Modulate Disease Risk. Clin. Microbiol. Rev. 2010;23(4)713-739. doi: 10.1128/CMR.00011-10. http://cmr.asm.org/content/23/4/713.full (accessed 11 July 2013).

[8] Konturek PC, Konturek SJ, Brzozowski T. Helicobacter pylori infection in gastric cancerogenesis. J Physiol Pharmacol. 2009;60(3):3-21.

[9] Venerito M, Selgrad M, Malfertheiner P. Helicobacter pylori: Gastric Cancer and Extragastric Malignancies - Clinical aspects. Helicobacter. 2013;18(Suppl 1):39-43.

[10] Wotherspoon AC, Ortiz-Hidalgo C, Falzon MR, Isaacson PG. Helicobacter pylori-associated gastritis and primary B-cell gastric lymphoma. Lancet 1991;338:1175-1176.

[11] Gisbert JP, Calvet X. Review article: common misconceptions in the management of Helicobacter pylori-associated gastric MALT-lymphoma. Aliment Pharmacol Ther. 2011;34(9):1047-1062. doi: 10.1111/j.1365-2036.2011.04839.x. http://onlinelibrary.wiley.com/doi/10.1111/j.1365-2036.2011.04839.x/full (accessed 10 July 2013).

[12] Pellicano R, Franceschi F, Saracco G, Fagoonee S, Roccarina D, Gasbarrini A. Helicobacters and extragastric diseases. Helicobacter. 2009;14(Suppl 1):58-68.

[13] Qu XH, Huang XL, Xiong P, Zhu CY, Huang YL, Lu LG, et al. Does Helicobacter pylori infection play a role in iron deficiency anemia? A meta-analysis. World J Gastroenterol. 2010;16(7):886-896.

[14] Figura N, Franceschi F, Santucci A, Bernardini G, Gasbarrini G, Gasbarrini A. Extragastric manifestations of Helicobacter pylori infection. Helicobacter. 2010;15(Suppl 1):60-68.

[15] Banić M, Franceschi F, Babić Z, Gasbarrini A. Extragastric manifestations of Helicobacter pylori infection. Helicobacter. 2012;17(Suppl 1):49-55.

[16] Pellicano R, Franceschi F, Saracco G, Fagoonee S, Roccarina D, Gasbarrini A. Helicobacters and extragastric diseases. Helicobacter. 2009;14(Suppl 1):58-68.

[17] Kowalski M, Konturek PC, Pieniazek P, Karczewska E, Kluczka A, Grove R, et al. Prevalence of Helicobacter pylori infection in coronary artery disease and effect of its eradication on coronary lumen reduction after percutaneous coronary angioplasty. Dig Liver Dis. 2001;33(3):222-229.

[18] Pieniazek P, Karczewska E, Duda A, Tracz W, Pasowicz M, Konturek SJ. Association of Helicobacter pylori infection with coronary heart disease. J Physiol Pharmacol. 1999;50(5):743-751.

[19] Miendje Deyi VY, Vanderpas J, Bontems P, Van den Borre C, De Koster E, Cadranel S, et al. Marching cohort of Helicobacter pylori infection over two decades (1988-2007): combined effects of secular trend and population migration. Epidemiol Infect. 2011;139(4):572-580.

[20] Tonkic A, Tonkic M, Lehours P, Mégraud F. Epidemiology and diagnosis of Helicobacter pylori infection. Helicobacter. 2012;17(Suppl 1):1-8.

[21] Bureš J, Kopáčová M, Koupil I, Seifert B, Skodová Fendrichová M, Spirková J, et al. Significant decrease in prevalence of Helicobacter pylori in the Czech Republic. World J Gastroenterol. 2012;18(32):4412-4418. doi: 10.3748/wjg.v18.i32.4412. http://www.wjgnet.com/1007-9327/full/v18/i32/4412.htm (accessed 11 July 2013).

[22] Dzieniszewski J, Jarosz M, Grupa Robocza PTG-E do spraw zakażenia Helicobacter pylori. Ustalenia Grupy Roboczej PTG-E dotyczące postępowania w zakażeniu Helicobacter pylori - consensus 2008. Gastroenterologia Polska 2008;15(5):323-331; Article In Polish.

[23] Karczewska E, Klesiewicz K, Skiba I, Wojtas-Bonior I, Sito E, Czajecki K, et al. Variability in Prevalence of Helicobacter pylori Strains Resistant to Clarithromycin and Levofloxacin in Southern Poland. Gastroenterol Res Pract. 2012;2012:418010. doi: 10.1155/2012/418010. http://www.hindawi.com/journals/grp/2012/418010/ (accessed 10 July 2013).

[24] Jaguszyn-Krynicka EK, Gajkowska A, Godlewska R. Virulence factors of Helicobacter pylori. Mikrobiol Med 1999;3(20):3-13 Article In Polish.

[25] Jagusztyn-Krynicka EK, Godlewska R, Laniewski P. Helicobacter pylori - patogen roku 2005. Kosmos 2005;54:307-319. Article In Polish.

[26] Malfertheiner P, Sipponen P, Naumann M, Moayyedi P, Mégraud F, Xiao SD, et al. H. pylori-Gastric Cancer Task Force. Helicobacter pylori eradication has the potential to prevent gastric cancer: a state-of-the-art critique. Am J Gastroenterol. 2005;100(9): 2100-2115.

[27] Peek RM Jr, Crabtree JE. Helicobacter infection and gastric neoplasia. J Pathol. 2006;208(2):233-248.

[28] Konturek PC, Konturek SJ, Brzozowski T. Gastric cancer and Helicobacter pylori infection. J Physiol Pharmacol. 2006;57(Suppl 3):51-65.

[29] Karczewska E, Wojtas I, Sito E, Trojanowska D, Budak A, Zwolinska-Wcislo M, et al. Assessment of co-existence of Helicobacter pylori and Candida fungi in diseases of the upper gastrointestinal tract. J Physiol Pharmacol. 2009;60(Suppl 6):33-39.

[30] Palli D, Masala G, Del Giudice G, Plebani M, Basso D, Berti D, et al. CagA+ Helicobacter pylori infection and gastric cancer risk in the EPIC-EURGAST study. Int J Cancer. 2007;120(4):859-867.

[31] Portal-Celhay C, Perez-Perez GI. Immune responses to Helicobacter pylori colonization: mechanisms and clinical outcomes. Clin Sci (Lond). 2006;110(3):305-314.

[32] Essawi T, Hammoudeh W, Sabri I, Sweidan W, Farraj MA. Determination of Helicobacter pylori Virulence Genes in Gastric Biopsies by PCR. ISRN Gastroenterol. 2013;2013:606258. doi: 10.1155/2013/606258. http://www.hindawi.com/isrn/gastroenterology/2013/606258/ (accessed 15 July 2013).

[33] Crabtree JE, Covacci A, Farmery SM, Xiang Z, Tompkins DS, Perry S, et al. Helicobacter pylori induced interleukin-8 expression in gastric epithelial cells is associated with CagA positive phenotype. J Clin Pathol. 1995;48(1):41-5.

[34] Gocki J, Bartuzi Z, Dziedziczko A. Cytotoxity genes of Helicobacter pylori. Annales Academiae Medicae Bydgostiensis. 2003, 17(2):65-70. Article In Polish.

[35] Duklińska U, Łasica AM, Jagusztyn-Krynicka EK. Białko CagA Helicobacter pylori-pierwsza zidentyfikowana bakteryjna onkoproteina. Post. Mikrobiol 2011;50(2): 97-106. Article In Polish.

[36] Figueiredo C, Machado JC, Yamaoka Y. Pathogenesis of Helicobacter pylori Infection. Helicobacter. 2005;10(Suppl 1):14-20.

[37] Wen S, Moss SF. Helicobacter pylori virulence factors in gastric carcinogenesis. Cancer Lett. 2009;282(1):1-8.

[38] Delahay RM, Rugge M. Pathogenesis of Helicobacter pylori infection. Helicobacter. 2012;17(Suppl 1):9-15. doi: 10.1111/j.1523-5378.2012.00976.x.

[39] Atherton JC, Cao P, Peek RM Jr, Tummuru MK, Blaser MJ, Cover TL. Mosaicism in vacuolating cytotoxin alleles of Helicobacter pylori. Association of specific vacA types with cytotoxin production and peptic ulceration. J Biol Chem. 1995;270(30): 17771-17777.

[40] Atherton JC, Peek RM Jr, Tham KT, Cover TL, Blaser MJ. Clinical and pathological importance of heterogeneity in vacA, the vacuolating cytotoxin gene of Helicobacter pylori. Gastroenterology. 1997;112(1):92-99.

[41] Wen S, Moss SF. Helicobacter pylori virulence factors in gastric carcinogenesis. Cancer Lett. 2009;282(1):1-8. doi: 10.1016/j.canlet.2008.11.016.

[42] Garner JA, Cover TL. Analysis of genetic diversity in cytotoxin-producing and non-cytotoxin-producing Helicobacter pylori strains. J Infect Dis. 1995;172(1):290-293.

[43] Skouloubris S, Labigne A, De Reuse H. Identification and characterization of an aliphatic amidase in Helicobacter pylori. Mol Microbiol. 1997;25(5):989-998.

[44] Langton SR, Cesareo SD. Helicobacter pylori associated phospholipase A2 activity: a factor in peptic ulcer production? J Clin Pathol 1992;45:221-224.

[45] Slomiany BL, Murty VL, Piotrowski J, Liau YH, Sundaram P, Slomiany A. Glycosulfatase activity of Helicobacter pylori toward gastric mucin. Biochem Biophys Res Comm 1992;183:506-513.

[46] Dzierżanowska-Fangrat K, Dzierżanowska D. Helicobacter pylori: Microbiology and Interactions with Gastrointestinal Microflora. J Physiol Pharmacol. 2006;57(Suppl 3): 5-14.

[47] Spigelhalder CB, Gerstenecker A, Kersten, Schiltz E, Kist M. Purification of Helicobacter pylori superoxide dismutase and cloning and sequencing of the gene. Infect Immun 1993;61:5315-5325.

[48] Hazell SL, Evans DJ Jr, Graham DY. Helicobacter pylori catalase. J Gen Microbiol 1991;137:57-61.

[49] Sidebotham RL, Batten JJ, Karim QN, Spencer J, Baron JH. Breakdown of gastric mucus in presence of Helicobacter pylori. J Clin Pathol. 1991;44(1):52-57.

[50] Evans DJ Jr, Evans DG. Helicobacter pylori adhesins: review and perspectives. Helicobacter. 2000;5(4):183-195.

[51] Testerman TL, McGee DJ, Mobley HLT. Adherence and Colonization. In: Mobley HLT, Mendz GL, Hazell SL, editors. Helicobacter pylori: Physiology and Genetics. Washington (DC): ASM Press; 2001. Chapter 34. Available from: http://www.ncbi.nlm.nih.gov/books/NBK2437/ (accessed 20 July 2013).

[52] Cid TP, Fernández MC, Benito Martínez S, Jones NL. Pathogenesis of Helicobacter pylori Infection. Helicobacter. 2013;18(Suppl 1):12-17. doi: 10.1111/hel.12076.

[53] D Scott, D Weeks, K Melchers, G Sachs. The life and death of Helicobacter pylori. Gut. 1998;43(Suppl 1):56-60.

[54] Matsuura M. Structural Modifications of Bacterial Lipopolysaccharide that Facilitate Gram-Negative Bacteria Evasion of Host Innate Immunity. Front Immunol. 2013;4:109. doi: 10.3389/fimmu.2013.00109. http://www.frontiersin.org/Journal/10.3389/fimmu.2013.00109/full (accessed 25 July 2013).

[55] Moran AP. Relevance of fucosylation and Lewis antigen expression in the bacterial gastroduodenal pathogen Helicobacter pylori. Carbohydr Res. 2008;343(12): 1952-1965. doi: 10.1016/j.carres.2007.12.012.

[56] Dzieniszewski J, Jarosz M, Grupa Robocza PTG-E. Postępowanie w zakażeniu Helicobacter pylori (Rok 2004). Wytyczne opracowane przez Grupę Roboczą Polskiego Towarzystwa Gastroenterologii Gastroenterol Pol. 2004;11:41-48. Article In Polish.

[57] Grupa Robocza PTG-E do spraw zakażenia Helicobacter pylori: http://www.ptg-e.org.pl/helico.php

[58] European Helicobacter Study Group Current European concepts in the management of Helicobacter pylori infection. The Maastricht Consensus Report. Gut 1997;41:8-13.

[59] Malfertheiner P, Mégraud F, O'Morain C, Hungin AP, Jones R, Axon A, et al. European Helicobacter Pylori Study Group (EHPSG). Current concepts in the management of Helicobacter pylori infection-the Maastricht 2-2000 Consensus Report. Aliment Pharmacol Ther. 2002;16(2):167-180.

[60] Mégraud F. H pylori antibiotic resistance: prevalence, importance, and advances in testing. Gut. 2004;53(9):1374-1384.

[61] Megraud F, Coenen S, Versporten A, Kist M, Lopez-Brea M, Hirschl AM, Andersen LP, Goossens H, Glupczynski Y; Study Group participants. Helicobacter pylori resistance to antibiotics in Europe and its relationship to antibiotic consumption. Gut. 2013;62(1):34-42. doi: 10.1136/gutjnl-2012-302254. http://gut.bmj.com/content/62/1/34.long (accessed 13 July 2013).

[62] Karczewska E, Wojtas-Bonior I, Sito E, Zwolińska-Wcisło M, Budak A. Primary and secondary clarithromycin, metronidazole, amoxicillin and levofloxacin resistance to Helicobacter pylori in southern Poland. Pharmacol Rep. 2011;63(3):799-807.

[63] Agudo S, Pérez-Pérez G, Alarcón T, López-Brea M. Rapid detection of clarithromycin resistant Helicobacter pylori strains in Spanish patients by polymerase chain reaction-restriction fragment length polymorphism. Rev Esp Quimioter. 2011;24(1):32-36.

[64] Yang YJ, Wu JJ, Sheu BS, Kao AW, Huang AH. The rdxA gene plays a more major role than frxA gene mutation in high-level metronidazole resistance of Helicobacter pylori in Taiwan. Helicobacter. 2004;9(5):400-407.

[65] Rimbara E, Noguchi N, Kawai T, Sasatsu M. Fluoroquinolone resistance in Helicobacter pylori: role of mutations at position 87 and 91 of GyrA on the level of resistance and identification of a resistance conferring mutation in GyrB. Helicobacter. 2012;17(1):36-42.

[66] Gisbert JP, Calvet X. Review article: rifabutin in the treatment of refractory Helicobacter pylori infection. Aliment Pharmacol Ther. 2012;35(2):209-221.

[67] Gisbert JP. Rescue Therapy for Helicobacter pylori Infection 2012. Gastroenterol Res Pract. 2012;2012:974594. doi: 10.1155/2012/974594. http://www.hindawi.com/journals/grp/2012/974594/ (accessed 10 July 2013).

[68] European Committee on Antimicrobial Susceptibility Testing. Breakpoint tables for interpretation of MICs and zone diameters. Version 3.1. Available from: http://www.eucast.org/fileadmin/src/media/PDFs/EUCAST_files/Breakpoint_tables/Breakp (accessed 10 July 2013).

[69] Kargar M, Ghorbani-Dalini S, Doosti A, Souod N. Real-time PCR for Helicobacter pylori quantification and detection of clarithromycin resistance in gastric tissue from patients with gastrointestinal disorders. Res Microbiol. 2012;163(2):109-113.

[70] Chen XJ, Yan J, Shen YF. Dominant cagA/vacA genotypes and coinfection frequency of H. pylori in peptic ulcer or chronic gastritis patients in Zhejiang Province and correlations among different genotypes, coinfection and severity of the diseases. Chin Med J (Engl). 2005;118(6):460-467. http://www.cmj.org/ch/reader/view_abstract.aspx?volume=118&issue=6&start_page=460 (accessed 15 July 2013).

[71] Chisholm SA, Owen RJ, Teare EL, Saverymuttu S. PCR-Based Diagnosis of Helicobacter pylori Infection and Real-Time Determination of Clarithromycin Resistance Directly from Human Gastric Biopsy Samples. J Clin Microbiol. 2001;39(4):1217-1220.

[72] Occhialini A, Urdaci M, Doucet-Populaire F, Bébéar CM, Lamouliatte H, Mégraud F. Macrolide resistance in Helicobacter pylori: rapid detection of point mutations and assays of macrolide binding to ribosomes. Antimicrob Agents Chemother. 1997;41(12):2724-2728.

[73] van Doorn LJ. Detection of Helicobacter pylori virulence-associated genes. Expert Rev Mol Diagn. 2001;1(3):290-298.

[74] Palframan SL, Kwok T, Gabriel K. Vacuolating cytotoxin A (VacA), a key toxin for Helicobacter pylori pathogenesis. Front Cell Infect Microbiol. 2012;2:92. doi: 10.3389/fcimb.2012.00092.

Chapter 13

The Mechanisms of Action and Resistance to Fluoroquinolone in Helicobacter pylori Infection

Carolina Negrei and Daniel Boda

Additional information is available at the end of the chapter

http://dx.doi.org/10.5772/57081

1. Introduction

The discovery of the *Helicobacter pylori* (*H. pylori*) infection and its role in various diseases (from chronic gastritis to gastric cancer) has been a radical change in the therapeutic conduct of patients suffering from this condition [1, 2].

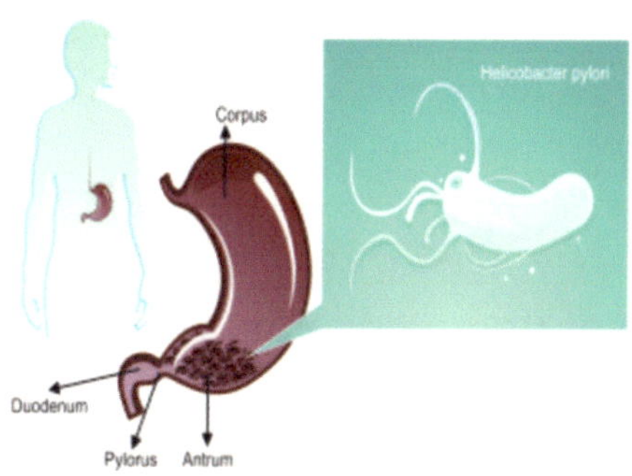

Figure 1. *Helicobacter pylori* infection

Unfortunately though, the purpose of inducing a cure of all first intention treated patients, as is the case in most ordinary infectious diseases, has not occurred in the *H. pylori* infection (Figure 1).

Current guidelines recommend triple therapy of a double dose proton pump inhibitor and two antibiotics chosen from among amoxicillin, clarithromycin and metronidazole for four to seven days, which is conducive to an eradication rate between 70-80%. Resistance to antibiotics, to clarithromycin and metronidazole in particular, is a major factor contributing to failure of the therapy [3, 4]; resistance to clarithromycin may lead to a decrease in efficiency to 70%, whereas the infection may persist up to about 20% of patients under treatment [5]. Such limitations have resulted in development of alternative therapies - "rescue" therapies – using medicines which have not been used as a first or second intention, such as fluoroquinolones (moxifloxacin, levofloxacin) and rifabutin (a derivative of rifamycin), which are commonly used in treatment of mycobacterial infections and are also highly efficient against *H. pylori* [5, 6].

Quinolones have been the focus of considerable scientific and clinical interest, since their very development in the early 1960s. This happened because such drugs possess many of the attributes of an ideal antibiotic, combining high potency, a broad spectrum of activity, good bioavailability, oral and intravenous formulations, high serum levels, a large volume of distribution, indicating concentration on a tissue level and potential low incidence of adverse reactions.

Nalidixic acid was the first quinolone to be developed. Subsequent medicines have been derived by manipulation at the level of their side chain and nucleus [7]. Development of the fluoroquinolone class may be described in terms of generations, each generation sharing similar characteristics or antimicrobial spectrum. The activity of first-generation medicines is more effective against gram-negative aerobic bacteria and less effective against gram-positive aerobic bacteria or anaerobic bacteria. Original fluoroquinolones are second-generation agents and they owe their name to the addition of a fluorine atom in the C6 position; they provide improved coverage against gram-negative bacteria and moderately improved coverage against gram-positive ones. Third-generation agents have greater efficacy against gram-positive bacteria, particularly against pneumococci, which is combined with good activity against anaerobic bacteria. Fourth generation fluoroquinolones provide superior coverage against pneumococci and anaerobic bacteria [8].

2. Clinical indications of fluoroquinolones

Fluoroquinolones such as levofloxacin are indicated in: acute bacterial sinusitis (diagnosed according to national guidelines on treatment of infections of the respiratory tract and where use of antibacterial agents commonly recommended for initial treatment of this infection is considered inappropriate or in case of their failure to cure the infection), acute bacterial exacerbations of chronic bronchitis (diagnosed according to national guidelines on treatment of respiratory tract infections and where use of antibacterial agents commonly recommended for initial treatment of this infection is considered inappropriate or in case of their failure to cure the infection), community acquired pneumonia (where use of antibacterial agents commonly recommended for initial treatment of this infection is considered inappropriate), uncomplicated urinary tract infections (including pyelonephritis), chronic bacterial prostatitis and skin and soft tissue infections.

http://dx.doi.org/10.5772/57081

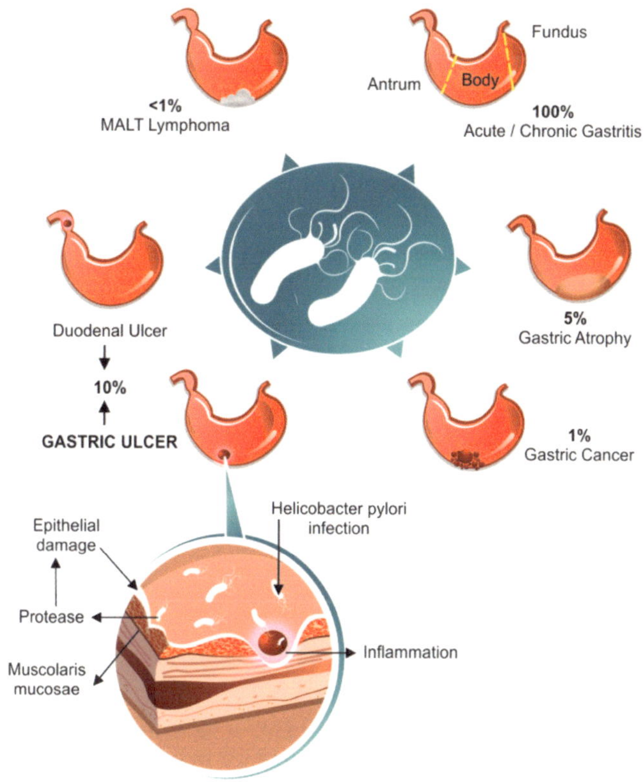

Figure 2. Diseases involving *Helicobacter pylori*

At the same time, as mentioned before, fluoroquinolones are implicated in *H. pylori* eradication. Indications for a *H. pylori* eradication therapy are defined in consensus guidelines. These indications include peptic ulcer disease, low-grade gastric mucosa-associated lymphoid tissue lymphoma, atrophic gastritis and after resection of early gastric cancer (Figure 2).

The following are included in the *H. pylori* elimination:

First-line treatment: should be considered as the first-line therapy in areas with high prevalence of *H. pylori* resistance to clarithromycin, in the frame of the new sequential ten-day scheme. Sequential therapy includes a dual therapy (proton pump inhibitor and amoxicillin for five days), followed by triple therapy with a proton pump inhibitor, clarithromycin and metronidazole for five days. The eradication rate achieved by sequential therapy has shown higher values, than those obtained with standard therapy [9, 10]. However, sequential therapy has been shown ineffective in eradicating *H. pylori* in patients with dual resistance to clarithromycin and metronidazole [11, 12]. A new aspect of the scheme as concomitant therapy is a fourth medicine – a non-bismuth-containing regimen (proton pump inhibitor, clarithromycin, amoxicillin and metronidazole), which seems more appropriate for patients in highly endemic areas and with dual resistance. Clinically speaking, this is much easier than sequential therapy and can improve compliance, because medicines are administered concurrently, instead of changed in mid therapy An intention-to-treat analysis demonstrated that sequential or concomitant therapy with a PPI, amoxicillin, clarithromycin and an imidazole agent has similar rates for eradication of *H. pylori* infection [10]. As far as dual resistance is concerned, several attempts have been made such as extension of sequential therapy and continuation with amoxicillin therapy for all 14 days, in order to improve effectiveness of standard triple therapy and proton pump inhibitors. A hybrid sequential-concomitant therapy has been recently designed by Hsu et al. [13]. Data have shown promising success rate: 99% by per-protocol analysis and 97% by intention-to-treat analysis. However, it should be noted this may not be effective in all geographic areas and results will have to be confirmed in areas where different patterns of resistance are present.

Second-line therapy: bismuth is a component of quadruple therapy and/or rescue therapy recommended by the Maastricht IV/Florence Consensus Report [7]. Several multicentre studies regarding quadruple therapy using a single triple medicine (bismuth, metronidazole and tetracycline), in a capsule pharmaceutical formulation together with a proton pump inhibitor have shown good efficacy in *H. pylori* eradication [14-16]. With regard to adverse reactions, bismuth induced toxic effects are still one of the unnecessary safety concerns in relation to quadruple therapy [17]; therefore, a reasonable bismuth dose regimen needs to be established to ensure maximum eradication. In patients where first-line treatment has failed, e.g., clarithromycin-based triple therapy, levofloxacine-based triple therapy (levofloxacin, amoxicillin and a proton pump inhibitor), a meta-analysis has shown this therapy to be superior to quadruple therapy and be accompanied by fewer adverse reactions than rescue therapy [18]. In addition, the study has shown that antibiotics (e.g., levofloxacin) in this triple therapy should not be changed randomly and then switched to first-line treatment. As far as antibiotic resistance is concerned, growth rates of levofloxacin resistance, particularly in developing countries, are to be taken into account, since resistance to quinolones is related to the status of patients having used fluoroquinolones for other indications [19].

Third-line treatment: the third-line treatment standard for refractory *H. pylori* infection has not been established. The Maastricht IV/Florence Consensus Report recommends conducting anti-*H. pylori* therapy according to results of susceptibility testing after failure of second-line therapy, whenever possible [7]. Unfortunately, antimicrobial sensitivity data for patients in whom eradication therapy has failed are not yet widely available in clinical practice.

Practitioners need a few simple strategies for empirical management. A prospective study has assessed the efficacy and safety of levofloxacin, amoxicillin, bismuth and rabeprazole, as a quadruple therapy, with regard to third-line treatment in patients where eradication of *H. pylori* infection has failed. In this study, the ten-day quadruple rescue therapy, based on levofloxacin and amoxicillin, ensured better eradication with a significant additional clinical benefit involving improvement of tolerability due to fewer adverse reactions [18]. Other alternative agents that are candidates for third-line treatment are rifabutin and quinolones, which also have promising results [20-22], although the optimal dose and the combination require further study (Table 1).

http://dx.doi.org/10.5772/57081

Treatment			Regimens A	C	M	T	L	R	F	B	PPI	Duration of treatment
First line therapy	Standard triple therapy		1g b.i.d.	0. 5g b.i.d.							SD b.i.d.	7-14 days
	Concomitant therapy		1g b.i.d.	0. 5g b.i.d.	0. 5g b.i.d.						SD b.i.d.	7-10 days
	Bismuth-containing quadruple therapy				0. 25g q.i.d.	0. 5g q.i.d.				0. 48g q.i.d.	SD b.i.d.	10-14 days
	Sequential therapy	First phase	1g b.i.d.								SD b.i.d.	5 days
		Second phase		0. 5g b.i.d.	0. 5g b.i.d.						SD b.i.d.	5 days
	Hybrid therapy	First phase	1g b.i.d								SD b.i.d.	7 days
		Second phase	1g b.i.d.	0. 5g b.i.d.	0. 5g b.i.d.						SD b.i.d.	7 days
Second line therapy	Bismuth-containing quadruple therapy				0. 5g t.i.d.	0. 5g q.i.d.				0. 48g q.i.d.	SD b.i.d.	10-14 days
	Levofloxacin-based triple therapy		0. 5g b.i.d.				0. 5g q.i.d.				SD b.i.d.	10 days
Third line therapy	Culture guided therapy		Sensitivity tests – two antibiotics selected							0. 48 q.i.d.	SD b.i.d.	NA
	Levofloxacin-based quadruple therapy		0. 5g q.i.d.				0. 5g q.i.d.			0. 48 q.i.d.	SD b.i.d.	10 days
	Rifabutin-based triple therapy		1g b.i.d.					0. 15g b.i.d.			SD b.i.d.	14 days
	Furazolidone-based quadruple therapy					1g b.i.d.			0. 2g b.i.d.	0. 24g b.i.d.	SD b.i.d.	NA

A = amoxicillin, C = clarithromycin, M = metronidazole, T = tetracycline, L = levofloxacin, R = rifabutin, F = furazolidone, SD = standard dose, B = bismuth, PPI = proton pump inhibitor

Table 1. Recommended regimens for the treatment of *H. pylori* infections in adults

3. Safety of fluoroquinolones

3.1. Overview

As a class of medicines, fluoroquinolones are generally well tolerated; most adverse reactions are mild, self-limiting and rarely require treatment discontinuation [23]. The most frequently occurring adverse reactions class consists of gastrointestinal trouble (nausea, vomiting, diarrhoea, constipation and abdominal pain, about 7% of all adverse reactions). Less common are adverse reactions include those involving the central nervous system (less than 5%), kidney disorders (approximately 4. 5%), skin hypersensitivity reactions and photosensitivity reactions (approximately 2%). In rare cases, convulsions, psychosis and tendonitis have been reported [24]. Some of these events may not be directly attributed to fluoroquinolone therapy, but to other underlying conditions in the patient, including additional therapies not related to the microbial infection but still contributing to adverse reactions. Phototoxicity could be observed over a longer period in relation to administration of lomefloxacin, sparfloxacin and clinafloxacine, which has been determined to be a dose-dependent phenomenon requiring direct or indirect exposure to UVA rays and also closely correlated with the presence of a habide in the C8 position.

Serious adverse reactions have been developed following introduction to the use of the following three agents: temafloxacin, grepafloxacin and trovafloxacine.

Temafloxacin syndrome has been characterized by haemolytic anaemia, renal failure, hepatotoxicity, disseminated intravascular coagulation and hypoglycaemia [28]. Approximately two thirds of patients with "temafloxacin syndrome" develop acute renal failure. In addition, slight hepatobiliary changes have been observed in half of patients, whereas coagulopathy has been observed in a third of patients. Development of such adverse reactions resulted in withdrawal of temafloxacin from the market in 1992 [26]. Adverse reactions to temafloxacin not shown in the clinical trials conducted were observed at a rate of 1/3500 patients after placement on the market. In contrast, rare adverse reactions similar to those seen in temafloxacin have been reported with ciprofloxacin. This is significant, considering that ciprofloxacin has the largest database regarding fluoroquinolone safety information. Further analysis of such specific temafloxacin events have demonstrated that data involving norfloxacin and ofloxacin have been similar to those of ciprofloxacin. Specifically, such effects have been observed in 1/17000 patients treated with ciprofloxacin, in 1/25000 patients treated with norfloxacin and in 1/30000 patients treated with ofloxacin [25].

Grepafloxacin was placed on the market in 1997 and subsequently withdrawn in 1999 because of serious cardiovascular reports of adverse reactions in patients who had been administered this medicine [27]. The association between grepafloxacin and serious cardiovascular adverse reactions became evident after extended clinical use. Starting with grepafloxacin placement on the market to its withdrawal in 1999, torsades de pointes were observed in 7/3.7 million patients [27]. Trovafloxacin was authorized based on clinical efficacy trials conducted on batches including more than 6000 patients treated with this medicine. In these studies, 5% of patients discontinued trovafloxacin treatment because of adverse events, the most common of which included those on the central nervous system and gastrointestinal tract levels. As with temafloxacin, adverse reactions had not been clearly associated with use of the medicinal product before extended clinical use. Serious adverse reactions associated with trovafloxacin included liver eosinophilia and hypoglycaemia [29], observed post-marketing.

All the adverse reactions described above have resulted in limiting the use of these medicines to hospital use only, in cases of severe life-threatening infections [29]. Whereas withdrawal of temafloxacin and grepafloxacin from the market has raised concerns about the safety of fluoroquinolones, in considering the evaluation of their safety and efficacy, several aspects have required balancing. Despite rigorous preclinical studies, once a medicine is placed on the market for widespread clinical use, the likelihood of observing rare but serious adverse reactions is significantly increased [29]. It is important to recognize the low incidence of adverse reactions and serious adverse reactions in other agents of the same class, which generally demonstrates the relative safety of this class of medicines [23].

3.2. Categorization of adverse effects

Adverse reactions of levofloxacin consist of: disorders such as tachycardia, ventricular arrhythmia and torsades de pointes (reported predominantly in patients with risk factors for QT prolongation), ECG QT prolonged, leukopoenia, eosinophilia, thrombocytopenia, neutropoenia, dizziness, headaches, drowsiness, convulsion, tremors, paraesthesia, vertigo, impaired hearing, bronchospasm, dyspnoea, diarrhoea, nausea, vomiting, abdominal pain, dyspepsia, flatulence, constipation, increased blood creatinine, rashes, pruritis, urticaria, tendon disorders including tendinitis (e.g., in the Achilles tendon), arthralgia, myalgia, anorexia, fungal infections (and proliferation of other resistant microorganisms), hypotension, asthenia, increased hepatic enzymes (aspartate aminotransferase/alanine aminotransferas, alkaline phosphatise and gamma-glutamyl transpeptidase) and increased blood bilirubin [30].

Many of the fluoroquinolone adverse reactions are associated with quinolone pharmacore in positions one, seven and eight. In the following sections, the discussion focuses on class specific reactions regarding structural modifications in positions one, seven and eight [25].

Adverse reactions on the central nervous system level: although much information about the pathophysiology of fluoroquinolone induced central nervous system adverse reactions remain less well defined, one hypothesis suggests that drug interactions with the gamma-aminobutyric acid (GABA) receptor, an inhibitory neurotransmitter, may explain the stimulant effects at this level.

Affinity for the GABA receptor seems to be triggered by the R7 side chain substituent, unsubstituted piperazinyl and pyrrolidinyl moieties in particular. In this respect, agents with an unsubstituted piperazinyl ring (ciprofloxacin, enoxacine and norfloxacin) display high-affinity binding to GABA as well as interference with GABA binding to its receptor. It has been demonstrated that biphenyl acetic acid, which is an active metabolite of fenbufen, a nonsteroidal anti-inflammatory medicine, enhances binding of fluoroquinolones to GABA receptors.

Concurrent administration of fenbufen and fluoroquinolones has been shown to be capable of inducing seizures in mice; certain researchers however have observed that alterations in GABA receptor binding mediated by quinolone are weak and may not fully explain reactions at the central nervous system level [31]. It was noted that seven Japanese patients developed seizures following concurrent administration of enoxacine and fenbufen. Studies have also shown that penetration of quinolones at the CNS level does not seem to be correlated with the incidence of adverse reactions at this level [25]. A possible understanding of such discrepancies is that fluoroquinolones may also induce excitatory effects by means of direct activation of N-methyl-D-aspartate (NMDA) and adenosine-receptor mechanisms. It is therefore possible that the events mentioned may occur at this level only under special circumstances, when sufficient penetration is possible in the CNS, coupled with threshold antagonism of inhibitory pathways (GABA) and stimulation of excitatory pathways (NMDA, adenosine).

Ofloxacin and levofloxacin, its levorotatory isomer, have been observed to induce a number of adverse reactions at the central nervous system level, including headaches (9% ofloxacin, 6% levofloxacin), dizziness (5% ofloxacin, 3% levofloxacin) and less common events such as confusion, impaired thinking, insomnia and psychosis, in rare cases. Such reactions were induced even in the absence of concomitant medications such as NSAIDs [25] and they tend to occur more frequently with ofloxacin than levofloxacin.

Genetic Toxicology: quinolones have been shown to inhibit mammalian cell topoisomerase II, a mechanism correlating with the occurrence of in vitro cytotoxicity, on the level of these cells [30]. Substitutions and positions one, seven and eight have the greatest potential cytotoxicity and the effect is additive. However, chromosomal disruption or clastogenicity usually occurs only at very high concentrations of the medicine (300 to 10000 times the therapeutic dose) and in post-marketing studies was not shown to have carcinogenic potential.

Cardiovascular adverse reactions: cardiovascular adverse reactions, particularly prolongation of the heart rate corrected QT interval (the QTc interval) have been reported with quinolone therapy [30]. Sparfloxacin increases the QTc interval in up to 3% of patients [32]. Such significant results involving serious cardiac events have led to the withdrawal of grepafloxacin. Sparfloxacin is not recommended for administration in patients with a history of QT prolongation or patients receiving concomitant therapy likely to increase the interval, induce bradycardia or cause torsades de pointes (e.g., class Ia and III antiarrhythmics, bepridil, cisapride, erythromycin, terfenadine or tricyclic antidepressants). It seems possible that this effect may be more predictable with medicines administered concurrently with quinolones inhibiting cytochrome P450-mediated metabolizing, because of drug accumulation. So far, no specific structural change has been associated with adverse cardiovascular outcomes, including those possibly affecting cytochrome P450-involving metabolism. Currently, the only possible specific structural changes that may be associated with increased incidence of serious cardiovascular events in relation to grepafloxacin or sparfloxacin therapy consist of a methyl or amino moiety in position C5 (of grepafloxacin, sparfloxacin, respectively) [32]. In light of experience acquired with sparfloxacin and grepafloxacin concerning adverse cardiovascular outcomes, more recent members of this class of medicines have been studied with particular focus on these reactions [30].

4. Basic antimicrobial activity

4.1. Pharmacokinetics

Fluoroquinolones have favourable pharmacokinetic properties, which have encouraged their extensive use. They are well absorbed and show good tissue penetration, which favours their use in many clinical syndromes. Whereas ciprofloxacin requires frequent administration, the long half-life of new generation fluoroquinolones allows use in daily single doses.

Most fluoroquinolones are eliminated renally. Moxifloxacin elimination involves the liver and this is one of the fluoroquinolones lacking effectiveness in treatment of genitourinary infections. In general, because they are not as highly bound to plasma proteins and because of CYP1A2 enzyme-limited inhibition of CYP450, drug interactions are somewhat minimized [33-35]. Fluoroquinolones have been shown to interact with xanthines, theophylline and caffeine, which is matter of concern with older generation agents [36]. Concurrent use of fluoroquinolone and warfarin may result in excessive anticoagulation [37]. Probably the most common interactions involve cationic di- and trivalents. Administration with antacids may result in subtherapeutic fluoroquinolone levels, thus raising potential therapeutic failure. This may be particularly relevant in an "inpatient setting", because of the frequent fluoroquinolone and antacids association; co-administration of agents mentioned previously has raised the issue of emergence of resistance to fluoroquinolones [38, 39].

In terms of levofloxacin involved in *H. pylori* eradication therapy, oral administration is rapidly and almost completely followed by levofloxacin absorption, with a peak concentration achieved within one hour. Absolute bioavailability is approximately 100% and food has a low impact on levofloxacin absorption.

Approximately 30-40% of levofloxacin is bound to plasmatic proteins and a therapy involving a 500mg dose once daily for several days has shown non-significant accumulation. However, there is modest but predictable accumulation after therapy involving 500mg twice daily, with a balance reached within three days. Levofloxacin metabolism is very scarce and its metabolites are "desmethyl-levofloxacine" and "levofloxacin N-oxide". These metabolites contribute to less than 5% of the urine-excreted dose. Levofloxacin is stereochemically stable and undergoes no chiral inversion. Following oral or intravenous administration, levofloxacin is relatively slowly eliminated from plasma (t1/2 = 6-8 hours). The chief route of excretion is mainly renal (>85% of the dose administered). There are no major differences in levofloxacin pharmacokinetics in terms of oral versus intravenous administration, which leads to the conclusion that oral and intravenous administration are interchangeable.

4.2. Pharmacodynamics

Pharmacokinetics (PK) regards the time course of antimicrobial concentrations in the body; on the other hand, pharmacodyamics (PD) provides insight into the relationship between such concentrations and the effect on antimicrobial level.

Traditionally, doses of antibiotic therapeutic schemes only determined the pharmacokinetics; however, pharmacodynamics plays an equally, if not more important, role.

In this period of increased antimicrobial resistance, pharmacodynamics is becoming perhaps the most important because it can be used in the design of a dosage regimen to prevent resistance [40, 41].

The primary parameter of antibiotic activity is the minimum inhibitory concentration (MIC). MIC is the lowest concentration of an antibiotic able to completely inhibit in vitro microorganism growth. Whereas MIC is a reliable indicator of antibiotic potency, it has no relevance in terms of the time course of antimicrobial activity.

Pharmacokinetic parameters quantify the time course of an antibiotic level. The three pharmacokinetic parameters most important in evaluating effectiveness of the antibiotic are the peak serum level (Cmax), the minimum level (Cmin) and the area under the serum concentration time curve (AUC). Whereas these parameters quantify the serum level over a certain period of time, they describe the destruction activity of an antibiotic.

Integration of pharmacokinetic parameters and MIC provides three pharmacokinetic/ pharmacodynamic (PK/PD) parameters quantifying the activity of an antibiotic: the peak/MIC ratio, the T>MIC and the ratio 24h-AUC/MIC

- the peak / MIC ratio is Cmax divided by MIC
- the T>MIC (time above MIC) is the percentage of a dosing interval when the serum level reaches MIC
- the 24h-AUC/MIC ratio is determined by dividing the 24-hour-AUC by MIC [40, 41].

The three pharmacodynamic properties of antibiotics best describing the destruction activity are time-dependent, concentration-dependent and the presence of persistent effects. The destruction rate is determined by either the time needed for destruction (time-dependent) or the effect of increased concentration (concentration-dependent). Persistent effects include post-antibiotic effect, which is the persistence of suppression of bacterial growth after exposure to antibiotics.

For fluoroquinolones, the best dosing regimen would maximize the concentration, as higher concentrations cause a superior and faster degree of destruction, therefore the "24h-AUC/MIC ratio" and the "peak/MIC ratio" are important predictors for antibiotic efficacy.

In this case, as far as fluoroquinolones are concerned, the "24h-AUC/MIC ratio" for Gram-negative bacteria (*H. pylori* included) is about 125 and 40, respectively, for Gram-positive bacteria. For Gram-negative bacteria, however, the "24h-AUC/MIC ratio" for the group of medicines described above, the reports vary widely in the literature [40, 41].

4.3. Mechanisms of action

The process of fluoroquinolone interference in cell replication, transcription and DNA repair consists in disabling DNA gyrase (previously topoisomerase II) and topoisomerase IV, two processes essential to bacterial enzymes (Figure 3).

Essentially a tetramer of two A and two B subunits, DNA gyrase is subject to encoding performed by gyrA and gyrB [42]. It brings in negative DNA supercoils, also removing both positive and negative supercoils and acts on chromosomal material by catenating and decatenating it [43].

The other bacterial enzyme mentioned above is topoisomerase IV, which is a homologue of DNA gyrase. This consists of two E and two E subunits, both subject to parC- and parE-encoding [42]. Similarly to its homologue, topoisomerase IV this is also able to remove both negative and positive supercoils; however, its main involvement remains contribution to separating of the daughter chromosome [33, 43] (Figure 4).

http://dx.doi.org/10.5772/57081

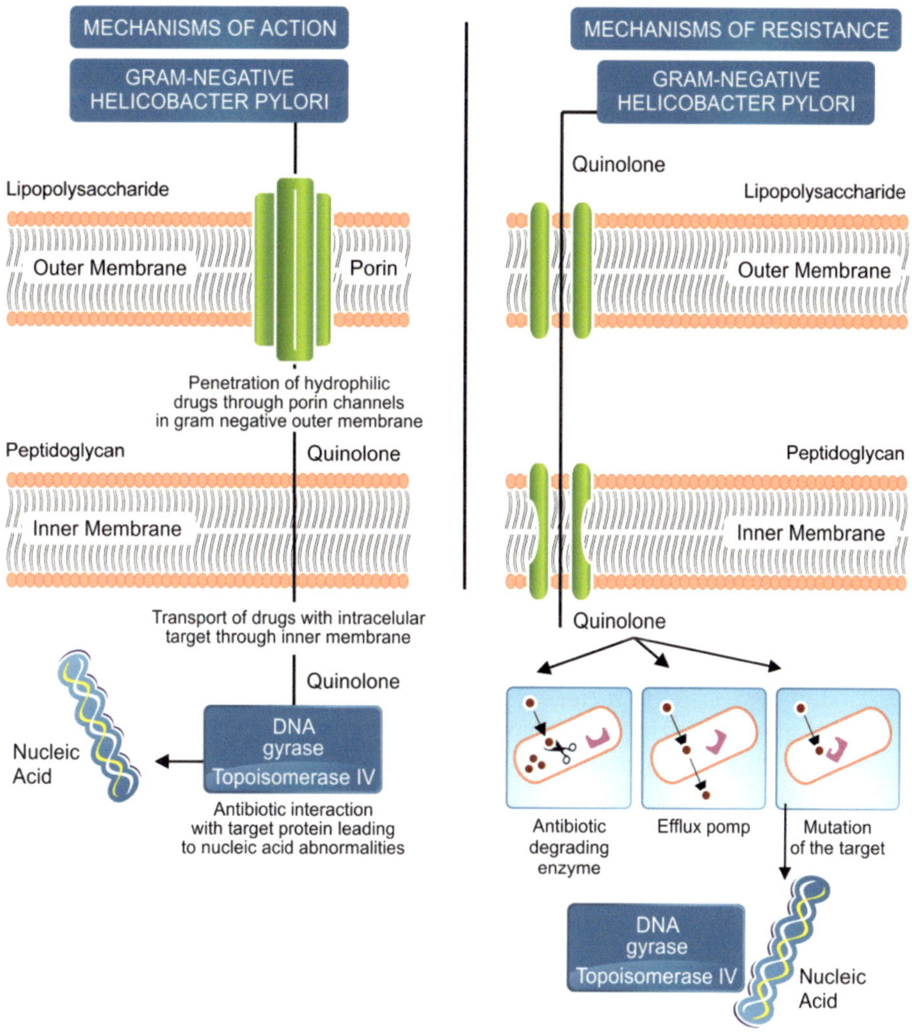

Figure 3. Mechanisms of action/Mechanisms of resistance

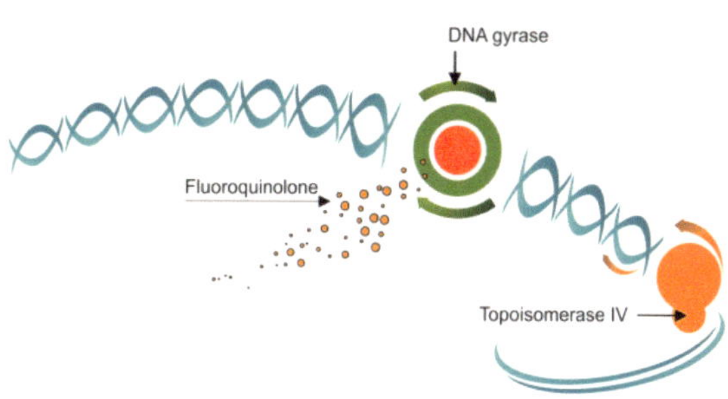

Figure 4. Fluoroquinolones bind the two nuclear enzymes, inhibiting DNA replication

The binding of fluoroquinolones to the complex made up of enzyme–DNA determines the change in enzyme conformation. This results in enzyme cleaving of the DNA, while ligation of broken DNA strands is prevented by the continued presence of the fluoroquinolone. Continuation of DNA replication is inhibited by the process in which the enzyme on the DNA is "trapped" by fluoroquinolone as a complex of fluoroquinolone–enzyme–DNA. DNA cleavage is generally held responsible for the destructive action of fluoroquinolones on bacteria [42, 43].

5. General mechanisms of fluoroquinolone resistance

Regarding quinolone resistance reported during treatment, it has been observed that, in the context of its rather extended use during the twenty years after its placement on the market, it was not commonly observed except for cases involving Staphylococcus aureus and notably P. aeruginosa and S. aureus, which were resistant to methicillin.

These two species have been observed to rapidly develop resistance to fluoroquinolones, which has been attributed to clonal spread occurring in immunocompromised patients and nursing home settings [44].

Starting around 1995 however, increased quinolone resistance has been noted in most Gram-negative (*H. pylori*) and Gram-positive species. At the same time, it has become evident that species were broadly varied (from ≤0.015 up to ≥128 mg/l [45-47]) by minimal concentrations (MICs) that inhibited 90% of the strains under study; this showed the common character of resistant subpopulations over the same period of time after placement on the market, which had however not been noticed.

In light of more recent studies involving surveillance of the issue, resistance rates have been shown to further increase and therefore have an impact on the management of patients.

5.1. Interaction with bacterial DNA gyrase and topoisomerase IV

From among antimicrobial agents in common clinical use, fluoroquinolones are the only class that directly inhibit synthesis of bacterial DNA. There are two bacterial enzymes with distinct and essential roles in DNA replication, called DNA gyrase and topoisomerase IV, which are inhibited by fluoroquinolones. The respective process involves binding quinolones to the complex with DNA of each such enzyme, which results in a ternary complex of topoisomerase-quinolone-DNA. Subsequently, this complex induces the generation of double-stranded breaks in DNA, further blocking progress of the DNA replication enzyme complex.

The final result of this action is damaged bacterial DNA and ultimately death of bacterial cells [48-51].

The responsibility for quinolones resistance lies with mutation in chromosomal genes. This occurs by means of two mechanisms: the altered target mechanism, on one hand, involving encoding DNA-gyrase and topoisomerase IV subunits and the altered permeation mechanism, on the other hand, regulating expression of proteins or cytoplasmic membrane efflux pumps, both of which make up the channels for outer membrane diffusion.

A further mechanism for the generation of low-level quinolone resistance has been considered, reduced target expression [52].

5.2. Response of the SOS gene network

Inhibition of bacterial type II topoisomerases activates repair mechanisms in response. This is because each piece of DNA damage activates an SOS gene network, which initiates the generation of repair proteins of various kinds [53-57]. There are over 40 genes making up this so-called SOS system, which is under the control of regulatory RecA and LexA proteins. The former is in charge of generating a signal triggering the SOS response, whereas the latter has a repressor function. The process consists of gene repressor LexA binding, which results in the unmasking of its autoproteolytic activity and subsequent ending of repression of the 40 SOS genes. The respective LexA binding takes place in the sequence up from qnrB (but not qnrS or qnrA). Therefore, in response to DNA damage, the SOS-system regulates qnrB as well [58]. Furthermore, the SOS response has recently been shown to promote qnrB expression [59].

Bacterial DNA-topoisomerases are protected from quinolone inhibition by the QnrB peptide, which also renders low-level resistance to quinolone. On the contrary, high-level resistance emerges with facilitation of the Qnr-determinants. It should also be noted that, in the case of *E. coli*, this particular effect directly depends on the increased ability for mutation due to action of nonessential polymerases Pol II, Pol IV and Pol V over the de-repression of the genes polB, dinB and umuDC, respectively, mediated by the LexA-cleavage.

In this way, the same signal of the SOS response triggers both increased mutation ability and qnrB-mediated quinolone resistance.

Because of the RecA/LexA-dependent manner in which ciprofloxacin upregulates the qnrB quinolone resistance gene, the development of quinolone resistance is integral to their action mode in bacteria harbouring qnrB.

LexA positive wild-type strains are much more liable to elicit ciprofloxacin resistant mutants than their mutant counterparts [60, 61]. The reverse is also true – prevention of LexA cleavage results in bacterial inability to develop fluoroquinolone resistance [60, 61].

The ability of the SOS response to induce persistent fluoroquinolone should also be mentioned [62].

From the above outcomes inference may occur in the role of fluoroquinolones as more than simply selectors of resistant variants, as well as on the active role of bacteria themselves in their own genomes' mutation.

Resistance to quinolone is acquired by means of both mutations in the target site and by the SOS system induced de-repression of genes, whose products increase rates of mutation.

The emergence of resistance may generally be reduced by interference with the response of bacterial stress [63].

In *E. coli*, ciprofloxacin has recently been shown to stimulate recombination of divergent DNA sequences that is independent from the SOS system.

Genetic variation may also be increased by fluoroquinolones by means of a second mechanism, which is SOS independent [64] and may also favour acquisition, evolution and the spread of resistance determinants.

Besides quinolones as DNA damaging agents, the SOS gene network response is triggered by other factors as well, such as beta-lactams interfering with penicillin binding protein 3 [65, 66], zidovudine or trimethoprim [67] and rifampicin [60].

As shown by these data, persistence and evolution of resistance in general is facilitated by induction of the SOS response by means of any of these medicines classes.

Given the above, speculation becomes possible concerning the ability of these agents to also affect quinolone activity and/or development of resistance via the expression of qnrB as promoted by the SOS system.

In turn, the SOS system further promotes horizontal dissemination of antibiotic-resistance genes [68] or mutations, thus contributing to the spread of antibiotic resistance.

5.3. Plasmid mediated resistance

Usually, genetic information for the efflux resistance mechanisms or the targeted site is chromosomally encoded.

In this context however, there have been reports of resistance to fluoroquinolones mediated by plasmids, which renders such resistance transferable (Figure 5).

This involves a number of mechanisms, such as:

1. Qnr
2. Aminoglycoside acetyltransferase AAC(6_)-Ib-cr
3. OqxAB, QepA [69-72]

Plasmid-mediated resistance to quinolone was first found in 1998, emerging in strains of Klebsiella pneumoniae in one US region [73]. The emergence was determined to be induced by one of the members of the pentapeptide repeat (PPR) family of proteins, Qnr (subsequently referred to as QnrA).

Later on, several related plasmid-mediated Qnr determinants were communicated in Enterobacteriaceae (QnrB, QnrC, Qnr D, QnrS) that were distantly related [74, 75].

These have been further found in the entire world and almost invariably in association with expanded spectrum β-lactamases production [76-78].

Gram-positive bacteria M. smegmatis Mycobacterium tuberculosis, M. avium [79], E. faecalis [80], C. perfringens, Listeria monocytogenes, C. difficile and E. faecium [81] have been found to display Qnr-like peptides (that share a 16 to 22% amino-acid identity with QnrA).

http://dx.doi.org/10.5772/57081

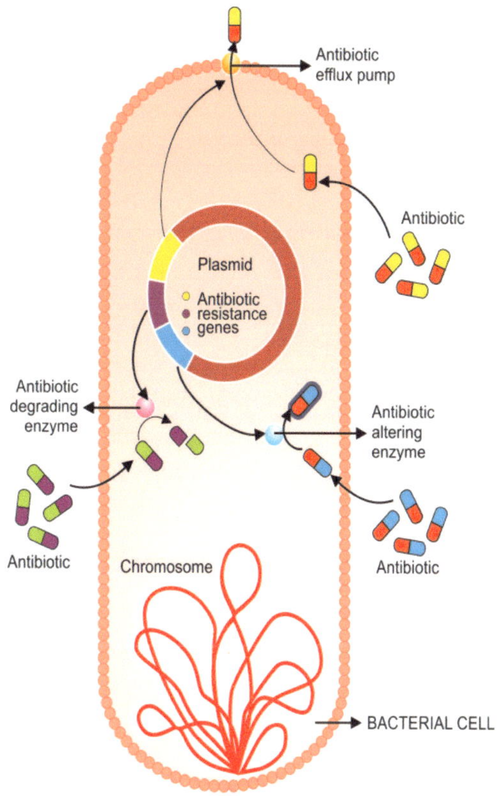

Figure 5. Plasmid mediated resistance

Stenotrophomonas maltophilia has recently shown the emergence of a new quinolone resistance gene of the PPR family that was chromosomally encoded, which has accordingly been called Smqnr [82]. Serratia marcescens has never been found to display the smaqnr gene[83].

Quinolone inhibition is prevented by the interaction of topoisomerase IV and DNA-gyrase with Qnr [69, 84].

The Qnr protein induces resistance to nalidixic acid and diminished susceptibility to fluoroquinolone resistance or low-levels of fluoroquinolone resistance [84].

Identification of Qnr-genes in isolates susceptible to ciprofloxacin and isolates displaying resistance to quinolones has made it possible to infer from laboratory results that because of chromosomal mutation, presence of Qnr-genes promotes higher-level resistance.

That is why there exists the possibility that development of quinolone resistance in clinically relevant species of both Gram-negative and Gram-positive bacteria can be fostered by presence of qnr genes.

In addition, the qnrA and qnrB genes usually make up integrons containing genes such as aminoglycoside inactivating enzymes or β-lactamases, which are responsible for resistance to other antibiotics.

Integrons do not contain qnrS genes, but these genes however associate with TEM-1 type β-lactamases-containing transposons [85].

As a result, the association of genes that encode resistance to both quinolone and other medicine classes like aminoglycosides and β-lactams are favourable to selection and subsequent dissemination by chemically unrelated medicines classes of strains that are resistant to fluoroquinolones.

The reverse is also found concerning fluoroquinolones selecting and disseminating aminoglycoside or β-lactam resistant strains (please see the sections related to resistance to fluoroquinolones for issues regarding the tight correlation between and quinolone resistance and production of extended spectrum β-lactamases (ESBL)).

The chromosome of Shewanella algae, a bacterium found in environmental water has also been found to display Qnr genes.

The discovery of other qnr homologs in the genome sequences characterizing several Photobacterium profundum and Vibrio spp. suggests the possibility of water-borne Vibrionaceae as a source of qnr genes and also a reservoir [86-88].

Recent in vitro tests have shown the possibility for transfer of the plasmid borne Shewanella algae qnr gene to Enterobacteriaceae [86].

A further discovery envisages a plasmid-encoded determinant of resistance to quinolones, a variant of the aac(6_)Ib gene that encodes an aminoglycoside acetyltransferase.

The process of acetylation of both medicine classes is catalysed by AAC(6_)-Ib-cr, the bifunctional fluoroquinolone and aminoglycoside active variant [89].

This variant enzyme has become able to acetylate norfloxacin and ciprofloxacin as well as to determine a fourfold reduction of ciprofloxacin activity [90, 91].

Because of the absence in position C-7 of a piperazinyl substituent, levofloxacin and moxifloxacin do not undergo acetylation.

Interestingly, S. marcescens, the first clinical isolate determined as ciprofloxacin resistant, was found prior to the introduction of quinolone treatment in a patient treated with an aminoglycoside and a β-lactam. In that context, ciprofloxacin MIC during pre-therapy was 0.06, whereas the respective post-therapy MIC was 4mg/L.

The strain in question underwent changes in the composition of its outer-membrane and produced an aminoglycoside acetyltransferase [92].

It is possible that Qnr- determinants are less widespread than AAC(6_)-Ib-cr.

ESBL production is associated with the production of both AAC(6_)-Ib-cr- and Qnr-, which may therefore be considered a second mechanism for co-selection of drug-resistance induced by exposure to agents that are chemically unrelated.

A third type of plasmid-mediated resistance to quinolones has been recently identified, consisting of the quinolone efflux pumps Qep and OqxAB, [70-72, 93, 94].

The QepA and OqxAB proteins are responsible for the induction of resistance to hydrophilic fluoroquinolones such as ciprofloxacin, norfloxacin and enrofloxacin, leading to a 32- to 64-fold MIC increase [93-96].

As far as QepA is concerned, in addition to quinolones, this extrudes a restricted range of agents such as ethidium bromide, erythromycin and acrifliavine.

In turn, OqxAB is responsible for the export of a wider range of agents among which are tetracyclines, chloramphenicol, ethidium bromide, olaquindox, trimethoprim and disinfectants such as triclosan [85, 96, 97].

However, the issue here is the presence of a transposable element also consisting of an aminoglycoside ribosome methyltransferase and the qepA gene [94]. This allows for the possibility for both aminoglycosides to select QepA determinants and for quinolones to select aminoglycoside resistance, which is also true in what concerns aac(6_)Ib gene mediated resistances.

A third mechanism for cross-resistance consists of extrusion by efflux-pumps of chemically unrelated agents.

To conclude, it appears that, even in the absence of exposure to this medicine, class resistance to fluoroquinolones can emerge. This can be explained by the action of several co-selection mechanisms, which all support emergence of quinolone resistance.

Identification in 50–70% of *E. coli* clinical isolates displaying high-level quinolone resistance (MICs up to 1500-fold higher than expected) of the multidrug efflux pump AcrAB, as well as of known plasmid- and chromosomally- mediated resistance mechanisms, makes it reasonable to infer the existence of additional mechanisms inducing quinolone resistance that have yet to be discovered

5.4. Other resistance mechanisms

In order to reach its target, all antibacterial agents that interact with an intracellular target have to cross the bacterial cell wall and then the cytoplasmic membrane. The process continues with active efflux of most antibacterial agents taken up.

This explains why permeation barriers and efflux pumps affect fluoroquinolones as well, whether accompanied by target modifications or just by themselves.

As indicated earlier, there are many, many Gram- positive and Gram-negative mutant strains resistant to fluoroquinolone, which did not display mutation in the region determining quinolone resistance (QRDR).

For instance, absence of classical QRDR mutations was observed in 70% of *E. coli* mutant variants recovered from besifloxacin selection plates [99]. At the same time, 39% of wild type *E. coli* accumulated higher levels of ciprofloxacin than high-level ciprofloxacine-resistant isolates. To this, one must add the gyrA mutations detected in all [100].

In addition, fluoroquinolone susceptibilities of *E. coli* were also affected by chemically unrelated substances such as salicylate, tetracycline and cyclohexane.

In this respect, it was determined that 21 of 57 clinical isolates of *E. coli* showing high level fluoroquinolone-resistance displayed tolerance to cyclohexane, which suggests a presence of elevated broad spectrum efflux activity [101]. Efflux of a wide range of chemically unrelated compounds, among which are different medicine classes of antibacterials, is determined by the so-called mar (multiple antibiotic resistance) genes [102], which suffer the influence of an assortment of chemically unrelated substances.

The role of the mar genes is the regulation of accumulation of quinolones and thus their intracellular concentrations, which is achieved by changing the expression of efflux pumps and porins [100, 102].

To this, one must add the extrusion of quinolones out of the bacteria by AcrAB, a different efflux pump.

The mar gene exerts partial control over the pump, which seems the most important mechanism of resistance for mar mutant variants [103].

Salicylate stimulates fluoroquinolone resistance selection because the production of MarA, a positive regulator of acrAB transcription, is induced by salicylate and tetracycline.

Resistance is visible in either mar expression alone or if combined with type II topoisomerase mutations [102]. The combination of topoisomerase mutations with AcrAB over-expression results in high-level resistance to fluoroquinolone. In this respect, increased production of AcrA has been noted in over 60% of high-level ciprofloxacine-resistant isolates [104-106].

Patterns of quinolone resistance may be altered by further nontopoisomerase resistance mechanisms, over which the mar exerts no control. The quinolone entry into the cell is decreased because of the nfxB gene action to code for a modified outer cell membrane protein F [107].

Fluoroquinolone activity is further affected by the action of soxRS gene products involved in bacterial adaptation to superoxide stress [101].

Fluoroquinolone-resistant *E. coli,* other Enterobacteriaceae and nonfermenters display a relatively wide range of diminished antibiotic accumulation, efflux and target enzyme modification [100, 108].

Because of their limited substrate specificity, increased expression of efflux pumps is associated with cross-resistance between fluoroquinolones and antibacterials of chemically unrelated medicine classes. This is the case of, for instance, MexAB, which induces resistance to nonfluorinated and fluoroquinolones, chloramphenicol and tetracycline in MexCD, rendering resistance to fluoroquinolones, trimethoprim, triclosan and erythromycin in MexEF and providing resistance to triclosan, imipenem, chloramphenicol and triclosan in MexXY, which gives resistance to fluoroquinolones, aminoglycosides and erythromycin.

There are a number of reviews available, which provide a comprehensive view on the impact of fluoroquinolone resistance and extrusion [108-111].

A fourth type of cross-resistance can be represented by the selection of a fluoroquinolone resistant or even multidrug-resistant phenotype by exposure to a broad range of chemically unrelated drug classes. All the above are illustrations which underline the complex character of mechanisms inducing resistance to fluoroquinolone, selection by fluoroquinolones and co-selection of resistance by chemically unrelated classes of antibacterials and antiseptics.

All general mechanisms of fluoroquinolone resistance have been presented for an overview of the issue. Regarding fluoroquinolone resistance in the case of *H. pylori* infection, this is due mainly (99%) to mutations in the QRDR of gyrA (Figure 3).

Antibiotic bacterial resistance is a result of the inhibition of binding between the enzyme and the antibiotic, determined by point mutations in QRDR of gyrA. In various studies, the following *H. pylori* loci have been found to be involved: (1) position 88 (Ala88Val), (2) position 91 (Asp91Gly, Asn, Ala, or Tyr) and (3) position 87 (Asn87Lys). In 100% of levofloxacin resistant isolates there have been observed mutations in both position 91 and 87. In addition, a new mutation has been identified, which consists of Tyr substituting Asn in position 87. Position 86 (Asp86Asn) is involved in infrequent mutations; the same position usually associates with mutations at positions 87 and 91, which diminishes its role in MIC values. In a similar manner, it is most likely that gyrB constantly associating with gyrA 87-91 mutations reduce to a minimum the role gyrB mutations hold in emergence of quinolone resistance. Actually, the involvement of gyrA and gyrB gene mutations has been observed in levofloxacin resistance as 83.8% and 4.4%, respectively.

There are also other factors that are involved in levofloxacin resistance, such as occurrence in codon 87 of gyrA of an amino acidic polymorphism, which consists of the presence of various asparagine-threonine residues. Specifically, presence of threonine in the J99 strain and asparagine residues in the 26695 strain associated with a higher antibiotic susceptibility has been identified due to the complete sequencing genome of two strains, namely the J99 and the 26695. Other Helicobacter types interestingly preserve the presence of threonine residue in codon 87, which therefore indicates the likelihood of the occurrence of a "philogenic" type evolution of the Helicobacter species.

6. Clinical and social implications of fluoroquinolone resistance

The increased incidence of fluoroquinolone resistance is a major reason for concern in medicine. Identification of and subsequent familiarisation with plasmid-mediated quinolone resistance (PMQR) has revealed a new and more dangerous mechanism of resistance allowing bacteria to adapt to and survive therapeutic concentrations of fluoroquinolones. As mentioned above, PMQR only provides low-level resistance, not enough to enable classification as clear resistance (MIC ≥4g/ml), according to the Clinical and Laboratory Standards Institute (CLSI) breakpoint criteria for quinolone resistance. With these low MICs, such isolates, although transporting mutations conferring low sensitivity to quinolones, are to be classified as sensitive (MIC ≥1g/ml), meaning that physicians can further prescribe this class of medicines.

This in itself is a dilemma, because PMQR allows such "sensitive" organisms to survive even under therapeutic concentrations, easily circulating their genes afterwards. Continued exposure to these antibiotics determines high selection for plasmid-carrying pathogens, then rapidly conducing to general development of high-level clinically significant degrees of resistance. It has been shown that PMRQ-conferred low resistance levels can still remain undetected by current CLSI criteria and therefore are still conducive to failure of therapy. This is reason for concern with regard to the safety of prescribing fluoroquinolones for treatment of PMRQ gene-bearing organisms, even if they do not qualify as "resistant".

In such cases, the problem arises whether clinical breakpoints should be reviewed with regard to plasmid-carrying pathogens.

There is a strong association between fluoroquinolone resistance and resistance to other antibiotics, particularly wide spectrum β-lactamases and aminoglycosides. This indicates that gene-carrying plasmid organisms conferring quinolone resistance increase the likelihood of developing multi-drug resistant bacteria and prescription of a quinolone may be selective of not only quinolone resistance but also resistance to other classes of medicines.

The discovery of plasmid-mediated resistance genes in some non-Typhi serotypes of Salmonella enterica in animals has raised a major public health concern. The presence of such resistance genes from plasmid-mediated resistance genes in some non-Typhi serotypes of Salmonella enterica suggests an unsettling potential for horizontal transmission of resistance genes among animals and of infection-causing human pathogens, by means of food. Fluoroquinolone resistance prolongs hospitalisation and may further determine complications because of the selected therapy. The following can be mentioned among strategies implemented in some geographic areas: prohibited use as animal food and restricted use of fluoroquinolones in agriculture and their use for therapeutic purposes only, development of programmes for antibiotics management in hospitals (by drug rotation, cycling and restriction) as well as carrying out educational campaigns addressing physicians and patients, whose aim should be to increase awareness of inappropriate antibiotics.

The current breakpoints allow continuation of the quinolone treatment, whereas the organisms carrying these plasmid-mediated resistance genes remain undetected, which results in further dissemination of these plasmids, because of the selection pressure. The aim is a review of CLSI quinolone and fluoroquinolone breakpoints, against the background of the new mechanism (PMQR). Lower clinical breakpoints will help physicians to detect the low-level-resistance phenotype as rendered by such genes as well as avoidance of resumed prescription of quinolones as a treatment.

Identification of the PMQR mechanism is indicative of an increased risk of spreading resistance not only to fluoroquinolones but also, because of co-transmission, to other significant antimi-

http://dx.doi.org/10.5772/57081

crobial classes. Tackling this issue by judicious use of antibacterials and re-evaluation of clinical breakpoints will constitute an important step in preserving the efficiency of this important class of medicines.

Concerning the *H. pylori* infection, an encouraging strategy to approach cases of multiple failures in prior *H. pylori* eradication is quinolone-based treatment as a rescue therapy. According to European guidelines, before selecting a third-line treatment, which is based on microbial sensitivity to antibiotics, culture is recommended. Quinolones for third-line therapy should be selected based on results of drug susceptibility tests or analysis of gyrA.

If available, further alternatives have also been suggested for rescue therapy, consisting of furazolidone-based therapy, triple rifabutin-based therapy or high-dose amoxicillin/PPI therapy.

Author details

Carolina Negrei[1*] and Daniel Boda[2]

*Address all correspondence to: carol_n2002@hotmail.com

1 Department of Toxicology, "Carol Davila" University of Medicine and Pharmacy, Bucharest, Romania

2 Dermato-oncology Excellence Research Center "Carol Davila" University of Medicine and Pharmacy, Bucharest, Romania

References

[1] Go M. F. Natural history and epidemiology of *Helicobacter pylori* infection. Alimentary Pharmacology and Therapeutics 2002; 16 (Suppl. 1): 3–15.

[2] Suerbaum S., Michetti P. *Helicobacter pylori* infection. New England Journal of Medicine 2002; 347: 1175–1186.

[3] Dore M. P., Leandro G., Realdi G., Sepulveda A. R., Graham D. Y. Effect of pretreatment antibiotic resistance to metronidazole and clarithromycin on outcome of *Helicobacter pylori* therapy: a meta-analytical approach. Digestive Diseases and Sciences 2000; 45: 68–76.

[4] Jenks P. J. Causes of failure of eradication of *Helicobacter pylori*. British Medical Journal 2002; 325: 3–4.

[5] Gisbert J. P., Pajares J. M. *Helicobacter pylori* "rescue" therapy after failure of two eradication treatments. Helicobacter 2005; 10: 363–372.

[6] Toracchio S., Capodicasa S., Soraja D.B., Cellini L., Marzio L. Rifabutin based triple therapy for eradication of *H. pylori* primary and secondary resistant to tinidazole and clarithromycin. Digestive and Liver Disease 2005; 37: 33–38.

[7] Malfertheiner P., Megraud F., O'Morain C. A., Atherton J., Axon A. T., Bazzoli F., Gensini G. F., Gisbert J. P., Graham D. Y., Rokkas T., El-Omar E. M., Kuipers E. J. Management of *Helicobacter pylori* infection–the Maastricht IV/ Florence Consensus Report. Gut 2012; 61: 646–664.

[8] Hsu P. I., Wu D., Chen A. et al. Quadruple rescue therapy for *Helicobacter pylori* infection after two treatment failures, European Journal of Clinical Investigation 2008; 38(6):404-409.

[9] Gisbert J. P, Calvet X., O'Connor A., Megraud F., O'Morain C.A. Sequential therapy for *Helicobacter pylori* eradication: a critical review, Journal of Clinical Gastroenterology 2010; 44(5): 313-325.

[10] Vaira D., Zullo A., Vakil N. et al. Sequential therapy versus standard triple-drug therapy for *Helicobacter pylori* eradication: a randomized trial, Annals of Internal Medicine 2007; 146(8): 556-563.

[11] Megraud F. *H. pylori* antibiotic resistance: prevalence, importance and advances in testing," Gut 2004; 53(9): 1374-1384.

[12] Wu D. C., Hsu P. I., Wu J. Y. et al. Sequential and concomitant therapy with four drugs is equally effective for eradication of H pylori infection, Clinical Gastroenterology and Hepatology 2010; 8(1): 36-41.

[13] Hsu P. I., Wu D. C., Wu J. Y., Graham D. Y. Modified Sequential *Helicobacter pylori* therapy: proton pump inhibitor and amoxicillin for 14 days with clarithromycin and metronidazole added as a quadruple (hybrid) therapy for the final 7 days, Helicobacter 2011; 16(2): 139-145.

[14] O'Morain C., Borody T., Farley A. et al. Efficacy and safety of single-triple capsules of bismuth biskalcitrate, metronidazole and tetracycline, given with omeprazole, for the eradication of *Helicobacter pylori*: an international multicentre study, Alimentary Pharmacology and Therapeutics 2003; 17(3): 415-420.

[15] Laine L., Hunt, R., EI-Zimaity H., Nguyen B., Osato M., Spenard J. Bismuth-based quadruple therapy using a single capsule of bismuth biskalcitrate, metronidazole, and tetracycline given with omeprazole versus omeprazole, amoxicillin, and clarithromycin for eradication of *Helicobacter pylori* in duodenal ulcer patients: a prospective, randomized, multicenter, North American trial, American Journal of Gastroenterology 2003; 98(3): 562-567.

[16] Malfertheiner P., Bazzoli F., Delchier J. C. et al. *Helicobacter pylori* eradication with a capsule containing bismuth subcitrate potassium, metronidazole, and tetracycline

given with omeprazole versus clarithromycin-based triple therapy: a randomised, open-label, non-inferiority, phase 3 trial, The Lancet 2011; 377(9769): 905-913.

[17] Phillips R. H., Whitehead M. W., Doig L. A. et al. Is eradication of *Helicobacter pylori* with colloidal Bismuth subcitrate quadruple therapy safe? Helicobacter 2001; 6(2): 151-156.

[18] Liou J. M., Lin J. T., Chang C. Y. et al. Levofloxacin-based and clarithromycin-based triple therapies as first-line and secondline treatments for *Helicobacter pylori* infection: a randomised comparative trial with crossover design, Gut 2010; 59(5): 572-578.

[19] Chey W. D., Wong B. C. Y. American College of Gastroenterology guideline on the management of *Helicobacter pylori* infection. The American Journal of Gastroenterology 2007; 102(8): 1808-1825.

[20] Nishizawa T., Suzuki H., Hibi T. Quinolone-based thirdline therapy for *Helicobacter pylori* eradication. Journal of Clinical Biochemistry and Nutrition 2009; 44(2): 119-124.

[21] Van Der Poorten D., Katelaris P. H. The effectiveness of rifabutin triple therapy for patients with difficult-to-eradicate *Helicobacter pylori* in clinical practice. Alimentary Pharmacology and Therapeutics 2007; 26(11-12): 1537-1542.

[22] Toracchio S., Capodicasa S., Soraja D. B., Cellini L., Marzio L. Rifabutin based triple therapy for eradication of *H. pylori* primary and secondary resistant to tinidazole and clarithromycin. Digestive and Liver Disease 2005; 37(1): 33-38.

[23] Ball P., Mandell L., Niki Y., Tillotson G. Comparative tolerability of the newer fluoroquinolone antibacterials. Drug Safety 1999; 21: 407-21.

[24] Childs S. Safety of the fluoroquinolone antibiotics; focus on the molecular structure. Infections in Urology 2000; 13: 3-10.

[25] Mandell L., Tillotson G. Safety of fluoroquinolones: An update. Canadian Journal of Infectious Diseases 2002; 13(1): 54-61.

[26] Finch R. G. The withdrawal of temafloxacin; Are there implications for other quinolones? Drug Safety 1993; 8: 9-11.

[27] GlaxoWellcome voluntarily withdraws Raxar (grepafloxacin). Press Release, October 26, 1999, http://www. fda. gov/medwatch/safety/1999/raxar. html.

[28] Trovafloxacin (Trovan) package insert. New York: Pfizer, 1998

[29] Chen J. L., MacLean J. A. Trovafloxacin associated eosinophilic hepatitis. New England Journal of Medicine 2000; 342: 359-60.

[30] The electronic Medicines Compendium (eMC), Levofloxacin, http://www. medicines. org. uk/emc/ (accessed 1 June 2013).

[31] Hori S., Shimada J., Saito A. Comparison of the inhibitory effects of new quinolones on gamma-aminobutyric-acid receptor binding in the presence of anti-inflammatory drugs. Reviews of infectious diseases 1989; 5: 1397-1398.

[32] Fish D. N. Fluoroquinolone Adverse Effects and Drug Interactions. Pharmacotherapy. 2001; 21: 10.

[33] O'Donnell J. A., Gelone S. P. The newer fluoroquinolones. Infectious Disease Clinics of North America 2004; 18(3): 691–716.

[34] Ball P. The quinolones: history and overview. In: Andriole VT. (ed) The quinolones. 3rd edition. San Diego (CA): Academic Press; 2000; 1–33.

[35] Stahlman R., Lode H. Safety overview: toxicity, adverse effects, and drug interactions. In: Andriole, V. T. (ed) The quinolones. 3rd edition. San Diego (CA): Academic Press; 2000; 397–453.

[36] Niki Y., Hashiguchi K., Okimoto N. et al. Quinolone antimicrobial agents and theophylline [letter]. Chest 1992; 101(3): 881.

[37] Carroll D. N., Carroll D. G. Interactions between warfarin and three commonly prescribed fluoroquinolones. Annals of Pharmacotherapy 2008; 42(5): 680–5.

[38] Barton T. D., Fishman N. O., Weiner M. G. et al. High rate of coadministration of di- or trivalent cation-containing compounds with oral fluoroquinolones: risk factors and potential implications. Infection Control and Hospital Epidemiology 2005; 26(1): 93–9.

[39] Cohen K. A., Lautenbach E, Weiner M. G. et al. Coadministration of oral levofloxacin with agents that impair absorption: impact on antibiotic resistance. Infection Control and Hospital Epidemiology 2008; 29(10): 975–7.

[40] Bolon M. K. The Newer Fluoroquinolones. Medical Clinics of North America 2011; 95: 793–817.

[41] Andriole V. T. The Quinolones: Past, Present, and Future Clinical Infectious Diseases 2005; 41: S113–9.

[42] Hawkey P. M. Mechanisms of quinolone action and microbial response Journal of Antimicrobial Chemotherapy 2003; 51(Suppl 1): 29–35.

[43] Jacoby G. A. Mechanisms of resistance to quinolones. Clinical Infectious Diseases 2005; 41(Suppl 2): S120–6.

[44] Dalhoff A. Quinolone resistance in Pseudomonas aeruginosa and Staphylococcus aureus. Development during therapy and clinical significance. Infection 1994; 22(2): S111–S121.

[45] Thauvin-Eliopoulos C., Eliopoulos G. M. Activity in vitro of the quinolones, in: Hooper D.C., Rubinstein E., Quinolone Antimicrobial Agents, 3rd edition, (ed.) ASM Press, Washington, DC, USA. 2003; 91-111.

[46] Dalhoff A. In vitro activities of quinolones. Expert Opinion on Investigational Drugs 1999; 8(2): 123-137.

[47] Dalhoff A, Schmitz F. J. In vitro antibacterial activity and pharmacodynamics of new quinolones. European Journal of Clinical Microbiology and Infectious Diseases 2003; 22(4): 203-221.

[48] Drlica K., Malik M., Kerns R. J., Zhao X. Quinolonemediated bacterial death. Antimicrobial Agents and Chemotherapy 2008; 52(2): 385-392.

[49] Drlica K., Zhao X, DNA gyrase, topoisomerase IV, and the 4-quinolones. Microbiology and Molecular Biology Reviews 1997; 61(3): 377-392.

[50] Zhao X., Xu C., Domagala J., Drlica K. DNA topoisomerase targets of the fluoroquinolones: a strategy for avoiding bacterial resistance. Proceedings of the National Academy of Sciences of the United States of America 1997; 94(25): 13991–13996.

[51] Hooper D.C. Mechanisms of fluoroquinolone resistance. Drug Resistance Updates 1999; 2(1): 38–55.

[52] Ince D., Hooper D. C. Quinolone resistance due to reduced target enzyme expression. Journal of Bacteriology 2003; 185(23): 6883–6892.

[53] Walker G. C. Mutagenesis and inducible responses to deoxyribonucleic acid damage in Escherichia coli. Microbiological Reviews 1984; 48(1): 60–93.

[54] Fernandez De Henestrosa A. R, Ogi T, Aoyagi S. et al. Identification of additional genes belonging to the LexA regulon in Escherichia coli. Molecular Microbiology 2000; 35(6): 1560–1572.

[55] Courcelle J., Kodursky A., Pete, B., Brown P., Hanawalt P. Comparative gene expression profiles following UV exposure in wild-type and SOS-deficient Escherichia coli. Genetics 2001; 158(1): 41–64.

[56] Ysern P., Clerch B., Castano M., Gibert I., Barbe J., Llagostera M. Induction of SOS genes in Escherichia coli and mutagenesis in Salmonella typhimurium by fluoroquinolones. Mutagenesis 1990; 5(1): 63–66.

[57] Malik M., Zhao X., Drlica K. Lethal fragmentation of bacterial chromosomes mediated by DNA gyrase and quinolones. Molecular Microbiology 2006; 61(3): 810–825.

[58] Wang M., Jacoby G. A., Mills D. M., Hooper. D. C. SOS regulation of qnrB expression. Antimicrobial Agents and Chemotherapy 2009; 53(2): 821–823.

[59] Da Re S., Garnier F., Guerin E., Campoy S., Denis F., Ploy M. C. The SOS response promotes qnrB quinoloneresistance determinant expression. EMBO Reports 2009; 10(8): 929–933.

[60] Cirz R. T., Chin J. K., Andes D. R., de Crecy-Lagard V., Craig. W. R. Inhibition of mutation and combating the evolution of antibiotic resistance. PLoS Biology 2005; 3(6): 175.

[61] Cirz R. T., Jones M. B., Gingles N. A. et al. Complete and SOS-mediated response of Staphylococcus aureus to the antibiotic ciprofloxacin. Journal of Bacteriology 2007; 189(2): 531–539.

[62] Dorr T., Lewis. K., Vulic M. SOS response induces persistence to fluoroquinolones in Escherichia coli. PLoS Genetics 2009; 5(12):1-9 e1000760. http://www. northeastern. edu/adc/publications/sostobidorr. pdf (accessed 9 June 2013).

[63] Avison M. B. New approaches to combating antimicrobial drug resistance. Genome Biology 2005; 6(13): 243.

[64] Lopez E., Elez M., Matic I., Bl´azquez J. Antibioticmediated recombination: ciprofloxacin stimulates SOS independent recombination of divergent sequences in Escherichia coli. Molecular Microbiology 2007; 64(1): 83–93.

[65] Miller C., Thomsen L. E., Gaggero C., Mosseri R., Ingmer H., Cohen S.N. SOS response induction by β-lactams and bacterial defence against antibiotic lethality. Science 2004; 305(5690): 1629–1631.

[66] Maiques E., U´ beda C., Campoy S. et al. β-lactam antibiotics induce the SOS response and horizontal transfer of virulence factors in Staphylococcus aureus. Journal of Bacteriology 2006; 188(7): 2726–2729.

[67] Lewin C. S., Amyes S. G. B. The role of the SOS response in bacteria exposed to zidovudine or trimethoprim. Journal of Medical Microbiology 1991; 34(6): 329–332.

[68] Beaber J. W., Hochhut B., Waldor M. K. SOS response promotes horizontal dissemination of antibiotic resistance genes. Nature 2004; 427(6969): 72–74.

[69] Tran J. H., Jacoby G. A. Mechanism of plasmid-mediated quinolone resistance. Proceedings of the National Academy of Sciences of the United States of America 2002; 99(8):5638–5642.

[70] Strahilevitz J., Jacoby G. A, Hooper D. C., Robicsek A. Plasmid-mediated quinolone resistance: a multifaceted threat. Clinical Microbiology Reviews 2009; 22(4): 664–689.

[71] Poirel L., Cattoir V., Nordmann P., Plasmid-mediated quinolone-resistance; interactions between human, animal, and environmental ecologies. Frontiers in Microbiology 2012; 3: 1-7.

[72] Rodriguez-Martinez J. M., Cano M. E., Velasco C., Martinez-Martinez L., Pascual A. Plasmid-mediated quinolone resistance: an update. Journal of Infection and Chemotherapy 2011; 17(2): 149-182.

[73] Martinez-Martinez L., Pascual A., Jacoby G.A. Quinolone resistance from a transferable plasmid. The Lancet 1998; 351(9105): 797-799.

[74] Jacoby G., Cattoir V., Hooper D. et al. qnr gene nomenclature. Antimicrobial Agents and Chemotherapy 2008; 52(7): 2297-2299.

[75] Baquirin M. H. C., Barlow M. Evolution and recombination of the plasmidic qnr alleles. Journal of Molecular Evolution 2008; 67(1): 103-110.

[76] Robicsek A., Jacoby G. A., Hooper D.C. The worldwide emergence of plasmid-mediated quinolone resistance. The Lancet Infectious Diseases 2006; 6(10): 629-640.

[77] Poirel L., Rodriguez-Martinez J. M., Mammeri H., Liard A., Nordmann P. Origin of plasmid-mediated quinolone resistance determinant QnrA. Antimicrobial Agents and Chemotherapy 2005; 49(8): 3523-3525.

[78] Poirel L., Van De Loo M., Mammeri H., Nordmann P. Association of plasmid-mediated quinolone resistance with extended-spectrum β-lactamase VEB-1. Antimicrobial Agents and Chemotherapy 2005; 49(7): 3091-3094.

[79] Montero C., Mateu G., Rodriguez R., Takiff H. Intrinsic resistance of Mycobacterium smegmatis to fluoroquinolones may be influenced by new pentapeptide protein MfpA. Antimicrobial Agents and Chemotherapy 2001; 45(12): 3387-3392.

[80] Arsene S., Leclercq R. Role of a qnr-like gene in the intrinsic resistance of Enterococcus faecalis to fluoroquinolones. Antimicrobial Agents and Chemotherapy 2007; 51(9): 3254-3258.

[81] Rodriguez-Martinez J. M., Velasco C., Briales A., Garcia I., Conejo M. C., Pascual A. Qnr-like pentapeptide repeat proteins in Gram-positive bacteria. Journal of Antimicrobial Chemotherapy 2008; 61(6): 1240-1243.

[82] Shimizu K., Kikuchi K., Sasaki T. et al. Smqnr, a new chromosome-carried quinolone resistance gene in Stenotrophomonasmaltophilia. Antimicrobial Agents and Chemotherapy 2008; 52(10): 3823-3825.

[83] Velasco C., Rodriguez-Martinez J. M., Briales A., Diaz de Alba P., Calvo J., Pascual A. Smaqnr, a new chromosome-encoded quinolone resistance determinant in Serratia marcescens. The Journal of antimicrobial chemotherapy 2010; 65(2): 239-242.

[84] Nordmann P., Poirel L. Emergence of plasmid-mediated resistance to quinolones in Enterobacteriaceae. Journal of Antimicrobial Chemotherapy 2005; 56(3): 463-469.

[85] Hernandez A., Sanchez M. B., Martinez J. L. Quinolone-resistance: much more than predicted. Frontiers in Microbiology 2011; 2: 1-6.

[86] Lascols, C., Podglajen I., Verdet C. et al. A plasmid-borne Shewanella algae gene, qnrA3, and its possible transfer in vivo between Kluyvera ascorbata and Klebsiella pneumoniae. Journal of Bacteriology 2008; 190(15):5217-5223.

[87] Cattoir V., Poirel L., Aubert C., Soussy C.J., Nordmann P. Unexpected occurrence of plasmid-mediated quinolone resistance determinants in environmental Aeromonas spp.. Emerging Infectious Diseases 2008; 14(2): 231-237.

[88] Poirel L., Liard A., Rodriguez-Martinez J.M., Nordmann P. Vibrionaceae as a possible source of Qnr-like quinolone resistance determinants. Journal of Antimicrobial Chemotherapy 2005; 56(6): 1118–1121.

[89] Vetting M. W., Chi H. P., Hegde S. S., Jacoby G. A., Hooper D. C., Blanchard J. S. Mechanistic and structural analysis of aminoglycoside N-acetyltransferase AAC(6_)-Ib and its bifunctional, fluoroquinolone-active AAC(6_)-Ib-cr variant. Biochemistry 2008; 47(37): 9825–9835.

[90] Ruiz E., Ocampo-Sosa A. A., Alcoba-Florez J. et al. Changes in ciprofloxacin resistance levels in Enterobacter aerogenes isolates associated with variable expression of the aac(6_)-Ibcr gene. Antimicrobial Agents and Chemotherapy 2012; 56(2): 1097–1100.

[91] Frasson I., Cavallaro A., Bergo C., Richter S. N., Palu G. Prevalence of aac(6_)-Ib-cr plasmid-mediated and chromosome-encoded fluoroquinolone resistance in Enterobacteriaceae in Italy. Gut Pathogens 2011; 3(1):12 doi:10. 1186/1757-4749-3-12. http:// www. gutpathogens. com/content/3/1/12 (accessed 9 June 2013).

[92] Sanders C. C., Watanakunakorn C. Emergence of resistance to β-lactams, aminoglycosides, and quinolones during combination therapy for infection due to Serratia marcescens. Journal of Infectious Diseases 1986; 153(3): 617–619.

[93] Perichon B., Courvalin P., Galimand M. Transferable resistance to aminoglycosides by methylation of G1405 in 16S rRNA and to hydrophilic fluoroquinolones by QepA-mediated efflux in Escherichia coli. Antimicrobial Agents and Chemotherapy 2007; 51(7):2464–2469.

[94] Yamane K., Wachino J. I., Suzuki S. et al. New plasmid-mediated fluoroquinolone efflux pump, QepA, found in an Escherichia coli clinical isolate. Antimicrobial Agents and Chemotherapy 2007; 51(9): 3354–3360.

[95] Kim H. B., Wang M., Park C. H., Jacoby G. A., Hooper D. C. oqxAB encoding a multidrug efflux pump in human clinical isolates of Enterobacteriaceae. Antimicrobial Agents and Chemotherapy 2009; 53(8): 3582–3584.

[96] Hansen L. H., Jensen L. B., Sørensen H. I., Sørensen S. J. Substrate specificity of the OqxAB multidrug resistance pump in Escherichia coli and selected enteric bacteria. Journal of Antimicrobial Chemotherapy 2007; 60(1): 145–147.

[97] Hansen L. H., Johannesen E., Burmølle M., Sørensen A. H., Sørensen S. J. Plasmid-encoded multidrug efflux pump conferring resistance to olaquindox in Escherichia coli. Antimicrobial Agents and Chemotherapy 2004; 48(9): 3332–3337.

[98] Morgan-Linnell S. K., Boyd L. B., Steffen D., Zechiedrich L. Mechanisms accounting for fluoroquinolone resistance in Escherichia coli clinical isolates. Antimicrobial Agents and Chemotherapy 2009; 53(1): 235–241.

[99] Cambau E., Matrat S., Pan X. S. et al. Target specificity of the new fluoroquinolone besifloxacin in Streptococcus pneumoniae, Staphylococcus aureus and Escherichia coli. Journal of Antimicrobial Chemotherapy 2009; 63(3): 443–450.

[100] Everett M. J., Jin Y. F., Ricci V., Piddock L. J. V. Contributions of individual mechanisms to fluoroquinolone resistance in 36 Escherichia coli strains isolated from humans and animals. Antimicrobial Agents and Chemotherapy 1996; 40(10): 2380–2386.

[101] Oethinger M., Podglajen I., Kern W. V., Levy S. B. Overexpression of the marA or soxS regulatory gene in clinical topoisomerasemutants of Escherichia coli. Antimicrobial Agents and Chemotherapy 1998; 42(8): 2089–2094.

[102] Goldman J. D., White D. G., Levy S. B. Multiple antibiotic resistance (mar) locus protects Escherichia coli from rapid cell killing by fluoroquinolones. Antimicrobial Agents and Chemotherapy 1996; 40(5): 1266–1269.

[103] Okusu H., Ma D., Nikaido H. AcrAB efflux pump plays a major role in the antibiotic resistance phenotype of Escherichia coli multiple-antibiotic-resistance (Mar) mutants. Journal of Bacteriology 1996; 178(1): 306–308.

[104] Mazzariol A., Tokue Y., Kanegawa T. M., Cornaglia G., Nikaido H. High-level fluoroquinolone-resistant clinical isolates of Escherichia coli overproduce multidrug efflux protein AcrA. Antimicrobial Agents and Chemotherapy 2000; 44(12): 3441–3443.

[105] Oethinger M., Kern W. V., Jellen-Ritter A.S., McMurry L. M., Levy S. B. Ineffectiveness of topoisomerase mutations in mediating clinically significant fluoroquinolone resistance in Escherichia coli in the absence of the AcrAB efflux pump. Antimicrobial Agents and Chemotherapy 2000; 44(1): 10–13.

[106] Wang H., Dzink-Fox J. L., Chen M., Levy S. B. Genetic characterization of highly fluoroquinolone-resistant clinical Escherichia coli strains from China: role of acrR mutations. Antimicrobial Agents and Chemotherapy 2001; 45(5): 1515–1521.

[107] Truong Q. C., Van Nguyen J. C., Shlaes D., Gutmann L., Moreau N. J. A novel, double mutation in DNA gyrase A of Escherichia coli conferring resistance to quinolone antibiotics. Antimicrobial Agents and Chemotherapy 1997; 41(1): 85–90.

[108] Hooper D. C. Mechanism of quinolones resistance, in Hooper, D. C., Rubinstein E. Quinolone Antimicrobial Agents, 3rd edition. (ed.) ASM Press, Washington, DC, USA; 2003; 41–67.

[109] Hooper D. C. Efflux pumps and nosocomial antibiotic resistance: a primer for hospital epidemiologists. Clinical Infectious Diseases 2005; 40(12): 1811–1817.

[110] Van Bambeke F., Pages, J. M., Lee, V. J. Inhibitors of bacterial efflux pumps as adjuvants in antibacterial therapy and diagnostic tools for detection of resistance by efflux. Frontiers in Anti-Infective Drug Discovery 2010; 1: 138–175.

[111] Piddock L. J. V. Multidrug-resistance efflux pumps—not just for resistance. Nature Reviews Microbiology 2006; 4(8): 629–636.